PEDIATRIC CONSULTATION LIAISON PSYCHIATRY

PEDIATRIC CONSULTATION LIAISON PSYCHIATRY

Edited by
Charles E. Hollingsworth, M.D.
Child Psychiatrist
Ventura County Mental Health Services

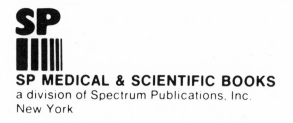

SP MEDICAL & SCIENTIFIC BOOKS
a division of Spectrum Publications, Inc.
New York

SPECTRUM PUBLICATIONS, INC.
175-20 Wexford Terrace
Jamaica, NY 11432

Library of Congress Cataloging in Publication Data
Main entry under title:

Pediatric consultation liaison psychiatry.

  Includes index.
  1. Child psychiatry. 2. Psychiatric consultation.
3. Pediatrics—Psychological aspects. I. Hollingsworth,
Charles E. [DNLM: 1. Mental disorders—In infancy and
childhood. 2. Psychophysiologic disorders—In infancy
and childhood. 3. Referral and consultation.
WS 350 P371]
RJ499.P423   1983   618.92'89   82-10744
ISBN 0-89335-177-6

Printed in the United States of America

Small children reason very childishly,
but their feelings are the same as adults—
joy, happiness, and trust tempered by sadness,
loneliness, fright, guilt, and mistrust.

Charles E. Hollingsworth

DEDICATION

To my father,

Wiley Jacob Hollingsworth

1903-

who taught his seven children

to love, honor, and obey

Contributors

PAT AZARNOFF, M.Ed.
Director, Pediatric Projects Inc.
Santa Monica, California

KENNETH F. CRUMLEY, M.D.
Department of Psychiatry
University of New Mexico Medical School
Albuquerque, New Mexico

SUSAN EDELSTEIN, M.S.A., L.C.S.W.
Clinical Social Worker III
UCLA Hospital and Clinics
University of California, Los Angeles

MARY ANN FELICE, M.D.
Assistant Professor Pediatrics
University of California at San Diego
School of Medicine
Director, Division of Adolescent Medicine
UCSD Medical Center
San Diego, California

CHRIS HAGEN, Ph.D.
Chairman, Speech, Language, Pathology
Department
Speech, Hearing and Neurosensory Center
Children's Hospital and Health Center
San Diego, California

CHARLES E. HOLLINGSWORTH, M.D.
Ventura County Mental Health
300 N. Hillmont Avenue
Ventura, California

MARY KAWAR, O.T.R.
Registered Occupational Therapist
Children's Hospital and Health Center
San Diego, California

MORRIS PAULSON, Ph.D.
Professor of Psychiatry and Biobehavioral
Sciences
Department of Psychiatry
School of Medicine
University of California, Los Angeles

LYNN REINEMAN, O.T.R.
Registered Occupational Therapist
Children's Hospital and Health Center
San Diego, California

JAMES Q. SIMMONS III, M.D.
Professor and Chief of Child Psychiatry
Acting Director of the Neuropsychiatric
Institute Hospital and Clinic
School of Medicine
University of California, Los Angeles

MARY SPENCER, M.D.
Assistant Professor of Pediatrics
Chief, Division of Ambulatory Pediatrics
School of Medicine
University of California, Los Angeles

DOROTHY STONE
Research Associate
Department of Psychiatry
UCLA Neuropsychiatric Institute
University of California, Los Angeles

Table of Contents

Foreword

"Pediatric Consultation Liaison Psychiatry" meets the current need for more emphasis on the biosocial and developmental aspects of pediatrics and the interface between pediatrics and child psychiatry. The Task Force on Pediatric Education in its report, "The Future of Pediatric Education" (Task Force on Pediatric Education, 1979) singled out these areas as the most underemphasized subjects in pediatric training programs.

"By 'biosocial problems' the Task Force means those health problems which are socially induced or complicated by social and environmental factors. These problems are sometimes referred to as 'psychosocial' or 'behavioral' but the task force prefers the term 'biosocial' because it indicates that these aspects of child health are just as much a part of human biology as those to which the term 'biomedical' is commonly applied. The 'developmental' aspects of pediatrics often involve both biomedical and biosocial concerns" (Task Force on Pediatric Education, 1979).

The subjects covered in "Pediatric Consultation Liaison Psychiatry" fill many of the gaps in pediatric and child psychiatric education and training. In addition one of the strengths of this volume lies in the willingness of Dr. Hollingsworth and his talented, knowledgeable contributors to go beyond the cognitive elements of their subjects into the affective components as they relate to the pediatrician and other health and mental health professionals.

In today's world parents are expected to do an impossible task. They are asked to raise children and fit them into an uncertain society. They are asked to serve as mediators and advocates for children within that society. They are asked to walk the fine line between under and over involvement with the children they are raising. They are expected to do all this with little or no training and little or no support from the community in which they live. Some trends in our society compound this "impossible task":

1. Approximately one-half of today's mothers work outside the home.

2. Most parents do not have their own parents, relatives, close friends or other supportive people sharing the responsibility of child rearing.

3. Few families are integrated into and active in their home communities.

4. Families are small and their is little opportunity for children to learn parenting skills by caring for their own siblings.

5. Many mothers are searching for a wider range of role alternatives and want to follow these alternatives free of guilt or depression.

6. Many fathers feel threatened by the challenge of modified parental roles within the family.

Pediatricians and other health and mental health professionals who counsel parents, if they are to be effective counsellors, must be cognizant of parent development, societal trends and changing parental roles (Friedman and Friedman, 1977). They must develop knowledge, skill and understanding in the areas of human psychology and family dynamics. They must also be aware of the community outside the world of their homes and offices. This community may include many parent-support services which supplement and complement family counselling. These services include parent discussion groups, parent education classes, child care alternatives, family community centers and a variety of health and mental health referral resources.

However knowledge, skill and understanding will not suffice if clinicians are not attuned to their own input into the professional-patient relationship. Counsellors must be aware of the feelings, attitudes and prejudices which they bring to the professional-child and professional-parent relationship. They must understand themselves in relation to their patients and their patients' families (Russak and Friedman, 1970).

In the training of pediatricians and other health and mental health professionals the resolution of the issues involved in three particular problem areas appear to be critical. Professionals who work through and cope with their feelings relative to these issues usually emerge as empathic, effective clinicians and counsellors. Professionals who fail to resolve these problems often tend to depersonalize patients and families, to counsel inappropriately and to distance themselves from human issues (Werner and Korsch, 1976). The three problem areas are:

1. Coping with the feelings of overwhelming responsibility engendered by work with sick and disabled children

2. Coping with feelings aroused by work with hopelessly ill and dying children and their families

3. Coping with almost universal propensity of immature clinicians to see themselves or members of their own families in every patient and parent encounter

Clinicians who have not resolved the issues involved in the first two problem areas often cope with their feelings by dealing in more and more detail with the mechanical, structural and molecular aspects of disease, illness and disability. They tend to retreat from the broader concept of health and disease which includes biological, social and psychological considerations.

Clinicians who have not resolved the issues involved in the third problem area tend to base problem-solving in their practices on their own limited experiences. They often demonstrate little or no personal insight. Counsellors who loved or hated their own siblings may relate those feelings to their young patients rather than dealing with reality. Counsellors who had good, ambivalent or poor relationships with their own parents may bring those feelings to encounters with parents in their practices.

Effective clinician-counsellors must make a satisfactory resolution of the issues involved in these three problem areas and come to an understanding of themselves and their own feelings. Only then can they serve as an optimal model for the families in their practices. Only then can they develop empathy for and a mutual respectful relationship with the children and the families they serve.

"Pediatric Consultation Liaison Psychiatry" deals with these issues and treats both the cognitive and affective elements of the bio-psycho-social subjects covered. The result is a strong, effective, creative text which should be read by everyone who works with children and their families.

David Belais Friedman, M.D., FAAP
Emeritus Professor of Pediatrics
University of Southern California
School of Medicine
Los Angeles, California

BIBLIOGRAPHY

Task Force on Pediatric Education, *The Future of Pediatric Education*, American Academy of Pediatrics, Evanston, Illinois, 1979

Friedman, A.S. and Friedman, D.B., *Parenting: A Developmental Process*, Pediatric Annals, 6:9, Sept. 1977

Russak, S. and Friedman, D., *Family Interviewing and Pediatric Training*, Clinical Pediatrics, 98:10, 594–598, October 1970

Werner, E.R. and Korsch, B.M., *The Vulnerability of the Medical Student: Posthumous Presentation of L.L. Stephens' Ideas*, Pediatrics, 57:3, 321–328, March 1976

Introduction

Charles E. Hollingsworth

The child is a beautiful, honest, intense being capable of giving much love, but vulnerable to hurt. Fortunately, many people are willing to take the risk of becoming parents knowing the possibility of being intensely grieved should something happen to the child. If we can help diminish the hurt for these parents and their children, our goal will be achieved.

This book is specifically for the disciplines who work with children as they interface with the health care system. Parents will also find this book of value in understanding their child's emotional responses to being hospitalized, evaluated, treated, and convalescing.

For a decade we have awaited a comprehensive book on pediatric consultation-liaison psychiatry, but this relatively new field has little literature—a few texts that vary considerably in their approach to the subject and to the population. Therefore, I have asked several of my colleagues to contribute a pertinent chapter from their area of expertise. Please refer to the list of additional references in pediatric consultation-liaison psychiatry in Appendix I at the end of this book.

The health care provider must recognize the interaction between physical and emotional factors in every illness, symptom, and complaint. It was a great mistake in the past to attempt to separate these two variables. The child should be viewed as a changing being—developing day by day. The emotions are constantly affecting his/her health and/or illness. Those attending to the child's physical health must accept responsibility also for the child's mental health. This cannot be abdicated. The environment sets the stage and gives the child a direct message about how he or she should behave.

Mental health professionals can and often should be called in as consultants and as active members of the team providing care, but the responsibility for the care of the child should not be flippantly passed from one service to another. We must use a true interdisciplinary team approach in providing the maximum comprehensive service to the child and his or her family. Family dynamics are often totally overlooked, although their involvement with and relationship to the child are critical to the child's recovery and convalescence. Occasionally, family dynamics precipitate or worsen an illness in a child. We have all seen children with asthma who will have a serious asthmatic attack at a time of serious family stress. Few hospitals provide a comfortable place for at least one parent to spend the night alongside the young child in the hospital. Even fewer hospitals allow sibling visitation, regardless of age. I strongly advocate liberal sibling visitation policies, as well as individualized visitation hours appropriate for the condition of the patient.

Hospitals should be family oriented—the child is not an island but is part of a constantly changing galaxy of beings whose interactions are the determinant of his response to his environment, his illness, and his coping skills. The thoughtful hospital must remember that they begin in the admitting office to set the tone for the family's impression of the quality of care their child will receive. The tone, attitude, and professionalism in the admitting office are very important and should not be overlooked. I also recommend that before a child comes to the hospital for an elective admission or procedure, he/she should make a prehospitalization visit. This includes an orientation to the ward, explanation of the use of the call light, location of bathrooms, taking of vital signs such as temperature and blood pressure, as well as an introduction to the primary nurse if this is possible.

This book is a compilation of chapters by workers in the field of pediatrics, obstetrics, child psychiatry, social service, and other allied health fields. The topics included are pertinent from both a developmental framework as well as by diseases of various body systems. We have focused particularly on what can be done to maximize the quality of care for the child and family when they are our wards—our trusting, compassionate clients. They can also let us know how *we* can work together to make their experience more tolerable for them during difficult circumstances.

Pediatric hospitals came a long way in the 1970s in providing more humane care, but the challenge for the 1980s must be faced with even more vigor. This is the decade for us to "practice what has been preached" in the best interest of children who have been afflicted.

The child's remarkable capacity to cope has always amazed me—during my pediatric training I was often horrified at procedures children had to undergo. I felt that we did not understand, or even try to understand, the child's emotional reaction to all these procedures; therefore, I made a pledge to myself to complete training in child psychiatry and to specialize in pediatric consultation-liaison psychiatry. Enough preaching—let me get on with the practice.

Acknowledgments

I greatly appreciate the editorial assistance of Sylva Grossman. Many thanks also for the secretarial support of Debi Taylor, Jan Golliet, Debbie Ness, Carole Hall, and to all the secretaries who prepared chapters for the contributors. Most importantly, I would like to thank my 11 colleagues who contributed their time, talent, wisdom, and acquired knowledge. We may now share their knowledge as a result of their valuable contribution of pertinent, concise information from their areas of expertise.

PEDIATRIC CONSULTATION LIAISON PSYCHIATRY

The Pediatric Consultation Liaison Program

Charles E. Hollingsworth

The child psychiatrist who ventures into the pediatric sphere as a consultant wisely spends some time gaining the trust and confidence of the various disciplines involved in providing care for those children. The pediatrician often asks for informal consults and often provides invaluable counseling to families in stress. The child psychiatrist helps educate the pediatrician to know which cases would benefit from the pediatrician's counsel and which cases would benefit from referral to child psychiatry. The busy pediatric practitioner has limited time to spend with each patient who needs extra emotional support, and can counsel only a few such families and refer the others.

If a psychiatric consultation is to be done, we strongly encourage the pediatrician to be honest when explaining to the parents that he is requesting a child *psychiatrist* for consultation. The parents must give consent before the psychiatrist can see the child; therefore, they should be correctly informed that we are psychiatrists. Too often we find pediatricians who are uncomfortable or embarrassed to tell the parents that Dr. Jones is a psychiatrist. We psychiatrists are proud of our profession and the skills we have to offer. After permission is granted, the pediatrician will speak directly with the child psychiatrist to explain exactly why he is requesting a consultation and what questions he wants answered by the consultant. If at all possible, the pediatrician or the ward staff will introduce the child psychiatrist to the pediatric patient and the parents.

A quiet room is selected for the interview. Some part of the interview will be with the child alone, if his condition and developmental level allows this. A careful developmental history is obtained from the parents. If the consultation is to be dictated, a brief handwritten note with any specific recommendations can be entered in the chart with a statement that the full consult will follow. A phone call or personal meeting with the pediatrician should be arranged in order for the child psychiatrist to communicate his observations and recommendations. In many cases, a conference with other ward personnel is also helpful in providing care for a difficult child with multiple problems, chronic illness, or ones who require special ward behavioral management.

We have found that there must be a balance between the hours of consultation and the hours of liaison activities. Liaison work will initially generate more referrals for consultation; but after months of psychiatric conferences, the staff becomes more sophisticated at handling difficult children at stressful times. The pediatric consultation-liaison psychiatry team is made up of mental health professionals including child psychiatric social workers, child psychologists, child psychiatrists, child activity workers from occupational therapy, nurses, and pediatricians.

A weekly psychosocial progress rounds meeting is held on each ward on each service to discuss the families' emotional reaction to the illness and hospitalization and to other stresses in their homes. This meeting is attended by representatives from each discipline, including nurses and pediatricians.

For the very complicated case, we suggest a predischarge family conference to allow the entire family to hear representatives from each discipline discuss the posthospital convalescence for the child (Hollingsworth and Sokol, 1978). The liaison psychiatrist can be a valuable addition to the team for educating parents, nurses, and pediatricians. This consultant is trained in interviewing techniques that allow him to facilitate open communication between members of the health care team and the child's family. There is a national trend for pediatricians to utilize child psychiatrists more frequently, and we hope that our professional expertise will continue to warrant this increased trust.

PEDIATRIC CONSULTATION-LIAISON PSYCHIATRY SERVICE

Procedure for requesting consultation from Child Psychiatry:
A. Obtain permission from attending physician for psychiatric consultation.
B. Have attending physician or pediatric resident inform family and patient that a child psychiatric consultation has been requested. Parental consent must be obtained before a consultation is initiated.
C. A written order requesting psychiatric consultation must be written in the patient's chart by the attending physician or the pediatric resident. It is imperative that the order be written. Insurance companies will not pay for consultations unless specific orders for such appear in the chart.
D. Call the Pediatric Consultation-Liaison Psychiatry Service's secretary to request a consultation. She will need the following information: name, sex, age of the child; admission date; name of person requesting the consultation; location of the child; brief statement of reason for request; how urgent is the consult; and insurance coverage information. The secretary and nursing staff will coordinate the time for the

consultation so that the family can be available when the child psychiatrist comes to do the consultation.

E. The secretary will then notify the child psychiatrist who will contact the person requesting the consultation.

F. Consultations are not free to the patient and/or family. Billing for these services will be handled by the billing office.

G. There are some time restrictions on our schedules. We will always attempt to do a consultation within 24 hours after a request is made. We will always attempt to have a typewritten consultation note in the chart within 24 hours after a consultation is done. Handwritten notes and follow-up notes will also appear in the chart. We will make every effort to discuss the case with the person requesting the consultation before we see the patient. That person or some other member of the staff should be available to introduce the consulting child psychiatrist or fellow in child psychiatry to the patient and family. After the consultation is done, we will discuss each case with the person who requested the consultation and other interested staff members. As much as possible, we will continue to follow the patient's progress throughout his hospitalization. In a model pediatric liaison psychiatry program, the following conferences are held on the pediatric service each week:

1. *Psychosocial patient progress rounds* are held on Mondays from 3:00 to 4:30 P.M. in the treatment room on the medical service of Children's Hospital, pediatric floor. This meeting is attended by social workers, occupational and physical therapists, nurses, and a pediatric liaison psychiatrist to discuss the psychosocial aspects of certain identified patients. Discussion includes family history, as well as the child's adjustment to hospitalization, injury, immobilization, and/or acute or chronic illness. Discharge planning is also discussed, as well as the nurses' feelings about working with the patient and the family.

2. *A pediatric case conference* is held in the dining room of Children's Hospital on Tuesdays from 12:30 to 1:30 P.M. This conference is attended by many pediatricians from the local community as well as pediatric residents, medical students, radiologists, pediatric surgeons, and a child psychiatrist. The conference is medically oriented, centered on the medical and clinical presentation, and frequently involves little discussion of the psychological effects of the illness. The child psychiatrist attends and encourages emphasis on psychosocial issues.

3. *Psychosocial rounds on the surgical service* are held in the head nurse's office on the pediatric surgical service on Tuesdays from

2:00 to 3:00 P.M. The meeting is attended by social workers, a nurse coordinator, head nurse, primary nurses, occupational and physical therapists, and a child psychiatrist. Certain patients are discussed concerning their family history, social history, adjustment to hospitalization, fears and fantasies concerning surgery, and their preparation for surgery. Discharge planning is discussed, as are the nurses' feelings related to working with certain identified patients. Many of the patients on this ward have had open heart surgery or are having Herrington Rods put in for orthopedic defects of the spine.

4. *Social worker's conference and supervision* meetings are held on Wednesdays at 11:00 A.M. in the Social Work Department of the hospital. Social workers and social work trainees from the hospital attend this meeting with the child psychiatrist. The social worker presents an interesting case, and the child psychiatrist discusses with the other social workers the various aspects of each case. This time is also used for social workers to discuss the stress involved in their work within the hospital.

5. *Psychosocial rounds on the rehabilitation service* are held in the conference room on the rehab section of Children's Hospital. This would be an excellent opportunity for students to see the interdisciplinary team approach. This meeting is also attended by the rehabilitation doctor and, occasionally, by a pediatric neurologist. Also in attendance are all the rehab nurses and representatives from occupational therapy, physical therapy, speech and hearing, and child psychiatry. There are usually only two to four cases on the rehab service at any time, and this gives adequate time for discussing the child from a multidisciplinary aspect.

6. *Pediatric grand rounds* are held at the hospital in the large dining room from 8:15 to 9:00 A.M. on Fridays. A monthly list of topics is mailed out. Child psychiatry, general pediatrics, and each of the pediatric sub-specialties present topics of interest for continuing medical education credit.

The enclosed forms (Appendices, pp. 6–16) will prove useful to anyone working in the field of pediatric consultation-liaison psychiatry or pediatrics.

Parents of children with chronic illness should make a copy of the child's medical history and have copies readily available when the child is seen by a new physician or at a different medical facility. This will save a great deal of time and will guarantee that all areas of interest are covered. The physician can quickly review it, and then ask pertinent questions to update the child's medical history.

REFERENCE

Hollingsworth, C.E., and Sokol, B. Predischarge family conference. *Journal of the American Medical Association, 239;* 740–741 (1978).

APPENDICES

Psychotropic Medication Policies
Child's Medical History
Form C (Revised Medication Evaluation Form)

Psychotropic Medication Policies

1. Each physician in the clinic will be provided or will purchase the following stamp, which will be used each time a patient is seen for medication evaluation and each time a prescription is being refilled. This vital information must be noted and recorded when prescribing or renewing prescriptions.

(Physician's Name)   (Date)   (Child's Name)

Height _____ Weight _____ Blood Pressure _____ Pulse _____

(Indicate + for yes; 0 for no)

Rash _____   Icterus _____

Abnormal Movements: Tics _____ Akesthesia _____ Akinesia _____

                                   Tardive Dyskinesia _____ Other _____

Appetite Change _____   Sleep Change _____

Therapeutic Value of Medication _____

☐ Possible side effects of medication were discussed with patient and/or parents.

2. When an ongoing case is reassigned to a new physician for medication management, the new physician should see the patient and do at least a brief clinical evaluation before renewing ongoing prescriptions.

3. Informed consent about side effects: please do not unnecessarily frighten the child or parents. Tell them there can be allergic reactions and side effects with any medication, even aspirin. Advise them that if the child has any unusual symptoms that the parents feel might be related to the medication, to please call you and you will let them know if the symptoms may possibly be due to the medicine. Use your own clinical judgment in explaining other possible side effects.

4. Parents should be informed that in a very small percentage of children who are hyperactive, the drugs used to treat hyperactivity may have a paradoxical effect—speed the child up, make him "wild," and in rare cases it may cause crying spells for no apparent reason. If any of these occur, they usually occur during the first week on the medication, and parents should call the physician or therapist. The hyperexcitable state and the depressed state will reverse in 24 hours after discontinuing the medication.

5. Frequency of visits:

a) Initial psychotropic medication evaluation: fill out revised medication evaluation form (Form C).

b) See child again one week after beginning the medication program to evaluate the benefits of medication and to question parents about any possible side effects. (Use stamp for chemotherapy follow-up visit or write out the same information in the patient's chart.)

6. Equipment for medical evaluation of patients: each clinic should be equipped with scales for height and weight and two sizes of blood pressure cuffs, ophthalmoscopes, otoscopes, and stethoscopes. A treatment examining room should be available.

7. We strongly encourage physicians to do their own physical and neurological exams on patients whom they are following for psychotropic medication, or to make arrangements for another physician to do physical exams on the patient if you are doing psychotherapy with that patient.

8. The American Academy of Pediatrics recommends that physical exams should be done annually on all children. When a child is initially seen for a behavioral disorder, it is important that a careful physical and neurological exam rule out any organic disease that might be contributing to the behavioral disorder. In some cases, it will be possible to have this done early in the diagnostic process; in others it will be necessary to establish some rapport with the family and proceed in the diagnostic evaluation with plans to have the physical exam done within two to three months after a case is opened.

The physical exam can be done by one of the following people: family physician, pediatrician, or nurse practitioner.

9. The attached physical exam form is to be used for our patients. It is conveniently printed so that three copies are made by writing firmly on the paper. For physicians outside the Child Psychiatry Clinic, a stamped, self-addressed return envelope is provided. The physician will keep on copy for his/her records, give one copy to the parents to return to us, and mail one copy in the return envelope to us. In this way, if the parents lose their copy, we will get one by mail, or if the physician's office fails to mail it back, we will still get the copy from the parents. Requests for CBC, RUA, and/or liver enzymes should be checked only when clinically indicated. The American Academy of Pediatrics recommends the CBC and RUA once a year.

10. Policy on mailing prescriptions to parents: this is *not* encouraged. However, there are some situations in which this is acceptable: (1) if a child has been followed in the clinic for some time and will run out of medication before the next visit is scheduled or (2) if the patient missed a scheduled appointment and needs enough medicine to last until the date of the next scheduled visit, you mail a prescription for no more than a 10-day supply of medication and a notice giving the rescheduled appointment time. Documentation of the telephone

conversation with the parents and the details of the prescription should be noted in the patient's chart. If a patient misses the next appointment, you may mail one more prescription for a 10-day supply of medication and once again re-schedule the appointment within one week. There should be no more prescriptions by mail after that.

11. Policy on:

a) Phenothiazines: Patients on major tranquilizers must be seen every month, and prescriptions should not be written for larger quantities than a one month's supply. A prescription by mail should be made for no more than a 10-day supply. If the child is on thioridazine (Mellaril®) s/he should have a complete ophthalmological exam once or twice a year.

b) Pemoline (Cylert®): Follow the child clinically once a month, since this drug is new and we know little about the long-term side effects. Inform families that it takes four to six weeks before beneficial effects are seen from this drug.

c) Imipramine (Tofranil®): Give a warning to keep this medication out of the reach of all children. It is very dangerous if a child ingests a large over-dose, and can cause cardiac arrhythmias. Do not prescribe more than a one month's supply at any one time.

12. After doing your evaluation of a child, you may recommend a trial on medication, such as a stimulant for hyperkinesis. If you do, we encourage you to advise the parents to get the prescription filled and give the medication to the child one hour before you see the child for his second visit so that you can evaluate any effects the medication may have on him. This will not always be possible, but we would encourage this as a valuable learning experience.

13. If, for any reason, you feel it is clinically indicated to deviate from this clinic policy, please explain this in the patient's chart and discuss it with a supervisor or team consulting physician.

Child's Medical History

Please complete the following to the best of your ability as it will help in our evaluation of your child, and return it to the above physician prior to your child's visit. Thank you.

Name of child _____ Sex _____ Birth date _____

Address: Street _____ Telephone _____

City _____ State _____ Zip _____

Parent's name: Father _____ Mother _____

Occupation _____

Name of school child attends _____

For what complaint(s) is child being evaluated? _____

_____

Names and ages of brothers and/or sisters _____

_____

Prior history of miscarriage: Yes or No _____ Number _____

PRENATAL	Yes	No	Don't know
Illness during pregnancy _____			
9 month pregnancy			
Excessive weight gain			
High blood pressure			
Bleeding or spotting			
Infections or contact with infection			
Medication during pregnancy (if yes, name drug) _____			
Exposure to toxins, x-ray or others _____			
Accidents during pregnancy _____			
Any increase in fetal activity compared to other pregnancies?			
BIRTH			
Did you go into labor by yourself?			
Did your membranes rupture prior to onset of labor?			
If so, how long before? _____			
How long did your labor last? _____			
Medication during labor _____			
Method of delivery: (check one)			
Spontaneous vaginal delivery			
Forceps vaginal delivery ____ High or Low Forceps? ___			
Caesarian delivery			
If Caesarian, give reason: _____			

NEONATAL

Baby's birth weight _____

	Yes	No	Don't know
Did baby cry immediately after birth?			
Was oxygen required for baby?			
Was your child premature?			
During hospital stay, did baby have:			
Jaundice			
Rash			
Blue spells			
Twitching			
Convulsions			
Did the baby stay longer than you in the hospital?			
Did the baby have difficulty with sucking or crying when he was first brought to you?			
Did infant have any congenital abnormality or birthmarks?			
If so, state: _____			

DEVELOPMENT

	Yes	No	Don't know
Was weight gain satisfactory?			
Did the infant have any trouble sucking, swallowing or retaining feedings?			
Did the infant have colic?			
Was the sleeping pattern normal?			
Any excessive crying?			
Was baby excessively quiet?			

At what age did your child first: (approximate age)

	Years	Months	Don't know
Hold head up			
Roll over			
Grasp objects			
Laugh			
Sit alone			
Walk			
Say words			
Toilet train			
Drink from a cup			
Feed himself/herself			
Ride tricycle and bicycle			
Give up bottle			
Throw a ball			
Catch a ball			
Use scissors			
Color with crayons			
Color within lines			

	Yes	No	Don't know
Was your child overly active?			
Did s/he climb excessively?			
Does child wet bed?			
How often? _____			
Days			
Nights			
Is the child able to enunciate sounds correctly?			
Is s/he afraid to talk?			
Does s/he often repeat sounds or words (stutter/stammer)?			
Does the child seem to have trouble hearing?			
Does s/he say "what, what?" all the time?			
Has s/he had frequent colds?			
Has s/he had frequent ear infections?			
Is s/he a mouth breather?			
Is the child "a loner"?			
Does the child turn on TV at a very high volume?			
Does s/he sit very close to the TV screen?			
Does s/he squint when looking intently at something?			
Does s/he regularly hold objects up very close to his/her eyes?			
Do his/her eyes tend to cross, or do they appear to move away from center?			
Does your child feed neatly?			
Can child dress self?			
Does child go up and down stairs alternating feet?			
Can child zip zippers?			
Can child button buttons?			
Can child tie shoe laces?			
Do you consider child to be clumsy?			
Is your child accident prone?			
Does child fall often?			
Handedness: (circle) right left alternates			
Footedness: (circle) right left alternates			
Does child sit fiddling with small objects?			
Does s/he hum and make other odd noises?			
Coordination poor?			
Day dreams?			
Quarrelsome?			
Can s/he hold a pencil properly?			
Does s/he run as fast as other children his/her age?			
Is s/he generally a happy child?			
Does s/he like to play with other children?			

	Yes	No	Don't know
Is s/he able to play alone?			
Does s/he cry easily?			
Does s/he often have temper tantrums?			
Does s/he usually follow directions?			
Does s/he have a very short attention span?			
Does s/he appear unaccepted by group?			
Does s/he get along with opposite sex?			
Does s/he get along with same sex?			

PAST MEDICAL HISTORY (underline appropriate conditions)

Childhood infections: measles, chickenpox, german measles, mumps, roseola, whooping cough, scarlet fever, rheumatic fever

Has your child had any serious medical condition, if so what and when? _____
_____

Has your child had an operation, if so what and when? _____
_____

Has your child had any head injuries which have rendered him/her unconscious, if so when? _____

Has your child had any hospitalization, if so when and for what? _____
_____

Has your child had any of the following: (underline if YES): seizures, recurrent headaches and/or abdominal pains, sleepwalking, night terrors, dizziness, staring attacks, muscle jerks, fainting attacks, breath holding spells or other: _____

Has the child lost any functions and/or abilities which he previously possessed?

Yes _____ At what age? _____ No _____

School History	Age	Name of School
Nursery School		
Kindergarten		
First Grade		
Second Grade		
Third Grade		
Fourth Grade		
Fifth Grade		
Sixth Grade		
Seventh Grade		
Eighth Grade		
Ninth Grade		

Did your child ever attend any of the following facilities? If so, please check:

Preschool Nursery for Retarded Children _____

Transition class _____

Special Class, Class for Emotionally Disturbed
Children, School for Learning Disabilities _____

	Yes	No	Don't know
Has your child ever received tutoring?			
Does your child have problems with any particular subject?			
If so, what? _____			
In what subject or subjects does your child excel?			
_____			
Does the school feel your child has any problems?			
If so, what? _____			

SPECIFIC TESTING

	Yes	No	Don't know
Has your child had his eyes examined?			
Does s/he wear glasses?			
Has your child had his hearing tested?			
Has your child had any psychological testing?			

FAMILY HISTORY

MOTHER: Age: _____ Level of education completed: _____

One of how many children? _____

Any brothers or sisters deceased? _____

If so, cause of death _____

Any family history of (underline appropriate): seizures, migraine headaches, fainting attacks, blackout spells, learning disabilities, mental retardation, progressive neurological disease, other: _____

FATHER: Age: _____ Level of education completed: _____

One of how many children? _____

Any brothers or sisters deceased? _____

Any family history of (underline appropriate): seizures, migraine headaches, fainting attacks, blackout spells, learning disabilities, mental retardation, progressive neurological disease, other: _____

PATIENT'S BROTHERS AND/OR SISTERS: List any of the above conditions if present in any sibling)

Sex   Age

_____
_____
_____
_____

REFERRED BY: _____

Please list names and addresses of individuals to whom you wish reports sent:

_____
_____
_____

_____
Signature of Parent or Guardian

FORM C
Revised Medication Evaluation Form

Dear Physician or Nurse Practitioner:

The Child Psychiatry Clinic would very must appreciate your assistance in doing an annual physical examination as well as a CBC, RUA, and, when indicated, liver enzymes (SGOT, SGPT, Bili T/D). Some of our patients are on psychotropic medication and it is important for us to know the status of their physical condition. Please do the lab tests which have been √ checked on this form. We urge you to use this form; however, if you have a physical exam form which is thorough and legible, a copy of that form will be sufficient for our files.

_____

Child Psychiatry Clinic Therapist

_____

_____ _____ _____
(Child's Name)   (Age)   Telephone number

Brief statement of any pertinent findings in patient's medical history:
_____
_____
_____

Known allergies: _____
Current medications: _____
History of hospitalizations: _____
_____

Comments on patient's emotional adjustment: _____
_____

Report of x-rays, special procedures or significant lab data: _____
_____
_____
_____

Date of most recent physical examination: _____

Physical Examination: _____

Height _____ Weight _____ Blood Pressure _____ Pulse Rate _____

Respiratory Rate _____

(Check √ if normal, explain any abnormalities)
Skin: _____
Lymph Nodes: _____
Head: _____
Ears: _____
Eyes: _____ Fundi _____ Are conjunctive icteria? _____ YES _____ NO
          EOM _____
Nose: _____
Mouth: _____
Throat: _____
Neck: _____
Chest: _____
Heart: _____
Back: _____
Abdomen: _____ Is liver enlarged? _____ YES _____ NO
          Is spleen palpable? _____ YES _____ NO
Genitalia: _____
Rectal: _____
Extremities: _____
Neurological Exam: _____ Fundiscopic Exam: _____
Cranial nerves II–XII: _____
Cerebellar function: _____ Sensory: _____ Coordination: _____
          Gait: _____
Impression: (Please state if normal physical exam or note any abnormalities)

_____

_____

_____

_____

_____

***
_____
(Date)   (Name of Physician)   (Medical License No.)

Please do the lab work which has √ mark beside it.

Result of CBC: _____

Hgb _____, Hct _____, wbc _____, rbc _____,

diff: polys _____, bands _____, eosin _____, baso _____

          lymph _____, mono _____.

Indexes: MCB _____, MCH _____, MCHC _____

Result of routine urinalysis: _____

color _____, sp. gr. _____, pH _____, protein _____,

glucose _____, acetone _____, bile _____, blood _____.

Microscopic urine report:

wbc _____, rbc _____, casts _____, crystals _____

Result of liver enzymes: _____

Please do this portion only if this space ____ is checked by Child Guidance Clinic.

SGOT _____, SGPT _____, Bili T/D _____ _____

Thank you very much for your assistance. Please give this form to the patient's parent to return to the Child Psychiatry Clinic and mail the yellow copy to the Child Psychiatry Clinic in the enclosed self-addressed, stamped envelope. If our clinic can be of any further assistance to you in caring for this patient, please ask for the parent's permission to contact the therapist listed on this form. Our telephone number is _____. We look forward to working with you in providing services to this patient.

Sincerely,

Child Psychiatry Service

2

Psychiatric Aspects of Physical Illness

in Children

Kenneth F. Crumley, Charles E. Hollingsworth, James Q. Simmons III

INTRODUCTION

The evaluation and care of the physically ill child requires that medical students and primary care physicians be increasingly aware of the common psychological responses of children to acute and chronic illness, as well as the more profound abnormal responses that may also become manifest with physical illness. There are predictable psychological concomitants to physical disease, and effective treatment of the illness should include psychological considerations (Engel, 1960; Lipowski, 1974; Strain and Grossman, 1975). These concomitants range from relatively simple situations, such as the diabetic child who refuses to take his insulin, to the triggering of asthma by emotional stress and the complex interactions between stress and the various symptoms and sequelae of ulcerative colitis.

The "complete" physician traditionally has been considered one who treats disease in the context of the total person in his overall social-emotional milieu. Unfortunately, in the age of specialization individual physicians tend to focus on specific organs and systems, with frequent inattention to the interrelationships between systems. This chapter is directed toward the physician who will have direct responsibility for comprehensive care of children and their families. The aim is to emphasize the ultimate psychobiological integrity in sick children.

Children may respond to illness with disturbance or failure in growth, development, or adjustment. The intensity of this response is related to many factors, including the child's and family's previous experience with disease, the child's adaptive capacity, the nature of the illness, and the circumstances surrounding the disease. Physiological, psychological, and social changes occur that help maintain equilibrium. However, if successful adaptation does not occur, it may lead to temporary decompensation; chronic impairment in growth, development, or function; or acute severe emotional breakdown. Many of the symptoms or signs associated with any disease state may actually be the result of attempts by the organism to maintain psychosocial adaptation, rather than the specific results of the disease process itself. Finally, multiple forces of a physical, psychological, and social nature are simultaneously involved in the predisposition to and perpetuation of any disease (Engel, 1977). Thus it is essential that one evaluate the interplay of all of these factors in the clinical picture and prescribe treatment that takes each into consideration.

One example of this complex interaction may be seen when a child's illness brings about a family crisis. Families with healthy adaptive patterns usually respond in ways that optimize the child's ability to adapt to the stresses of the disease process. In less effective families, parental patterns of handling the child may be significantly impaired by anxiety or guilt. These patterns, in turn, may actually impair the ability of the child to manage the disease itself. In seriously disturbed families, the child who falls ill may become the focus of family tensions, may be treated unrealistically as a chronic invalid, or handled in ways that reflect a response to the child's illness in terms of parental needs. In a more general sense, families from different socioeconomic and ethnic backgrounds may respond quite differently to the illness of a child, particularly in relation to the problem of dependence on medical personnel or other helping agencies. To effectively treat a child, the physician should understand him in the context of his particular family and culture. Thus the child, his family, and culture represent the necessary milieu of study for the diagnosis and treatment of disease.

Within the context of the above-described unit, the effect of a child's illness or injury on his own adaptation or the family equilibrium depends on a variety of factors. These include the developmental level of the child, his previous adaptive capacity, the nature of the illness or injury, the degree of prostration or pain, the type of treatment, residual defect or handicap, and the meaning of the illness to the child and his family.

Children's reactions to illness vary in severity, but may not be totally related to the specific disease. In predisposed children, stress from various illnesses may exaggerate developmental deviations, precipitate psychoneurotic disorders, magnify chronic personality disorders, or result in regressive behavior. However, the nature of a given illness and the specific treatment associated with it may also exert a significant influence on the child's reactions. Finally, overwhelming illness is a profound stress and produces psychological disequilibrium even in emotionally healthy children. The psychological response to overwhelming disease has been described as consisting of an initial impact phase of recoil, which includes a lessening of repression and the appearance of mourning the loss of the self. This may lead to overt depression, or may be expressed through disturbances in vegetative functions or behavior. Finally, restitution is seen in mastery of the situation, at which time unique patterns related to the pre-illness personality emerge.

Physical illness itself is also affected by psychological events. Although the mechanisms are unclear, such stressful stimuli as competitive pressures or the loss of a parental figure appear in association with various illnesses, such as the common cold, tuberculosis, and streptoccocal infections (Prugh, 1963). Although the general responses of children and their families to physical illness vary considerably independent of condition, there are some characteristic responses that are a function of chronicity, degree of disability or disfigurement, need for hospitalization, significance and function of the organ or system involved, and the need for self-care. These will be described in more detail below.

EFFECTS OF ACUTE ILLNESS IN CHILDREN

Acute illness in children is usually accompanied by behavioral responses derived from two sources: the physical impact of the disease and the psychological response to it. Such phenomena as irritability, malaise, listlessness, prostration, disturbance in the rhythms of sleep and appetite, and alterations in bowel and bladder functions represent responses to the impact of the disease. These biological responses may generate a variety of reactions from anxious parents and from staff (Blom, 1958). Psychological response to illness and injury in children is much more varied in type and severity. It is usually seen in terms of some variation of the following primarily psychological phenomena: denial, regression, depression, misperception, anxiety, conversion reactions, dissociative reactions, and academic underachievement or/and other behavioral changes.

Denial represents a means to mitigate the impact of awareness of threatening illness. The spectrum of the manifestations of denial runs from hopeful statements about recovery from an illness of relatively grim prognosis to the refusal to admit the existence of symptoms that are objectively verifiable.

Regression is a return to behavior more appropriate at an earlier age or to a level of control more characteristic of a younger child. In older infants and preschool children it appears in the form of thumb sucking; return to the bottle; demanding, clinging, negativistic, or aggressive behavior; speech disturbances; and the loss of recently acquired habit patterns, such as bowel or bladder control. In older children regression is seen in the reappearance of immature social patterns, including greater dependency, particularly on the mother; demanding or aggressive behavior; limitations in the capacity to share with siblings or others; and difficulties in concentration and learning.

Depression is an affect disturbance that is often seen in conjunction with physical illness. It takes on different characteristics according to the child. It may arise partly as a primary effect of the illness in such disorders as infectious mononucleosis or infectious hepatitis. In other instances, it arises mainly from restriction of activity, the meaning of a particular disorder, its influence on body structure or function, or from separation from the parents, as in the case of hospitalization. Depression in children may be associated with behavioral changes such as eating and sleeping disturbances; changes in motor behavior, from hyperexcitability to withdrawal; or in antisocial behavior. In older children and adolescents, wide mood swings may indicate depression. Other common signs of depression include irritability, loss of usual interests and enthusiasm, and a sense of hopelessness about the future.

Misperception of the meaning of illness or injury is common, especially in the young child who employs magical thinking and has a limited capacity for rationalization. Young preschool children often view the pain or discomfort arising from illness or injury as punishment for real or imagined transgressions. In preschool and early school-age children, illness or injury may be viewed as threats of bodily mutilation. In adolescence, illness or injury may be seen as retribution for aggressive or sexual thoughts and behavior. Such fears are much more subject to distortion when sensitive areas such as the head or the genitals are involved.

Anxiety of varying degrees of intensity is frequently associated with psychological conflicts, which stem most often from the meaning of the illness or symptoms to the child. This anxiety is manifested by a subjective sense of fear or unease and by such objective phenomena as tachycardia, palpitations, hyperventilation, sweating, and gastrointestinal disturbances. These effects often serve to compound the problems of the physical illnesses.

Conversion reactions are neurological-like dysfunctions of rapid onset that may affect the voluntary muscles and sensory nerves. They are thought to be the behavioral manifestations of emotional conflict, and in most instances the area involved has symbolic significance. Conversion symptoms usually follow relatively acute psychological events, which in this context would relate to the experience of acute illness. Examples include conversion blindness, paralysis, sensory loss, aphonia, and astasia-abasia (ataxic-like gait). These reactions are to be distinguished from those disorders with significant psychological components that affect involuntary musculature of viscera and are usually without particular symbolic significance. Conversion symptoms may be seen in any personality type, but are more common in the classical hysterical personality. Most conversion reactions are resolved in a few days or weeks, but some persist in children with limited adaptive capacities or in families and/or environments that continue to reinforce the symptom patterns during convalescence.

Dissociative reactions include amnesia, fugue, depersonalization states, and delirium-like states without evidence of organic impairment; or other manifestations of an apparent loss of contact with the environment occurring in response to acute illness when the physical, psychological, or social circumstances are sufficiently stressful. Catatonic behavior without psychosis may also occur. These reactions are usually transient and can be differentiated from delirium or other CNS disorders by the absence of changes in sensorium, orientation, or other cognitive functions.

Behavioral changes are common, especially in young children. These may range from increased passivity and dependency, to aggression and resistance, to cooperating with procedures and treatments. These alterations in behavior may require many weeks after resolution of the illness to disappear completely. Their duration and intensity are decreased in association with good pre-illness family functioning and psychologically sound hospital child management programs.

Academic underachievement may be seen after return to school in children who have experienced the effects of serious disease, including a temporary disturbance in cerebral metabolism. If the relationship of this performance impairment to physical disease is not recognized, the learning difficulties may be compounded by environmental pressures and develop into a chronic and more pervasive pattern. When an illness is prolonged and interferes with school attendance or the performance of assigned work, the academic lag may be much more pronounced. Careful attention should be given to this effect of disease on chronic treatment planning, where early recognition can allow the parents and teachers to help the child gradually to return to full academic performance (Langford, 1961; Prugh et al., 1953; Prugh and Eckhardt, 1975).

In general, the psychological impact of acute illness or injury in children varies according to the organ and system involved, the severity of the disorder, and the nature of the treatment. However, those illnesses that affect social functioning have greater impact on the parents and child than illnesses that do not impair their peer contacts (Freud, 1952). The child who faces the loss of acquired developmental skills during illness or hospitalization experiences feelings of helplessness, embarrassment, and irritation. This is particularly true of the bedridden child, who especially resents the loss of recent gains in his development. The less ill he feels, the stronger the resentment. Anger, humiliation, and anxiety about dependency are frequently observed, and more often than not, the hospital staff and the parents become targets of defiant protests (Mattson and Gross, 1966). Some children may need help in regaining their performance level in motor and social functioning after an acute illness. These problems are magnified in chronic illness.

CHRONIC ILLNESS IN CHILDREN

Many of the considerations mentioned for acute problems are applicable to chronic illness and handicapping injury. Chronic disease frequently leads to severe impact on the child's personality development and family functioning, although some individuals make a surprisingly adequate adaptation to their disability. Although there are general reactions to any chronic disease, a child's previous adaptive capacity, his pre-illness personality, and the parent-child-family balance appear to be more important than the nature of the specific illness or handicap in determining the type and extent of psychological perturbation (Pless and Roghmann, 1972).

The concept of specific personality disorders resulting from particular diseases or handicaps has been largely abandoned. However, it is clear that the impact of a given handicap on a particular person, although determined by a variety of factors, often relates significantly to its psychological meaning. Virtually unnoticeable defects may have an extraordinary impact in some families. A visible cosmetic defect may be most troubling in one family, while in another a hidden metabolic defect may seem a greater threat, without relation to its actual severity. In certain situations the actual physical disability produces the greatest stress and challenge. The latter is particularly evident in children with blindness or deafness, with some differences in responses to congenital versus acquired defects; in the problems of sexual development in children with genital malformations or exstrophy of the bladder; and in the special difficulties in adaptation for the child whose movements are restricted in an orthopedic cast or the handicapped child who requires special prosthetic devices (Shirley, 1963).

The child with serious chronic disease has to cope with threats of periodic exacerbations, lasting physical impairment, and, possibly, a shortened life expectancy. Other common concerns for the child and his family relate to mounting medical expenses and the interference of the illness with schooling, leisure-time activities, vocational training, job opportunities, and later adult roles as a spouse and a parent. The clinical case below illustrates some of these problems in the young adult.

> Beth is a 20-year-old woman who developed systemic lupus erythematosus when she was 16 years of age. Over the course of the last four years, she has required treatment with steroids to manage the disease during its active phase. Because of the symptoms of decreased stamina, sensitivity to sunlight, and anxiety and depression about the disease itself, she saw her most important ambitions thwarted. She dropped out of school, gave up her plans to become a nurse, and had to discontinue most of her outside physical activities. She also suspended her plans for marriage to a boyfriend of many years. During the four years of treatment, she was almost always anxious and fearful concerning the actual symptoms of the disease and the effect of the disease on her life span. At the time of her most recent admission to the hospital, the psychiatric symptoms were more serious, with possible hallucinations, suicidal ideas, and, of course, her continuing depression and high state of anxiety. The question at the time was one of differential diagnosis concerning the relationship of steroid therapy

and the disease process to the psychiatric picture, or whether the psychiatric symptoms were purely a reaction to the limitations the disease was placing on her. Since disease activity required the administration of steroids, they had to be continued, and psychoactive medication was utilized to manage anxiety and depression regardless of their origin. Six months after discharge, she was doing well on low doses of amitriptylene and diazepam in this regimen. However, despite a lessening of the depression and anxiety, she still faced the continuing adjustment problems of career choice, marriage, and leisure-time activities.

In learning to live with a disability that demands continuous medical attention, often away from home, the growing child is expected to assume responsibility for his own care and accept certain limitations in his activities. The final outcome of a child's attempts to meet the continuous stress associated with chronic disease cannot be assessed until young adulthood. Each new step in emotional, intellectual, and social development modifies the psychological impact of the illness on his personality and on his family and, in the best-managed instances, usually endows the child with improved coping ability (Minde et al., 1972).

REACTIONS OF CHILDREN TO HOSPITALIZATION

Numerous studies have indicated the likelihood of serious emotional deprivation for children who experience long-term hospitalization or institutional care (Spitz and Cobliner, 1965; Bowlby, 1969; Robertson, 1970; Schaffer and Callender, 1959; Kanner, 1964). Fortunately, recognition of this possibility, coupled with more advanced technology, has led to treating chronically ill or handicapped children with a shorter hospital stay and outpatient follow-up, which allows them the advantages of living at home (James and Wheeler, 1969). The disadvantages of prolonged hospitalization are seen in the chronic depression and detachment often visible in children raised in large institutions. When prolonged, this often results in shallow social relationships, distorted time concepts, limited capacity for learning, lowered resistance to disease, and rebellious or antisocial behavior (Bowlby, 1969; Provence and Lipton, 1962). These and other observations concerning the effects of hospitalization (Robertson, 1970) have led to significant changes in the method of operating pediatric wards. Perhaps the best ones utilize nurses who have had psychiatric training, child development specialists who attend to both recreational and cognitive needs, school personnel who help avoid prolonged educational interruptions, foster grandparent programs that provide affection and attention, and more relaxed visiting hours and privileges, which allow the chronically ill child a relatively normal routine. In some hospitals, the very young child is cared for by the parents through a live-in arrangement (James and Wheeler, 1969).

Posthospitalization reactions in children are related to their pre-illness personality but are difficult to predict (Shrand, 1965). They sometimes occur in children who seemed able to maintain control throughout the hospital experience. However, once the child returns to the familiar home environment he may regress and show outbursts of anxiety and fears around procedures that were tolerated reasonably well during the actual hospitalization.

In many cases, especially during a long hospital stay, a child may form emotional attachments to certain key hospital personnel and may display sadness or depression after returning home. The child may act withdrawn and prefer to stay in his room, even when he is physically capable of doing more. The child may also have become so dependent on the hospital staff to care for him that he may expect such attention at home. Most hospital personnel try to prevent such dependency and regression, but when it occurs parents should recognize it and encourage more independent behavior and return to self-care. Overprotection or overrestriction by the parents, either as a continuation of the dependent situation of the hospital or as a result of their own fears, may significantly prolong the return to normal functioning (Senn, 1945). When handled realistically, most of these reactions are self-limited and subside within several weeks.

EFFECTS OF TREATMENT PROCEDURES ON CHILDREN

Injections, infusions, immobilization, surgery, isolation, and other procedures arouse anxiety beyond the physical discomfort involved because they reactivate the common childhood fears of bodily mutilation and disfigurement and the misperceived view of medical procedures as a punishment for actual or imagined misdeeds. Such fantasies generally cause fewer problems for the older grade-school child, because his level of cognitive development enables him to comprehend the causal and time relationships of an illness or injury better than the preschool child or toddler (Mattson and Weisberg, 1970).

Most acutely ill children find immobilization and restriction of activity emotionally stressful. They have relied on freedom of movement to discharge tension, to express dissatisfaction and aggression, and to explore and master the environment. Sudden or prolonged motor restraint, particularly of a preschool child, can cause him to panic, develop temper tantrums, and become a serious management problem. At other times, he might show the reaction of withdrawal into an apathetic, depressed state. The child with poor ability or lack of opportunity to verbalize his feelings is more prone to show major behavioral reactions to acute illness (Mattson, 1972). All of these represent factors that, when recognized, may be easily managed by medical personnel and parents.

EFFECTS OF DISFIGUREMENT ON CHILDREN

Among the most difficult physical disorders to manage are those that disfigure a child. These include such traumatic events as burns, amputations, and craniofacial trauma, and distortions of body image associated with certain medical treatments (radiation, chemotherapy for malignant disorders, cushingoid changes with adrenal steroid hormone treatment). With regard to amputation, parental awareness has a profound effect on the child's ability to verbalize mourning for the lost limb and anger associated with its loss or to mitigate the loss of self-esteem and depression seen after amputation. Although children experience phantom limb phenomena to a lesser degree than adults, it may also be a significant consideration in management (Plank and Horwood, 1961). An additional complication of disfiguring defects is seen in children's beliefs that the defect may be responsible for many unrelated events, such as scolding, disciplinary limitations, and loss of peer relationships. Anxiety associated with the surgical amputation procedure may be magnified by the concern that the child will not be appreciated if there is a change in his appearance. The outward expression of this may appear as feelings of fear and hatred toward adults, jealousy of other children, and motivation for revenge. These feelings often produce an intense guilt, which may find outlet in self-destructiveness and misinterpretation of reality.

Recognition of the actual change in body configuration is a prerequisite to the child's development and acceptance of a new body image. The child needs a reality-based concept of his body before the acceptance of a significant change is possible. This is obviously determined by a number of factors, but of all of these, the parent's attitude toward the child may be the most significant. In general, if a child has expressed self-consciousness, self-derogation, or anxiety in regard to his disfigurement, he may extend this attitude to other body parts or to his general body image. On the other hand, if the child has an attitude of acceptance of the modified limb configuration, he usually has a similar regard for other body parts and a higher general level of self-approval (Watson and Johnson, 1958). It is helpful if the child can picture himself with the limb missing before the amputation and begin to speak of the anticipated difference in appearance. This may be accompanied by anxiety, but it is helpful in later adjustment and acceptance of the modified body image. The most important intervention technique related to successful emotional adjustment after amputation is adequate preparation for all of the events surrounding the surgery and its effects. This usually involves a team consisting of the surgeon, child psychiatrist, social worker, amputation nurse, and an amputee volunteer (Buck and Lee, 1976; Pfefferbaum and Pasnau, 1976). The patient should be exposed to a prosthesis and be allowed to familiarize himself with it before surgery. All of these preparations must take into consideration that a healthy parent-child relationship is important both prior to surgery and during convalescence.

Burns in Children

Burns are fairly common in children and are generally seen in one of several contexts: a true accident, a situational crisis, or child abuse (Gil, 1970). Severe burns are extremely stressful experiences for both children and their families. Not only is physical recovery slow and painful, but there is frequent disfigurement, and the psychological trauma of the burn and the events surrounding it have long-lasting effects. Follow-up studies of children who recovered physically from severe burns have revealed that emotional disturbances exist in approximately 80 percent of the children and 60 percent of their mothers (Holter and Friedman, 1969; Woodward and Jackson, 1961; Bernstein, 1976). The majority of these mothers thought that the disturbances in their children were the result of the burn experience, pain, and the separation from home during hospitalization. However, Long and Cope (1961) reported a high incidence of psychopathology in the family unit antedating the burn incident, and Vigiliano, Hart, and Singer (1964) further suggested that chronic relationship problems may become overtly manifest only at the time of the burn incident. Holter and Friedman (1968) emphasized the importance of considering the "battered-child syndrome" in children with burns. In assessing the emotional makeup of the families of severely burned children, they found that 10 of the 13 families in their study had major psychological and social problems within the family unit prior to the burn incidents. In some cases, the gross emotional disturbances within the families may have propelled the children into tragic situations resulting in severe burns. Here again the degree of difficulty in managing children with burns depends to a considerable extent on the same family and child variables noted above in the discussion of surgical disfigurement. The treatment approach again is best carried out by a team of physicians, psychiatrists, and other personnel to handle the psychological problems encountered during recovery (Bernstein, 1976).

CHRONIC DISABILITIES

Most children with a chronic illness or handicap have difficulties with body image. These difficulties may be seen in children without physical disfigurement in terms of characteristics such as size, strength, and attractiveness, which play a significant role in the development of confidence and social skills. However, it is only in very severe deviations from the norm or in special family situations that these factors appear to be of major importance (Barker, Wright, and Gonick,

1953). In adolescents, who need acceptance by the peer group and are extremely sensitive to body configuration, reactions to an altered body image may interfere with the rehabilitation process. This is seen, for example, in the difficulty in getting adolescents to wear hearing aids because of the effect on their perceived body image. Coping techniques used by handicapped or chronically ill children vary considerably. At one extreme are the overdependent, overanxious, and passive or withdrawn patterns—with strong psychological gain from illness—and at the other extreme the overly independent, aggressive modes of behavior—with strong associated tendencies for total denial. The well-adapted child shows realistic dependence and acceptance of his limitations, with adequate social patterns and with a level of denial that doesn't interfere with carrying out therapeutic procedures and the maintenance of hope (Shirley, 1963). Again, the type of response is most closely associated with the pre-illness social adjustment of the child and the nature of the family support systems.

Parental reactions to handicapped or chronically ill children vary considerably. In some instances the patterns seen are those of marked anxiety, overprotectiveness, and overindulgence—manifested by difficulties in setting limits. In other instances there may be problems in acceptance of the child's disability, most often seen in denial of its extent, projection of anger onto the medical staff, reluctance to accept recommended treatment, and even rejection or isolation of the child within the family unit. The more effective parent may show a similar initial response, but soon is able to accept the child's limitations, permit his appropriate dependence, and help him to utilize his strengths in a constructive manner. Nevertheless, most parents display some degree of chronic sorrow or chronic mourning for the handicapped or chronically ill child that does influence their relationship (Olshansky, 1970).

TERMINAL ILLNESS IN CHILDREN

A child's concept of death is not fully developed, in the sense of realistic comprehension, until he is about 10 years old (Osborne, 1967). Thus young children may not express fears of death but, rather, show intense reactions to pain or treatment. Even in adolescents, these fears are often expressed in terms of pain or of need for someone to be with them during difficult moments, rather than in terms of death. The critical need is to have someone to whom the child and parents can express their feelings, rather than to be forced to maintain an unrealistic silence (Friedman, 1968). However, the ability to handle the expression of these feelings from the chronically ill or dying child or his parents requires special training in interviewing techniques (Grollman, 1967; Easson, 1970). Parents may show anticipatory grief and mourning prior to death and further reexperience depression or guilt after the child's death. Thus the most comprehensive care provides support both before and after the child's death (Hollingsworth and Pasnau, 1977). A further complication, especially in young parents, is the attempt to replace the lost child before adequate time has been invested in the work of mourning; this should be discussed in counseling (Poznanski, 1972). The influence of terminal illness is not limited to the child and his family. There is often considerable need for appropriate liaison psychiatry services to help manage the perturbations among health professionals who have worked closely with a dying child and his family (Hollingsworth and Pasnau, 1977).

SPECIFIC DISEASES AND THEIR PSYCHIATRIC ASPECTS

In most instances of physical disorders with a significant psychological dimension, both patients and parents, at least consciously, desire to have the physical problem eradicated, but often they do not perceive the emotional component. Thus they are not ready to accept treatment along psychological lines to manage what to them seems to be an obviously physical problem. Unfortunately, many physicians have a similar viewpoint. Physicians are often so busily engaged in treating the physical disorder that they tend to overlook the psychological problems, or at least place them low among treatment priorities. The key factor in avoiding this omission is awareness of the profound influence of physical disease on psychological functioning, particularly with regard to certain organs that have unique symbolic significance or unique function with respect to organic determinants of behavior (e.g., the brain). Therefore, the type of problems seen in cardiac disorders, with their limitations on activities, life span, and sense of well-being, differ from those seen in seizure disorders, with periodic, unexplained loss of control, or in asthma, where there is intense preoccupation with the ability to breathe.

Neurological Disorders

Utilizing epilepsy as one example of a brain disorder, some of the unique problems can be exemplified. It is quite important for the patient and the parents to understand that although epilepsy may be a chronic disorder, it is not necessarily a handicapping condition. But because of the unusual nature of the behavioral response to the neurophysiological aberration, they may need to be helped by the physician to express whatever their feelings may be about the disease. These feelings may include fear, anger, concern, and embarrassment. Most children with convulsive disorders fear the loss of consciousness, or uncontrollable strange behavior while having a seizure. Moreover, seizures may be socially stigmatizing, especially when they take place at school or among peers. When pharmacologic control of the seizures is achieved, the next critical step is a return to school and normal physical and social activities. During middle adolescence the epileptic may feel uniquely frustrated, since he cannot obtain a driver's license until he has been seizure-free for one or two years. Thus the disease manifestation interferes with the tasks of adolescence and prolongs his dependence on the parents for providing transportation for many school and leisure activities (Detre and Feldman, 1963). The physician's understanding of these complications, coupled with an empathic approach to the patient and his family care, are most important for the long-term management of the disease and the development of the individual. Some of the problems associated with seizure disorders are seen in the clinical case below, where correct diagnosis led to effective treatment and more effective social functioning.

Jason was eight years old when his mother brought him to the pediatric clinic. He was doing very poorly academically in school and his teacher had complained that he seemed tuned out, lacked motivation, and did not always appear to hear her. She felt he just was not interested. The pediatric house officer had Jason's vision and hearing checked and found both to be normal. He consulted the child psychiatrist for an evaluation of the child's school performance. The parents had divorced ten months previously, and the pediatric resident felt that the child might be depressed because his father had not continued to visit after the divorce. The psychiatrist obtained a history that Jason had frequent very brief episodes of staring into space, and would then ask, "What did you say?'" An EEG was done, which revealed the 3 per second spike and slow wave pattern of petit mal epilepsy. After treatment with Zarontin, Jason's school performance improved noticeably. His socialization also improved, and he became one of the most popular children in his class. His classmates did not know that he had a seizure disorder, and thus he was able to avoid the stigma of being labeled by his peers.

A secondary problem associated with seizure disorders concerns the effects of anticonvulsant medications. Although there is a dearth of clear and specific information in the research literature, there are a number of disquieting reports. The traditional drugs, such as phenobarbital and dilantin, have been associated with a variety of cognitive and emotional changes, including impairment in attention and learning, and mood alterations such as depression. These effects may be subtle and not always associated either with toxic blood levels or with neurological signs. Drug control of seizures may thus generate important mental changes, which also should be monitored (Trimble and Reynolds, 1976).

Cardiac Disease

The child with a chronic heart disease of infectious or congenital origin has the usual problem of coping with chronic disease, but is also confronted with considerations unique to the organ involved. He may find it difficult to comprehend the nature of his illness and the reasons for restrictions, extensive workups, and surgery. In addition, the knowledge of an affliction of one's heart is especially frightening because of the common symbolic references to the heart in everyday language and the awareness of its function in life maintenance (Glaser, Harrison, and Lynn, 1964). In view of the extensive problems, an active psychoeducational program is essential in the management of cardiac disease, particularly when there is considerable restriction of activity and interference with growth. This type of program is particularly important in the preparation for heart surgery, since states of profound apprehension and depression may complicate such surgery in childhood and adolescence (Toker, 1971; Barnes et al., 1972).

Respiratory Disorders

Cystic fibrosis, like cardiac disorders that involve the respiratory system, produces significant psychological effects because of the kinds of symptoms and the types of problems encountered. Impairment of breathing adds another dimension to that of the chronic disease process itself. In the child with cystic fibrosis, one sees the debilitating symptoms characteristic of many chronic physical disorders, such as poor appetite and decreased stamina, and such embarrassing symptoms as flatulence and stool odor. But his life is further complicated by the involved management of respiratory problems, including postural drainage and nebulization, and by the growing awareness that his illness is hereditary, progressive, and leads to early death. Few children with cystic fibrosis expect a cure, but maintain the hope that the disease might be controlled with the proper therapy. Tropauer, Franz, and Dilgard (1970) reported that one-third of the mothers of children with cystic fibrosis indicated that their children had voiced concerns about dying prematurely. For this and other reasons, some parents may attempt to hide the facts about the disease from their children, even to the extent of attempting to prevent the child from learning the diagnosis. In such cases it is imperative to work with the parents to secure their cooperation and avoid further confusion and fear that would be stimulated by conflicting information. It is of particular value to adolescents and young adults with cystic fibrosis to have the opportunity to discuss with their physician concerns about continuing education, employment, marriage, and parenthood, so that realistic future plans can be made (Tropauer, Franz, and Dilgard, 1970).

Asthma

In asthma there are common physiological mediating mechanisms that produce airway constriction and symptomatic wheezing. There appears to be a wide variety of stimuli that can trigger these mechanisms, including pollens, dust, exercise, and emotional changes. Children with family allergic histories and multiple allergic manifestations themselves often wheeze in response to emotional stimuli as well as to airborne allergens. Thus, the traditional dichotomy between "organic" versus "psychogenic" asthma appears to be untenable. Emotional factors, such as anger, fear, or excitement may precipitate or prolong any asthmatic episode. Also, the presence of such a chronic recurrent disorder can cause individual and family psychological problems.

Repeated asthmatic attacks and the additional limitations that may be imposed by medical management often compel these youngsters to reduce their activities and thus limit their opportunity to interact with peers and to participate in age-appropriate activities, including competitive athletics. In addition, asthmatic children often have other symptoms of the basic allergic disorder, such as atopic dermatitis, which may require dietary restriction and thus may further interfere with overall adjustment.

The threat of the asthmatic attack may also generate separation anxiety in both child and parents. Familiarity with the disease and stepwise plans for intervention may decrease anxiety and allow for more normal independence in the child.

Earlier psychodynamic theories of asthma, such as the wheezing representing a suppressed cry for mother or the disorder signifying maternal deprivation (Alexander, 1950; Dunbar, 1948), have not been substantiated by more recent research (Graham et al., 1967; Gauthier et al., 1977). Nor has it been possible to delineate specific personality types in asthmatic children. Various psychological difficulties are associated with the disorder and may be more marked in some children than in others. Certainly an asthmatic attack is a psychologically traumatic event. Inability to breathe is life threatening and is certain to produce varying degrees of anxiety. The conditioned fear of a subsequent attack may well serve as a triggering mechanism for producing a new attack. Significant adults in the child's environment may themselves become increasingly anxious and often serve to intensify this basic anxiety (Purcell and Weiss, 1970). Furthermore, the existence of a primary psychiatric disorder is only a bit more common in asthmatic children (10.5 percent) than in the general population (6.3 percent). A similar degree of difference is also noted in children suffering from a miscellaneous group of other physical disorders (Graham et al., 1967).

Thus the child with bronchial asthma requires a thorough physical and psychiatric evaluation. Such a total study often clarifies the biological and psychological factors involved, thus allowing appropriate therapeutic measures.

In some instances the immunological factors appear to be predominant. Children with high allergic potential demonstrate fewer problems that could be labelled as primarily psychiatric, and the asthmatic condition is less responsive to any psychiatric intervention. In children with lower allergic potential, environmental manipulation and psychiatric treatment may be effective, probably because of the significant contribution made by environmental events. There are, of course, children with combinations of both. Whatever the case, there are usually problems in adapting to this particular disorder that will require some degree of psychiatric intervention. When the child's emotional difficulties are predominant, therapeutic assistance to parents is essential, but this may also be necessary even when the child's asthma is primarily allergic in nature. The psychiatric treatment at times may be directed toward underlying emotional problems existing in the parents or, as in most instances, it may be directed toward helping the parents deal realistically with the asthmatic child to avoid the complications mentioned above. Direct work with the child may be centered on accepting the disease and its limitations and minimizing the psychological gain from the asthmatic attack.

Renal Disease

Advances in the state of the art in management of renal disease have introduced an increasing number of problems related to changes in life expectancy and the peculiarities of technical management. Kidney diseases themselves have many of the characteristics of other chronic diseases, including a reduction in stamina, appetite, and impairment in growth, as well as the usual psychological responses mentioned earlier in this chapter. In addition, an increasing number of children with chronic renal disease are treated with hemodialysis and kidney transplantation, which introduces several unique psychological considerations related to these procedures. The hemodialysis machine itself often creates frightening fantasies of bleeding to death or of the machine assuming control (Abram, 1970; Bernstein, 1971).

The use of immunosuppressive drugs in association with transplant procedures may further interfere with the child's growth and thus compound the problems associated with the preexisting kidney disease. These young patients often feel isolated and apart from their peers. The disease and its treatment puts them in a dependent position, which may be particularly difficult for the teenager who is seeking independence from his family and a sense of identity among his peers. After kidney transplantation, many children find that their parents tend to overprotect them in the same fashion as during the disease process. In other instances parents use threats of possible failure of the transplant as a means of controlling their activities. The overall picture is further complicated by anxiety generated in the child and the parent in relationship to minor physical symptoms. This has occurred as long as six years after a successful transplant (Bernstein, 1971). In cases of actual kidney rejection, requiring a return to hemodialysis, the young patient, like the adult, usually responds with depression and withdrawal. Children in particular tend to blame themselves for "destroying" the kidney given to them as a special gift. Despite the problems associated with this procedure, it should be noted that follow-up studies on children who have undergone renal transplant show that many are well adjusted as young adults and some of them have growth spurts as long as five years after surgery (Bernstein, 1971).

Hematopoietic Disorders

Chronic bleeding disorders, such as hemophilia, often cause the young child to be concerned about fatal bleeding resulting from physical trauma or certain medical procedures, such as venipuncture (Engel, 1960; Mattson and Gross, 1966). Over time, disfigurement occurs in hemophilia in the form of perpetual bruises and bleeding into joints. Much more stressful are the problems of neoplastic disorders of the bone marrow or such disorders as aplastic anemia. Both involve the same kind of medical treatments that are debilitating and, in the case of bone marrow transplant, carry a high risk for fatal outcome. The disease itself most often ends in a fatal outcome either acutely or, in some instances, after a period of agonizing for months or years. The psychological problems encountered during treatment are pervasive and involve the patient, family, and medical team to a degree rarely seen in other disorders. A clinical case will illustrate this point.

Leroy is an 11-year-old male who developed myelogenous leukemia 11 months prior to admission to UCLA for bone marrow transplant. Treatment with cytotoxins resulted in a transient remission, but also resulted in a total loss of hair. The latter led to significant teasing by peers while Leroy was attending school. His remission lasted three months and was followed by two more courses of chemotherapy without remission. Finally, bone marrow transplant was suggested as the only possible procedure that could prolong his life. The family dislocation associated with the necessity to live near the hospital was considerable. Although the patient himself handled most of the problems quite well, the mother and siblings showed a great deal of confusion and anxiety, manifested by loss of control of the children's behavior. The mother and children proved difficult to integrate into the treatment program while at the same time trying to maintain a medically controlled environment. After the transplant, the fluctuating course associated with symptoms secondary to total body radiation and to infections and fevers was extremely frustrating to the staff. Their hopes continually rose and fell as a function of the patient's condition. The psychiatrist on the team was constantly involved in helping to manage the psychological problems of the patient, the family, the nursing staff, and the medical team. Despite all of the effort expended, the patient died three months after discharge.

Endocrine Disorders

Disorders of the endocrine system are particularly noteworthy for psychological complications surrounding such issues as stature, sexual characteristics, body configuration, stamina, and eating. These general disturbances are often directly related to the endocrine dysfunction and, in some instances, to therapy utilizing hormones. Interest in the problems of short stature in children and teenagers, often complicated by delayed sexual maturation, has increased recently. It has become evident that a major problem of the undersized child is related to the tendency to treat him like a child of similar size who would be chronologically much younger (Rothchild and Owens, 1972). This particular response to the child may result in withdrawal and, in some instances, lead to a degree of inhibition of cognitive and emotional development (Money and Politt, 1966). Some short youngsters cope by an excessive denial of their outspoken and overtly assertive individuals. The following case demonstrates some of the problems seen in adolescents with short stature.

Frank was 15, but he looked more like 11. He had been followed in the clinic for short stature for four years. Now he was being unmercifully teased by peers, especially in the gym when dressing for physical education. He related that for years he had been the butt of his peers' jokes, but had been able to allow the jokes to pass by with the hope that if he did not react his "friends" would stop teasing him. He also complained that everyone, including his parents and physicians, related to him as if he were 11, not 15. Frank related that he was not genuinely depressed because he had only grown one inch in one year. The pediatrician showed him X-rays of his hands and knees that indicated that he would continue to grow, and commented that he would possibly end up around four to five feet and six inches in height. The ability of the pediatrician to be reassuring to this young man and to be candid in discussing Frank's incipient concerns was quite helpful. His voice had finally started to change and he felt very hopeful now. He was rather excited about a few pubic hairs that had recently appeared. The child psychiatrist, who was asked to consult, focused on Frank's feelings related to peer teasing, his interest in girls, and methods of coping with everyday problems, rather than constantly focusing on his short stature. Overall, Frank felt that the focus on the realities of his potential for growth by the pediatrician and methods of social management by the child psychiatrist had been quite useful to him.

Ulcerative Colitis

Ulcerative colitis is a chronic inflammatory disease of the large bowel characterized by ulceration, diarrhea, hemorrhage, and pain, with a somewhat variable course. The onset is usually in childhood or early adolescence. Once established, further attacks of ulcerative colitis often occur with emotional stress (Engel, 1958). The acute attack carries with it the dangers of a severe bleeding episode or bowel perforation. When the condition persists for years, general somatic growth may be seriously affected. A frequent complication of ulcerative colitis in both children and adults is (a high incidence of) carcinoma of the bowel (Devroede, 1971).

It has often been suggested that children with ulcerative colitis show a relatively distinct personality type. The typical history reveals that the child has been perfectionistic, rigid, and overly conscientious. This pseudomature adjustment is occasionally interrupted by brief episodes of infantile dependent behavior. Many of the children have peculiar eating habits, with intense dislikes for certain foods, based on their consistency or color. When the child develops an attack of ulcerative colitis, he characteristically becomes whiney, depressed, and demanding and generally withdraws from most of his ordinary activities. Depression during these attacks is quite prominent, and preoccupations with death is often seen. The difficulty in ascribing causality or uniqueness to these characteristics and symptoms lies in their frequent appearance in other conditions of chronic disease and in individuals without physical disease. In fact, the chronic symptoms characteristic of ulcerative colitis may shape and enhance many of the personality traits, including obsessive concerns with gastrointestinal functions.

A smaller number of children with ulcerative colitis have characteristics somewhat different from those described above. They are querulous, demanding, manipulative children, who are somewhat less likely to develop acute fulminating attacks of colitis. Their symptoms are usually less dramatic, but more persistent, and they often use the colitis in a manipulative fashion to force parents and others to attend to their excessive demands.

The parents of children with ulcerative colitis and similar conditions, such as Crohn's disease, often have exaggerated fears that certain foods will harm them. Their frequent inability to control defecation causes considerable embarrassment. The characteristic family preoccupation with the gastrointestinal functioning requires energetic management to separate it from the common psychological problems of growing up. Perhaps most significant of all is the frequent need for surgical intervention, which requires that the child and family be prepared for a temporary or permanent ileostomy when the stage of the disorder warrants it. Such a procedure entails major body changes, which are particularly stressful to adolescents during the time when they are beginning to establish intimate heterosexual friendships (Finch and Hess, 1962). Despite all of these complications, a successful ileostomy can be useful in supporting the young patient's adaptation. The final treatment plan is formulated by a joint decision of the medical team and communicated to patient and parent by the primary physician (Pasnau, 1964).

Recurrent Abdominal Pain

The recurrent abdominal pain syndrome may affect as many as 10 percent of all persons during some period in childhood or adolescence. Criteria for this disorder include at least three episodes of pain affecting activities and occurring over at least a three-month period. Medical evaluations reveal organic disorders only in about 8 percent of cases (Apley, 1968). Several psychiatric disorders are associated with this syndrome, including hyperventilation, anxiety, depression, phobias, and anorexia nervosa. In the parents and siblings there is an increased incidence of recurrent abdominal pain, also of headache and peptic ulcer disease. Specific stress situations often seem to precipitate attacks of pain. The families are frequently conflicted, and the parents are overprotecting and overinvolved with the child.

Another frequent finding is unwillingness to admit and resolve conflict, as well as real unawareness of conflict or strong emotion. Many of these families seem to exhibit alexithymia—the inability to give verbal expression to feeling (Sifneos, 1973).

There are dangers in the failure to diagnose the disorder. Surgical intervention can complicate the situation by producing adhesions. Repeated evaluations and hospitalizations can reinforce the symptom massively by focusing the attention of family and staff on the child as a medical-surgical problem and by allowing escape from aversive situations (e.g., school avoidance for a child with school difficulties).

Treatment involves education and reassurance, reinforcement of verbal expression and adaptive behavior, and treatment of any underlying psychiatric disorders.

Juvenile Diabetes Mellitus

Emotional problems play a rather large role in the juvenile diabetic (Swift and Seidman, 1964). First, there is the possibility that emotional stress is a triggering mechanism, related to the onset of the diabetes. Some children may have a constitutional predisposition in this direction, and with sufficient emotional tension the diabetes may become evident. More obvious, however, is the frequent finding that once the disease is established in children and adolescents, significant secondary problems develop that center on the need to accept the diabetes and the limitations it imposes.

Juvenile diabetes has often been referred to as "brittle" because it is usually more difficult to manage medically than the same disease in an adult (Kempe, Silver, and O'Brien, 1972). Fluctuations in the control of juvenile diabetes frequently seem related to emotional stress, which may exert its effect both through physiological mechanisms and through rebellious or hostile behavior and depressed states. The child is often unwilling to accept the disorder and may try to prove that it does not exist by ignoring the rules and regulations for management, or may abandon the diabetic regimen in angry and self-destructive retaliation (Swift and Seidman, 1964; Tietz and Vidmar, 1972). The latter type of response may indicate a more serious maladjustment than the somewhat more common use of the ailment as an escape from or a defense against the responsibilities and expectations of childhood (Mattson, 1972).

An extensive study by Tietz and Vidmar (1972) showed no correlation between effectiveness of control of diabetes and factors such as age of onset, duration of illness, number of siblings, intactness of family, psychopathology, intelligence of child and parents, knowledge about diabetes, birth rank, or ethnic and social class. However, a positive correlation was found between families with a history of diabetes and children being under good medical control. Children who appeared to be in the midst of an "adolescent growth spurt," however, clustered in the group with poor control. Clinical observations of individual patients and their families within this same study suggested that the reactions to the onset of diabetes were influenced by the styles of coping with fears, anxieties, and guilt. Both fear and anger activate physiological mechanisms that influence the disease course. Thus, mastery over fear enables better coping and control of the diabetes. At the other extreme, complete denial of the illness may also lead to ineffective control.

In terms of general emotional health McGavin et al. (1940) studied a group of 45 diabetic children and found that 32 were emotionally maladjusted. Among other things, the diabetic children perceived themselves as being significantly "different" from other children. This sense of difference often created feelings of inferiority and conflicts that expressed themselves in various types of reactions, including seclusiveness, aggressiveness, boastfulness, and show-off behavior. Some children expressed shame for having diabetes; others felt that children avoided them as if they could "catch the disease." Some began to withdraw from social contacts, and a few interpreted diabetes as punishment. Among adolescents, some resented having diabetes because it placed them outside the "marriage market," presumably because of the possibility of impotence or the genetic significance of having diabetes. A few rebelled against the disease by refusing to accept restrictions in diet, resulting in frequent attacks of acidosis.

Once juvenile diabetes is diagnosed, it is important that the disease be brought under some degree of control (Kempe, Silver, and O'Brien, 1972). This requires cooperation on the part of the parents as well as the child himself. The parents need a reasonably complete education concerning diabetes and its control. They should be allowed the opportunity to ask questions and receive informative answers. It is important that they understand that with proper control their child can lead an essentially normal life. Depending on the age of the child at the time of the diagnosis, the parents may have to assume the major responsibility for insulin administration as well as diet. Gradually, over time the youngster must take over increasing responsibility for these matters, consistent with increasing independence in general. Explanations of the disorder should be presented in language commensurate with his age. It is necessary at some point that the child recognize that adherence to the prescribed treatment regimen should enable him to minimize complications during his life. This is especially important now that endocrinological opinion again emphasizes the association between strictness of control and reduced complications.

When faced with behavioral disturbances in diabetes, it is essential for the primary care physician to differentiate between those cases where the behavior is related to diabetes or is linked to some other cause, including normal childhood and adolescent problems. In addition to the focus on problems in the child, the physician should be aware of the emotional impact of the disease on the family. Whenever psychiatric difficulties are identified in child or parent, they should be handled with the same degree of concern as directed toward other aspects of the disorder. The following clinical case gives some idea of the complexity of the problems in juvenile diabetes.

Angela, a 13-year-old, quiet, withdrawn girl, came to the pediatric clinic at her mother's insistence because of depression. She had been diagnosed as having diabetes mellitus one year previously, and had taken both regular NPH insulin for six months after the diagnosis had been made. Initially she had been very cooperative with the management of her disease. She did her own urine checks and administered her own insulin. Suddenly, six months ago, Angela became quite sad, withdrew from social contacts, and refused to check her urine or to give herself injections. She also refused to allow anyone else to give the insulin. She voiced concerns about the cost of the insulin and wanted her mother to spend the money for a gift each week for her two-year-old sister. The pediatric resident who saw Angela felt that she was being stubborn and self-destructive, and consulted a child psychiatrist for an evaluation of Angela's possible suicidal tendencies. Further history gathered by the child psychiatrist revealed that Angela's grandmother had died two years previously of complications of diabetes after bilateral above-the-knee amputations and after becoming blind from diabetic retinopathy. Angela's 18-year-old brother had been diagnosed as having diabetes at age 15 and had taken his insulin faithfully each day until a breakup with a girl friend, when he stopped taking his insulin.

Three days later, he lost consciousness while driving his car on the freeway and was killed in a four-car accident. This occurred three months prior to Angela stopping her insulin. Angela was very distraught after relating this information and said she wanted to join her brother. The final family stress that precipitated Angela's refusal to take insulin was her father's hospitalization for bleeding esophageal varices. He was near death for two weeks, and Angela had been so afraid that she would be left alone that she stopped caring for her diabetes in the hope that she too would die. She related that she had spent many nights in the past six months crying about this, but that she had not been able to talk with anyone about it. It was felt that Angela was a high suicide risk, and hospitalization was arranged for further evaluation of her mental status and to reestablish good control of her diabetes. Angela was discharged from the hospital after two weeks and was followed up by a psychiatrist twice a week for six months. Her outlook on life became somewhat brighter, and she acknowledged that if she carefully regulated her diabetes she could prevent the serious complications seen in other members of the family; thus it was not necessary to give up hope.

Anorexia Nervosa

Anorexia nervosa occurs more commonly in girls than boys and usually has its onset in mid-adolescence. The parents of these children show no uniform type of psychopathology (Bruch, 1966) but are often overprotective, and one or the other may be involved in an intensely ambivalent relationship with the child. Although there is a spectrum of severity, this disorder may require intensive long-term treatment, including psychiatric hospitalization, since in some instances it is life threatening. The initial problems of eating and weight gain are often fairly easily managed using behavioral techniques, but the peculiarities of thought relative to food and the difficulties encountered by the parents may require a more intensive intervention in the form of individual and family psychotherapy.

Important criteria for a diagnosis of anorexia nervosa include a vigorous pursuit of weight loss and thinness through diet and/or vomiting and the use of cathartics, a distortion of body image (perception of heaviness in the face of emaciation), loss of 25 percent of body weight, and amenorrhea in girls. Appetite may actually be intense, occasionally provoking eating binges, followed by anxiety and remorse.

Many of these adolescents have symptoms of depression. Family members have an increased incidence of depressive illness. The patients themselves frequently exhibit depressive disorders without the symptoms and signs of anorexia nervosa on follow-up (Sturzenberger et al., 1977). Thus, there seems to be a strong association of this disorder with affective illness.

Another concern is the hypothalmic dysfunction that has been documented. FSH and LH levels are reduced, growth hormone is increased, thyroid hormone may be slightly decreased. At least some of these changes seem to be associated with severe weight loss alone; they resolve as soon as relatively normal nutrition is restored. This underscores the importance of weight gain as the initial intervention.

Obesity

Obesity is a common problem in childhood that has significant impact on personality development and social adaptation. Certainly, some children become overweight purely because of endocrine difficulties; however, such cases are relatively rare and are usually identified by a thorough medical evaluation. Most often children are obese because of overeating and associated constitutional variables related to a family history of obesity (Mayer, 1975). Frequently, these children are quite demanding, and when such excessive demands are not met the child tries to satisfy them by an increase in food intake. It appears that many obese children come from families in which food is overvalued (Bruch, 1943). Thus there may be a tendency to feed the infant whenever he is uncomfortable, regardless of the reason for the discomfort. The older child and adolescent may overeat in response to insecurity or depression. Unfortunately, the resulting weight increase may further serve to reduce the child's already low self-esteem.

In addition to psychological factors there are genetic, constitutional, and biological determinants of obesity. There is an increased risk of later and more intractable obesity the earlier the onset and the stronger the family history of obesity. Nevertheless, some obese children are not particularly maladjusted, and their obesity can be kept under reasonable control without undue difficulty. In terms of management, the overall picture presented by each child requires examination to determine the contribution of each of these factors.

Failure to Thrive

Failure to thrive is a syndrome of infancy and early childhood, with severe impairment of physical growth and mental development (Bullard et al., 1967). This condition may result from chronic illness, environmental or emotional deprivation, or severe feeding problems. The majority have physical diseases, but approximately one third have no evidence of physical causality. This group is characterized by a high incidence of psychiatric disturbance in mother and child. The more stable the family the greater the likelihood or response to treatment.

SYMPTOMATIC DISORDERS

There are a number of symptomatic conditions that involve various body systems or functions but are primarily psychological in nature. These disorders stand in contrast to those described above in that organ pathology, when it exists, is usually secondary to the condition induced by psychological factors. They must be differentiated from organic disturbances that lead to the same symptomatology.

Headache

Headache is a symptom probably experienced by most children at one time or another. In some, the symptom picture is persistent and may be evidence of a defensive adaptation technique or an expression of some form of serious psychological disturbance. Ling, Oftedal, and Weinberg (1970) found that of 25 children presenting with headache, including migraine, ten were shown to have depressive illness that responded to antidepressant medication. Headache can also be seen as part of a delusional state, conversion reaction, or hypochondriacal state. Migraine, a complex psychophysiological problem is present in four percent of school-age children (Ling, Oftedal, and Weinberg, 1970). In addition to the physiologically based headache, this disorder is often accompanied by the type of psychological pain associated with any headache, and this must always be considered in managing the problem.

Encopresis

Encopresis is defined as the voluntary or involuntary deposition of fecal matter in an inappropriate place (e.g., pants, bedroom) after the age of toilet training. In primary encopresis toilet training never has been accomplished, whereas secondary encopresis represents a regression after at least a year of appropriate toileting behavior. Family or individual stresses or acute emotional changes frequently seem to be associated with the secondary type.

The majority of children with encopresis probably also exhibit fecal retention. As the fecal mass increases, a megacolon results, in which the colon seems to lose its normal sensitivity as well as motility. Overflow incontinence develops around the fecal mass; this produces a further withholding response, which perpetuates the retentive cycle. Children who retain stool, especially those who never accomplished toilet training, appear to respond best to a program of education, behavioral contingencies, and bowel stimulants such as mineral oil.

Children who do not retain but always empty stool into pants or other inappropriate receptacles appear to have more significant psychopathology in themselves and in their families. Other psychiatric disorders may accompany encopresis, including depression, attentional and learning disorders, and psychosis.

Particular personality types in parents, style of toilet training, and events of the toilet training period have not been shown to correlate with encopresis in general or with the specific subtypes. However, the impression exists that there are difficulties in the families and in parent-child relationships that contribute to onset and maintenance of the problem.

Encopresis is found more frequently in boys than in girls, in a 5:1 ratio, and is independent of socioeconomic class. The disorder is often persistent, but usually disappears by adolescence. It may be accompanied by significant feelings of being unwanted and a low sense of self-esteem (Henoch, 1970). Encopresis may be seen in association with other illnesses or symptoms, which include infantile autism, childhood schizophrenia, and mental retardation.

The proper management of encopresis requires a careful evaluation (including barium enema and rectal biopsy to rule out Hirschsprung's disease) and a comprehensive approach. There are often associated problems that must be addressed; their resolution often results in remission of the encopresis. Another important goal of intervention is to minimize the child's guilt and the parents' anger about the symptom.

Enuresis

Enuresis can be defined as bed-wetting or clothes wetting in persons over the age of three who fail to inhibit the reflex to urinate when the impulse is felt during waking hours and who do not arouse from sleep when urinating during the sleeping state. Eighty-eight percent of children are dry by age 4½, but after age five the incidence of enuresis rises to 15 percent. This includes those who have never been dry at night and the four percent who have been dry at night but began wetting again for a variety of reasons. By age 7½ the number of enuretics decreases to seven percent, and between 7½ and 18 years of age the percentage in the general population drops to about two percent (Klackenberg, 1971; Murphy and Chapman, 1970; Roach, 1969; Chen-chin and Yi-sen, 1969). The major psychological consideration is whether there is any relationship between enuresis and maladjustment. There is growing opinion that maturational or developmental factors are more critical considerations than are psychodynamic factors. Enuretics seems to show no significant differences, except for the symptom of enuresis, when matched with a group of nonenuretics (McKendryu, Williams, and Broughton, 1968; Werry and Cohrssen, 1965). Various treatment approaches have been tried with somewhat similar results: (1) placebos (Kardash, Hillman, and Werry, 1968); (2) conditioning devices, such as the bell and pad method (Turner, Young, and Rachman, 1970); (3) psychotherapy (Blum, 1970); (4) drugs (Tec, 1968); (5) bladder training by fluid restriction or gradual voluntary withholding (Shader, 1968); (6) sleep interruption (Shader, 1968); and (7) hypnosis (Baker, 1969). Psychotherapy alone, based on various theoretical considerations, has not been shown to be unusually effective in relieving the symptom.

SUMMARY

In children, most medical disorders and procedures or medications used to treat disease carry with them the possibility of significant psychological impact. This impact is usually seen in behavioral reactions, which either complicate the diagnosis, require treatment as major problems in themselves, or interfere with the treatment of the primary disorder. Children's reactions to disease and medical intervention range from total denial to profound depression and include such mechanisms as misperception, regression, conversion, and academic underachievement. Not only is the child faced with the symptoms of the disorder itself, but also the fantasy concerning what it means in terms of changes in body image, limitations of social capabilities, and retribution for imagined or real transgressions. Most serious medical situations in children are further complicated by the reactions of siblings and parents, often along the same dimensions as noted with the ill child.

Some conditions generally have a more than ordinary psychological impact on the child and family. These include disfiguring trauma and disease, where the problems focus heavily on body image disturbances; certain psychological disorders, where the patient and family become overinvolved in organ functioning; and those extremely tragic disorders where survival of the child himself is at issue. Effective management of physical illness in children requires the ability to recognize psychiatric problems in child and parent, and to understand their relationship to the disease process and its management. The reader is referred elsewhere for information about other situations and conditions. These include mental retardation (Mandelbaum, 1967), brain dysfunction and cerebral palsy (Gardner, 1968; Chess, Korn, and Fernandez, 1971), congenital amputees (Gurney, 1968; Roskies, 1970), orthopedia conditions (Myers, Friedman, and Weiner, 1970), cleft palate (Tisza and Gumperty, 1962), cryptorchidism (Cytryn, Cytryn, and Rieger, 1967), and metabolic conditions (Prugh, 1963; Apley and MacKeith, 1968). The focus of this chapter has been brief coverage of significant conditions. A number of the references cited in the text should prove useful for more detailed information.

REFERENCES

Abram, H. S. Survival by machine: The psychological stress of chronic hemodialysis. *Psychiatric Medicine, 1;* 37 (1970).

Alexander, F. *Psychosomatic Medicine.* W. W. Norton, New York (1950).

Apley, J. and MacKeith, R. *The Child and His Symptoms.* F.A. Davis, Philadelphia (1968), pp. 209–215; 216–240.

Baker, B. Symptom treatment and symptom substitution in enuresis. *Journal of Abnormal Psychology, 74;* 42 (1969).

Barker, R.G., Wright B. and Gonick, M. *Adjustment to Physical Handicap and Illness: A Survey of the Social Psychology of Physique and Disability.* Social Science Research Council, New York (1953).

Barnes, C.M., Kewnnyu, F.M., Call, T., and Reinhart, J.B. Measurement in management of anxiety in children for open heart surgery. *Pediatrics, 49;* 250 (1972).

Bernstein, D.M. After transplantation: the child's emotional reactions. *American Journal of Psychiatry, 127;* 1189 (1971).

Blom, G.E. The reactions of hospitalized children to illness. *Pediatrics, 22;* 590 1958).

Blum, H.P. Maternal psycho-therapy and nocturnal enuresis. *Psychoanalytic Quarterly, 39;* 609 (1970).

Bowlby, J. *Attachment and Loss: Attachment.* Basic Books, New York (1969).

Bruch, H. Psychiatric aspects of obesity in children. *American Journal of Psychiatry, 99;* 752 (1943).

———. Anorexia nervosa and its differential diagnosis. *Journal of Nervous and Mental Diseases, 141;* 555 (1966).

Buck, B., and Lee, A. Amputation: Two views. *Nursing Clinics of North America, 11;* 641–657 (1976).

Bullard, P.M., Glaser, H.H., Heagarty, M.C. and Pivchik, E.C. Failure to thrive in the neglected child. *American Journal of Orthopsychiatry, 37;* 680 (1967).

Chen-chin, H., and Yi-sen, C. An epidemiological study on enuresis among school age children: 2nd report: A study on the reliability of information obtained through questionnaires regarding presence and absence of enuresis. *Journal of the Formosan Medical Association, 68;* 85 (1969).

Chess, S., Korn, S.J., and Fernandez, P.B. *Psychiatric Disorders of Children with Congenital Rubella.* Brunner/Mazel, New York (1971).

Cytryn, L., Cytryn, E., and Rieger, R.E. Psychological implications of cryptorchism. *Journal of the American Academy of Child Psychiatry, 6;* 131 (1967).

Detre, T., and Feldman, R.G. Behavior disorder associated with seizure states. *Pharmacological and Psychosocial Management in EEG and Behavior,* In G. Glaser, ed. Basic Books, New York (1963), p. 366.

Devroede, G.J. Cancer risk and life expectancy of children with ulcerative colitis. *New England Journal of Medicine, 285;* 17 (1971).

Dunbar, F. *Psychosomatic Diagnosis.* Harper & Row, New York (1948).

Easson, W.M. *The Dying Child, the Management of the Child or Adolescent Who Is Dying.* Charles C. Thomas, Springfield (1970).

Engel, G.L. Studies of ulcerative colitis; Psychological aspects and their implications for treatment. *American Journal of Digestive Disease, 3;* 315 (1958).

–––. A unified concept of health and disease. *Perspectives in Biological Medicine, 3;* 459 (1960).

–––. The need for a new medical model. A challenge for Biomedicine. *Science, 196;* 129 (1977).

Finch, S.M., and Hess, J.H. Ulcerative colitis in children. *American Journal of Psychiatry, 118;* 819 (1962).

Freud, A. The role of bodily illness in the mental life of the child. *Psychoanalytic Study of the Child, 7;* 42 (1952).

Friedman, S.B. Management of fatal illness in children. *Ambulatory Pediatrics.* In M. Green and R.J. Haggerty, eds. W.B. Saunders, Philadelphia (1968), pp. 753–759.

Gardner, R.A. Psychogenic problems of brain-injured children and their parents. *Journal of the American Academy of Child Psychiatry, 7;* 471 (1968).

Gauthier, Y., Fortier, C., Drapeau, P., Breton, J.S., Gosselin, J., Quintal, L., Wersnagel, J., Tetreault, L., and Pinaud, G. The mother-child relationship and the development of autonomy and self-assertion in young asthmatic children. *Journal of the American Academy of Child Psychiatry, 16;* 109 1977).

Gil, D. *Violence Against Children: Physical Child Abuse in the United States.* Harvard University Press, Cambridge, Mass. (1970).

Glaser, H.H., Harrison, G.S., and Lynn, D.B. Emotional implications of congenital heart disease in children. *Pediatrics, 33;* 367 (1964).

Graham, P.J., Rutter, M.L., Yule, W., and Pless, I.B. Childhood asthma: A psychosomatic disorder? Some epidemiological considerations, *British Journal of Prevention and Social Medicine, 21;* 84 (1967).

Grollman, E.A. *Explaining Death to Children.* Beacon Press, Boston (1967).

Gurney, W. Congenital Amputee. In *Ambulatory Pediatrics,* M. Green and R.J. Haggerty, eds. W.B. Saunders, Philadelphia (1968), pp. 534–540.

Henoch, E.G. How Henoch treated children with encopresis. *Pediatrics, 46;* 802 (1970).

Hollingsworth, C.E., and Pasnau, R.O. *The Family in Mourning: A Guide for Health Professionals.* Grune & Stratton, New York (1977).

Holter, J.C., and Friedman, S.B. Child abuse. *Pediatrics, 42;* 128 (1968).

–––. Etiology and management of severely burned children: Psychosocial considerations. *American Journal of Diseases of Children, 118;* 680 (1969).

James, V.L., and Wheeler, W.E. The care by parent unit. *Pediatrics, 43;* 488 (1969).

Kanner, L. *A History of the Care and Study of the Mentally Retarded.* Charles C. Thomas, Springfield (1964).

Kardash, S., Hillman, E., and Werry, J. Efficacy of imipramine in childhood enuresis: A double-blind control study with placebo. *Canadian Medical Association Journal, 99;* 263 (1968).

Kempe, H., Silver, H.K., and O'Brien, D. *Current Pediatric Diagnosis and Treatment,* 2nd ed. (1972), pp. 629–637.

Klackenberg, C. A prospective longitudinal study of children: Data on psychic health and development up to eight years of age. *Acta Paediatrica Scandinavica, Supplement,* Vol. 224, pp. 1–239 (1971).

Langford, W.S. The child in the pediatric hospital: Adaption to illness and hospitalization. *American Journal of Orthopsychiatry, 31;* 667 (1961).

Ling, W., Oftedal, G., and Weinberg, W. Depression presenting as headache. *American Journal of Diseases of Children, 120;* 122 (1970).

Lipowski, Z.J. Consultation-liaison psychiatry: An Overview. *American Journal of Psychiatry, 131;* 623 (1974).

Long, R.T., and Cope, O. Emotional problems of burned children. *New England Journal of Medicine, 264;* 1121 (1961).

McGavin, A.P., Schultz, E., Peden, G.W., and Bowen, B.D. The physical growth, the degree of intelligence and the personality adjustment of a group of diabetic children. *New England Journal of Medicine, 233;* 125 (1940).

McKendry, J.B., Williams, H.A., and Broughton, C. A study of untreated patients. *Applied Therapy, 10;* 815 (1968).

Mandelbaum, A. The group process in helping parents of retarded children; *Children, 14;* 227 (1967).

Mattson, A. Long-term physical illness in childhood: A challenge to psychosocial adaptation. *Pediatrics, 50;* 801 (1972).

Mattson, A., and Gross, S. Adaptational and defensive behavior in young hemophiliacs and their parents. *American Journal of Psychiatry, 122;* 1349 (1966).

Mattson, A., and Weisberg, I. Behavioral reactions to minor illness in preschool children. *Pediatrics, 46;* 604 (1970).

Mayer, J. Introduction. In *Childhood Obesity,* P.J. Collipp, ed. John Wright Publisher, Lilleton, Mass. (1975), pp. vii–xv.

Minde, K.K., Hachett, J.D., Killon, D., and Silver, S. How they grow up: Forty-one physically handicapped children and their families. *American Journal of Psychiatry, 128;* 1554 (1972).

Money, J., and Pollitt, E. Studies in the psychology of dwarfism: II. Personality maturation and response to growth hormone treatment in hypopituitary dwarfs. *Journal of Pediatrics, 68;* 381 (1966).

Murphy, S., and Chapman, W. Adolescent enuresis: A urologic study. *Pediatrics, 45;* 426 (1970).

Myers, B.A., Friedman, S.B., and Weiner, I.B. Coping with a chronic disability: Psychosocial observations of girls with scoliosis treated with the Milwaukee brace. *American Journal of Diseases of Children, 120;* 175 (1970).

Olshansky, S. Chronic sorrow: A response to having a mentally defective child. In *Counseling Parents of the Mentally Retarded,* L.N. Robert, ed. Charles C. Thomas, Springfield (1970), pp. 49–54.

Osborne, E. *When you lose a loved one.* Public Affairs Pamphlet 269 (1967), pp. 16–28.

Pasnau, R.O. Therapy of ulcerative colitis in children: The combined pediatric psychiatric surgical approach. *Psychosomatics, 5;* 137 (1964).

Pfefferbaum, B.J., and Pasnau, R.O. Post-amputation grief. *Nursing Clinics of North America, 11;* 687–690 (1976).

Plank, E.N., and Horwood, C. Leg amputation in a four-year old: Reactions of the child, her family, and staff. *Psychoanalytic Study of the Child, 16;* 405 (1961).

Pless, I.B., and Roghmann, K.J. Chronic illness and its consequences: Observations based on three epidemiologic surveys. In *Annual Progress in Child Psychiatry and Child Development,* S. Chess and A. Thomas, eds. Brunner/Mazel, New York (1972), pp. 589–601.

Poznanski, E.O. The replacement child: A saga of unresolved parental grief. *Journal of Pediatrics, 81;* 1190 (1972).

Provence, S., and Lipton, R. *Infants in Institutions.* International University Press, New York (1962).

Prugh, D.G. Toward an understanding of psychosomatic concepts in relation to illness in children. In *Modern Perspectives in Child Development,* A.J. Solnit and S.A. Provence, eds. International Universities Press, New York (1963), pp. 246-367.

Prugh, D., and Eckhardt, L.O. Children's reactions to illness, hospitalization, and surgery. In *Comprehensive Textbook of Psychiatry,* Vol. 2, 2nd ed., H.I. Kaplan and B.J. Sadock, eds. Williams & Wilkins, Baltimore (1975), pp. 2100-2107.

Prugh, D.G., Staub, E.M., Sands, H., Kirschbaum, R., and Lenihan, E. A study of emotional reactions of children and families to illness and hospitalization. *American Journal of Orthopsychiatry, 23;* 78 (1953).

Purcell, K., and Weiss, J.H. *Symptoms of Psychopathology: A Handbook,* C.G. Costello, ed. Wiley, New York (1970), pp. 597-623.

Roach, N.E. Enuresis: A literature review. *Journal of the Kansas Medical Society, 70;* 15 (1969).

Robertson, J. *Young Children in Hospitals,* 2nd ed. Tavistock, London (1970).

Roskies, E. *Abnormality and Normality: The Mothering of Thalidomide Children.* Cornell University Press, Ithaca, N.Y. (1970).

Rothchild, E., and Owens, R.P. Adolescent girls who lack functioning ovaries. *Journal of the American Academy of Child Psychiatry, 11;* 88 (1972).

Schaffer, H.R., and Callender, W.M. Psychologic effects of hospitalization in infancy. *Pediatrics, 24;* 528 (1959).

Senn, M.J.E. Emotional aspects of convalescence. *Child, 10;* 24 (1945).

Shader, R.I. Behavioral treatment of enuresis nocturna. *Journal of Diseases of the Nervous System, 29;* 334 (1968).

Shirley, H.F. The physically handicapped child. *Pediatric Psychology,* 498 (1963).

Shrand, H. Behavior changes in sick children nursed at home. *Pediatrics, 36;* 604 (1965).

Sifneos, P. The prevalence of alexithymia: Characteristics in psychosomatic patients. *Psychotherapy and Psychosomatics, 22;* 255 (1973).

Spitz, R.A., and Cobliner, W.G. *The First Year of Life.* International Universities Press, New York (1965).

Strain, J.J., and Grossman, S. *Psychological Care of the Medically Ill: A Primer in Liaison Psychiatry.* Appleton-Century-Crofts, New York (1975), pp. 23-36.

Sturzenberger, S., Cantwell, D.P., Burroughs, J., Salkin, B., and Green, J. A follow-up study of adolescent psychiatric inpatients with anorexia nervosa. *Journal of the American Academy of Child Psychiatry, 16;* 703 (1977).

Swift, C.R., and Seidman, F.L. Adjustment problems of juvenile diabetes. *Journal of the American Academy of Child Psychiatry, 3;* 500 (1964).

Tec, L. The treatment of enuresis with imipramine. *American Journal of Psychiatry, 125;* 266 (1968).

Tietz, W., and Vidmar, T. The impact of coping styles on the control of juvenile diabetes. *Psychiatry in Medicine, 3;* 67 (1972).

Tisza, V.B., and Gumperty, E. The parents' reaction to the birth and early care of children with cleft palate. *Pediatrics, 30;* 86 (1962).

Toker, E. Psychiatric aspects of cardiac surgery in a child. *Journal of the American Academy of Child Psychiatry, 10;* 156 (1971).

Trimble, M.R., and Reynolds, E.A. Anticonvulsant drugs and mental symptoms: A review. *Psychological Medicine, 6;* 169–178 (1976).

Tropauer, A., Franz, M.N., and Dilgard, V.W. Psychological aspects of the care of children with cystic fibrosis. *American Journal of Diseases of Children, 119;* 424 (1970).

Turner, R., Young, G.C., and Rachman, S. Treatment of nocturnal enuresis by conditioning techniques. *Journal of Behavioral Research and Therapy, 8;* 367 (1970).

Vigliano, A., Hart, L.W., and Singer, F. Psychiatric sequelae of old burns in children and their parents. *American Journal of Orthopsychiatry, 34;* 753 (1964).

Watson, E.J., and Johnson, A.M. The emotional significance of acquired physical disfigurement in children. *American Journal of Orthopsychiatry, 28;* 85 (1958).

Werry, J.S., and Cohrssen, J. Enuresis: An etiologic and therapeutic study. *Journal of Pediatrics, 67;* 423 (1965).

Woodward, J.M., and Jackson, D.M. Emotional reactions in burned children and their mothers. *British Journal of Plastic Surgery, 13;* 316 (1961).

3

The Child Activity Program: Playing

for Health

Lynn Reineman

INTRODUCTION

Hospital—traditionally the word has brought to mind images of sterile, white hallways, antiseptic smells, and efficient, brisk, uniformed personnel. This is hardly an environment oriented toward meeting the psychosocial and developmental needs of children. And yet, in the past two decades, increasing awareness and import has been given to the impact of hospitalization upon children. With this new understanding, the use of play has emerged as a valuable tool in facilitating a child's adjustment to the hospital experience.

In this chapter, the writer will discuss play and its importance to optimal growth and development. The specific value of play in a hospital setting, practical issues in developing a play program in a pediatric setting, and the role of the child life activity worker will also be addressed.

IMPORTANCE OF PLAY

Defining play may well be the most difficult part of this writing, for play is an abstract, often vague behavior that eludes precise definition. We surely know what play is not, although we have trouble agreeing on exactly what it is. Most theorists do agree that an essential characteristic of play is satisfaction or pleasure in the activity itself, and play is a self-initiated, orderly way of learning characterized by satisfaction in the activity itself. Play theorists frequently have stated that play is a leisure-time activity that is complete in itself, not impelled by immediate necessity or delayed reward.

For children, play is an integral part of growth and development. The phrase, "Play is a child's work" is common enough, yet play can also be viewed as a child's "preparation for life," for play allows a child to initiate, practice, and master skills essential for adult life task performance.

A child's play also reflects his "response to life," for through play a child, whose verbal communication skills remain immature, is able to express emotions, feelings, and reactions to life.

Although no attempt will be made here to further examine the classical theories of play motivation, the specific value of play in a hospital setting will be discussed later in greater detail.

THREATS OF HOSPITALIZATION

To a child, the threats of hospitalization are numerous and well documented in the literature (Oremland and Oremland, 1973). A child's reaction is of course dependent upon many variables: his own past experience with hospitals, preparation by parents and hospital personnel, media biasing, discussions with peers, the hospital's philosophy and approach, and naturally, the child's own active imagination. The following seem to be among the most widely applicable reactions.

Fear of Separation

The threat of separation from a nurturing environment and "significant others," whether parents, grandparents, foster parents, etc., seems to have the greatest impact upon children of all ages. Toddlers and preschoolers may view each separation as permanent, while older children often view separation and hospitalization as rejection or punishment. To a youngster, whose conception of time is vague at best, short separations may be as difficult to tolerate as overnight absences.

Fear of Pain

The threat of pain is frequently the first thing a child associates with illness and hospitalization.

Children often perceive the pain they must experience with hospitalization as punishment for some wrongdoing, either real or imagined. By nature egocentric, they feel that all issues, good or bad, revolve around them. Therefore, a priority in any hospitalization is helping the patient to gain an accurate understanding of the reasons for his hospital stay. Honesty in preparing a child for procedures that may cause pain has the long-term effect of building trust between child and staff. For example, let a child know that his throat will hurt following a tonsillectomy, but that the hurt will lessen each day.

Fear of Helplessness and Loss of Control

The feeling of mastery, of increasing control is an important task of childhood. Loss of this developing feeling is a very real concern in the hospital environment. Upon admission, the child, who at home is assuming increasing responsibility with household chores, allowance, etc., is often placed in the role of passive sufferer. Here he is the helpless recipient of numerous invasive procedures, and choices, if any, are few.

The strangeness and unfamiliarity of the hospital setting serve to enhance the child's feelings of helplessness. Coming from a home situation where structure is set and limits fixed, he is faced with a foreign environment and unclear behavioral expectations. Feelings of helplessness and loss of control are the frequent result.

Fear of Disfigurement and Death

Often with children, the sole experience with a hospital is the death of a grandparent. Therefore, hospitalization is logically associated with death and loss. Again, understanding of the reasons for hospitalization and, if at all predictable, discussion of the probable length of stay does much to dispel a child's fantasy fears.

Fear of disfigurement and mutilation are often encountered in children preparing for surgery. Describing with honesty and compassion how surgery will change them and showing them in a mirror how they look after surgery will reassure and support them.

Concern over anesthesia is common. Children may fear they will wake too soon or not at all. Describing anesthesia as a special kind of sleep where the patient cannot feel any pain and where the doctor will awaken him at just the right time does much to ease a child's mind.

HOW CAN PLAY HELP?

How can play, that essential task of childhood, help a child deal with these very real and very alarming threats of hospitalization?

By its very nature, play enables the child to regain mastery and control. In play, he is no longer the passive sufferer, but can become again the active change agent, the "boss." Play is not prescriptive. In play the child maintains the ability to choose: type and quality of play, companions, toys, and props all remain the whim of the child.

Play in the hospital allows a normal part of growth and development to continue in an otherwise very abnormal environment. The play area can be a safe, familiar post in a confusing or overwhelming setting. Social development and peer interaction can continue through play. This companionship provides much needed support: the awareness that the peer can truly identify with the child's own feelings and emotions.

> Justin, eight years old, and Steve, seven years old, were both being followed in outpatient hematology clinic for treatment of acute lymphocytic leukemia. In the course of a group game, the play therapist questioned Steve as to why he was visiting the doctor. When Justin heard Steve's response, he exclaimed, "Leukemia! Why, I have leukemia too, and that's why I'm here!" Since that day the boys have been close friends, and have benefitted and grown a great deal from the heart-to-heart talks they share.

Play is a natural method of communication for children who are still unable to express feelings and emotions verbally. Play between staff and child, using drawings and dolls, can be effective in preparing a child for procedures. Learning, then rehearsing, through play helps increase awareness and decrease apprehension. Play may reveal a child's fears and misconceptions and give clues as to where further intervention is needed.

> Alex, age five, was in pediatric intensive care due to severe gastroenteritis. Severely dehydrated, he was on intravenous fluids. Repeated vessel collapse necessitated restarting the IV several times daily, a procedure which Alex understandably hated. Seriously depressed, he became almost nonresponsive. Puppet play, however, interested him, and in the course of conversation with his puppets, it became apparent that Alex viewed the IV therapy as punishment for the diarrhea he could not control.

Additionally, play is a vehicle that allows children to express feelings they may be suppressing for fear that they are not acceptable. In reality children need to know that these feelings of anger, confusion, and fear are not only "OK" but possibly quite common among the other patients.

Providing play helps children realize that hospital staff are concerned with them as people and that hospitals are caring places. It follows that trust between child and staff is increased. Parents also benefit, since their comfort and security are enhanced when their child's anxiety is diminished.

PLAY PROGRAMS IN PEDIATRIC SETTINGS

As the awareness and need for play in the hospital setting has increased, a new member of the health care team has emerged. Primarily concerned with the child's emotional adjustment to hospitalization, this team member has been called the play therapist, the child life specialist, the child activity worker, etc. The major focus of a child life activity program is to assist the pediatric patient to understand and cope with hospitalization. Entertainment and diversion, although not the central goals, can certainly be valuable.

Role Definitions

In establishing a therapeutic play program in a pediatric setting, consideration must be given to the selection of a program coordinator. Presently, individuals with backgrounds in many fields are directing programs throughout the United States: recreation therapists, occupational therapists, social workers, nurses, graduates of child development programs, psychologists educators, etc. Recently, efforts have been initiated to further define the profession of child life specialist and arrive at a more widely consistent college curriculum.

Some areas of background learning and competence are essential to effective therapeutic play programs. These include knowledge of: growth and development, the play phenomenon and its motivators and inhibitors, interpersonal communication and family dynamics, behavior management, children's illnesses and medical terminology, and children's reactions to hospitalization, as well as intervention strategies.

Certain standards cannot be taught; these include enjoyment of all children and sensitivity to their needs, emotional maturity, flexibility, and creativity.

As an occupational therapist, this author feels she has had an educational background particularly well suited toward child life activity work; however, she recognizes other members of the health care team may have equally good academic and experiential preparation.

A further point is that in this era of increasing specialization it is too easy to view the child life activity worker as the sole member of the hospital team dealing with the pediatric patient's psychosocial adjustment. This is a dangerous attitude, which not only fosters resentment among the medical team but also makes it impossible for the child to receive the best possible care.

A total team awareness, made possible by good communication of the psychosocial as well as medical needs of hospitalized children, is essential for optimal care.

Job descriptions of therapeutic play program coordinators will, of course, vary depending upon the hospital size, administrative setup, and program philosophy. Whether the coordinator works directly with children, or supervises a staff of child life workers and, possibly, trained volunteers, an important goal should remain good communication among all team members, focusing on emotional care of the hospitalized child. Providing ongoing education programs to nursing personnel and other staff, attending and contributing to psychosocial patient rounds, charting-in the medical record (at Children's Hospital and Health Center we are experimenting with an addition to the patient "Kardex," entitled the "Hospital Adjustment Record"), all contribute toward the therapeutic play program goal of helping the pediatric patient understand and adjust to the hospital experience.

Volunteers—Their Role in a Therapeutic Play Program

Much has been written, pro and con, regarding the role of volunteer assistants in play programs. We have found them to be of invaluable assistance, and credit this to careful recruitment, intensive training, close supervision and support, and ongoing educational opportunities.

Working with a total volunteer group of between 50 and 60, our child activity staff arranges for bimonthly discussion groups focused on topics as diverse as "the development of play behavior in children" and "working with children from different cultural backgrounds."

Our volunteers come weekly to an assigned shift: morning, afternoon, or evening. Meeting with them prior to their shift to discuss individual patients and some of their specific emotional needs and, at the end of their shift, to ask for feedback and talk over some of the volunteers' experiences is a valuable way to enhance the volunteers effectiveness and commitment.

Although it can be argued that volunteers cannot provide the consistent, ongoing contact the children require or the expertise called for in therapeutic play programs, they can certainly help provide the caring, nurturing environment valued in pediatric facilities. Child activity program staff can provide the expert knowledge and the consistency of contact; however, administrative reality often makes the use of volunteers to augment program personnel necessary. With proper preparation and support, they can become invaluable members of the health care team.

THE PLAY ENVIRONMENT

In a pediatric facility, the play environment should not be limited to one playroom but be in evidence throughout the hospital: in patient rooms, waiting areas, and any location where children are likely to be.

Yet it is often the playroom that remains the focal point of the therapeutic play program. It has been said of hospitals that "a playroom in the right place can make all the difference" (*To Prepare a Child,* 1976).

The size of the play area is generally dictated by the space available, and careful record keeping of utilization will probably be necessary to persuade the administration to enlarge or expand. Hopefully, the play area will be large enough to accommodate not only ambulatory patients, but wheelchairs, gurneys, and even patients' beds.

We have found that an overstimulating playroom can contribute to the sense of overwhelming strangeness a child may experience with hospitalization, in addition to distracting from purposeful play. Yet, a barren, unwelcoming room is equally inappropriate. Warm, inviting color schemes and plenty of enclosed cupboard space for toys not in use facilitates optimal play.

If only one playroom is available in a pediatric setting, care must be taken not to visually gear it toward one specific age group.

> Robert, age 12, refused to enter the playroom, commenting, "No way will I go in there; that's only for little kids."

If it is impossible to provide an area specifically for use by older patients (i.e., a teen lounge), then decorating techniques may help to visually divide a room.

Some pediatric facilities manage age distributions by setting times of the day when the playroom is reserved for children of specific ages. We feel, however, that if there is only one play area, it should be available whenever a patient of any age feels a need for a safe, comfortable place.

Siblings should be encouraged to use the play facilities with their hospitalized brother or sister. The intact family unit remains a priority in patient care, and many of the psychosocial issues affecting a child's adjustment to hospitalization will be mirrored, and possibly intensified, in a sibling.

To aid in infection control, we have found it very helpful to prominently post a sign on the playroom door asking visitors not to enter if they have been exposed to chicken pox, measles, rubella, mumps, whooping cough, or hepatitis; or display any of the following symptoms: runny nose, coughing, chills and fever, vomiting, diarrhea, or skin rashes.

THE PLAYROOM AS A SANCTUARY

Before discussing which toys and materials are appropriate for a hospital playroom, one additional point might be made. We view the playroom as a safe place—in fact, a sanctuary—for the children in the hospital. As such, we prohibit painful procedures (such as lab tests) from occurring there. Yet we encourage noninvasive, nonpainful procedures (e.g., measuring vital signs, discussion with the anesthesiologist prior to surgery) to take place in the playroom on the assumption that the patients will be better able to cope in a comfortable environment.

For Kristen, five years old, taking oral medications had become a battle of wills between nursing staff and herself. Parents were enlisted to help, yet the battle lines only extended. A concerned child life worker suggested attempting to give medication by mouth in the playroom. Her nurse readily agreed, and Kristen, to the relief of all, willingly took her medication.

PLAY MATERIALS

In addition to providing toys for infant and toddler, as well as books and magazines, we have found it helpful to think of toys as facilitating various types of play.

Safe and Familiar Play

An overstimulating, unfamiliar environment and resultant anxiety may make it initially impossible for a child to engage in play that reveals or releases feelings, or in creative and dramatic play. For the child at this time, nothing is so reassuring as a familiar wooden or jigsaw puzzle, board game, coloring books, crayons, cards, or checkers.

Toys to Encourage Creative Play

Arts and crafts materials, including construction paper, scissors, glue, and crafts media; and musical instruments, including drums, tambourines, piano, and record player, can be useful in giving satisfaction in a completed project, feelings of mastery and self-worth, as well as opportunities for self-expression. Taking a self-made project home from the hospital provides long-term positive associations.

Toys to Allow for Aggressive Play

To help a child vent some of his/her frustration, hostility, rage, and even excess energy in appropriate ways, we have used clay and play dough, punching bags, inflated "bounce-back" toys, socker-boppers, batacas, Velcro dart boards, blocks (to build up and knock down), and bean-bag target throwing.

Hospital Play

Frequently nothing is as appealing to the patient as the chance to explore the hospital experience through role-reversing hospital play. For trained staff members this can be a very revealing tool with which to further learn how children are comprehending hospitalization as well as a unique method of teaching and preparing the child. A play hospital, complete with operating rooms, X-ray, lab, etc., is useful, as are real and toy stethoscopes, blood pressure cuffs, "doctor kits" for physical examinations, caps, masks, gloves, syringes, alcohol wipes, Band-Aids, gauze dressings, tape, plaster of paris Redi-cast bandages, IV bottles, etc.

THE CHILD WHO CANNOT COME TO THE PLAYROOM

Special concern must be given the child who is unable to come to the playroom. Emotional support of the child in isolation or the critically ill child could well be the subject of an entire chapter! The threats of hospitalization are intensified when a child is restricted behind a glass-windowed door and when visitors must wear gowns and, possibly, gloves and masks. We have found several strategies to be helpful in working with children in isolation or on bed rest:

Asking families to bring familiar items from home (i.e., bedspreads, quilts, pillows, wall posters, photographs)

Keeping calendars and daily schedules with the children

Ensuring that the volunteers understand and are comfortable with isolation procedures (otherwise they may pass over these very needy children to spend time with a more available patient)

In general, we feel that these children need more time, attention, and care from the play program staff than patients for whom the play area is more accessible.

SPECIAL PROGRAMS IN THE PLAYROOM

In addition to the routine tasks of a therapeutic play program, working with the public relations or community services department of the hospital to schedule a "special event" is usually entertaining for the children and rewarding for the staff. Most likely, the community is full of amateur musicians, clowns, jugglers, etc., who would be delighted to put on a show for a pediatric facility. We have found that a carefully worded entertainment policy detailing and clarifying any restrictions (i.e., time limits, photographs, gifts, and candy) is very useful. Bringing the entertainers to the bedside of those patients who cannot attend the playroom show is yet another way to help these children cope with hospitalization.

ENVIRONMENTS FOR THE ADOLESCENT PATIENT

Meeting the needs of the teenage patient is a special challenge to the hospital staff. For the young adult struggling with the tasks of adolescence (emancipation, role definition, peer acceptance, intellectual development, and sexual and functional identity), the hospital is a particularly invasive and inhibiting environment (Hoffman, Becker, and Gabriel, 1976).

A separate or recreation program geared specifically toward the patient of 12 and over can aid hospital adjustment enormously. A special area or room, designated as the *teen lounge,* is ideal, and might contain such teenage favorites as record players, radios, game tables (such as pool or bumper pool), facilities for cooking, and more sophisticated crafts opportunities. Enlisting adolescent patients' help in decorating the room will not only ensure that the area will appeal to teenage taste but will also provide the decorators with a sense of purpose and completion. Supervision should be loose and undertaken by tactful staff members who are able to "keep the peace," while allowing the teenagers the privilege of being responsible for their own territory.

WHERE TO GO FOR HELP IN DEVELOPING A PLAY PROGRAM

People, programs, literature—support for pediatric play programs is large and growing.

A primary place to look for support is within your own facility. No matter what administrative department your play program is under, an interdisciplinary advisory group is helpful. At Children's Hospital and Health Center, our therapeutic play program is fortunate enough to have an advisory group composed of representatives from child psychiatry, psychology, nursing, medical social service, occupational therapy, volunteer services, and education. A fine support group, it is also a valuable place for initiating ideas and problem solving. Additionally, it helps to facilitate good communication and public relations among the diverse health care teams.

This author has found the Association for the Care of Children in Hospitals (ACCH) to be an extremely helpful and supportive organization in setting up and running a pediatric play program. Headquartered in Washington, D.C., it is an international organization with members primarily from the United States and Canada. Dedicated to the goal of promoting the health and well-being of children and their families in the health care setting, ACCH has numerous, useful publications. These include: *Guidelines for the Development of Hospital Program and for the Personnel Conducting Programs of Therapeutic Play for Pediatric Patients, Ideas for Activities with Hospitalized Children,* and *The Hospitalized Child Bibliography.* Additionally, the organization publishes a quarterly journal. A publication order from and additional information are available from ACCH headquarters.

Through a review of the literature, this author has found several authors to be particularly original and informative. Axline (1969), Azarnoff (1970), Bergman (1965), Bopp (1972), Petrillo and Sanger (1972), and Plank (1971) are names well known in child life circles.

CONCLUSION

In this new era of cost effectiveness and dollar consciousness, all programs not directly concerned with acute medical care are subject to discussion and close scrutiny.

Slowly, but with growing momentum, therapeutic play programs are being recognized as not simply a fringe benefit or superficial extra but as an essential part of the healing process. Increasingly, research studies are being undertaken that validate anecdotal evidence demonstrating the value of play programs in pediatric settings.

In a larger framework, it is our responsibility as adults to encourage others to examine their own attitudes about play. Is play merely regarded as a frivolous pastime, time taken for granted ("Oh, she's just outside playing"), or is it viewed as an essential step in development, as a child's "preparation for life"?

By implementing the three Cs of pediatric care—compassion, consistency, and communication—we will better enable children to understand and cope with the hospital experience. Let us work together to give our patients the opportunity of "playing for health."

REFERENCES

Axline, V. *Play Therapy*. Ballantine Books, New York (1969).

Azarnoff, P. A play program in a pediatric clinic. *Children, 17;* 218 (1970).

Bergman, T. *Children in the Hospital.* International University Press, New York (1965).

Bopp, J. *Guidelines for the Development of Hospital Programs and for the Personnel Conducting Programs of Therapeutic Play for Pediatric Patients.* Association for the Care of Children in Hospitals, Washington, D.C. (1972).

Hoffman, A., Becker, R.D., and Gabriel, H.P. *The Hospitalized Adolescent.* The Free Press, New York (1976).

Oremland, E., and Oremland, J. *The Effects of Hospitalization Upon Children.* Charles C. Thomas, Springfield (1973).

Petrillo, M., and Sanger, S. *Emotional Care of Hospitalized Children.* J.B. Lippincott, Philadelphia (1972), pp. 99-102.

Plank, E.N. *Working with Children in Hospitals.* Case Western Reserve University Press, Cleveland (1971).

To Prepare a Child. Film produced by Pierce Atkins Production and Peter Vogt and Associates, Washington, D.C. (1976).

4

Preparing the Pediatric Family

Pat Azarnoff

Preparation is an effort to help children to become emotionally ready to manage their feelings about potentially stressful events. It provides information, reassurance, and encouragement. Preparation has been called emotional inoculation because it creates stress in tolerable amounts prior to the greater stress. It is a stimulant to the mobilization of resources.

Preparation for hospitalization and surgery is important because being treated in the hospital is psychologically and physiologically distressing. For some there is temporary stress, ameliorated by being free of pain and restored to function, by getting well and going home. For others, however, the emotional effects remain for a considerable time. Significant disturbances in behavior not present prior to hospitalization have been found in studies of children of various ages hospitalized for various diagnostic classifications. Those children already stressed by life circumstances and those with a diagnosed emotional disturbance or with disabling physical conditions unrelated to the reasons for hospitalization, such as blindness or deafness, may have a particularly difficult time. Children may be stressed also when hospitalization follows soon after the birth of a sibling, the death of a relative, friend, or pet, or other emotional disruption in family relationships.

Preparing children for their encounters through a supportive, consistently available person can have a direct effect on the correction of the primary disorder. Studies of various preparation methods, such as group discussions, puppetry, story booklets, and films, show that prepared surgical patients are induced into anesthesia in a shorter time, return to normal vital signs faster after the operation, recuperate for a shorter time at home, and have fewer observed behavioral problems. In addition, informed and reassured children learn to trust medical center personnel—an important aspect for those in long-term care, such as children with diabetes or asthma—and develop positive attitudes that affect lifelong habits of self-care.

In some ways the family is already prepared by the time any health science or mental health professional sees them. They have had experiences with doctors, nurses, clinics, hospitals, and home illnesses. They have seen television medical shows in which doctors take a personal interest in the patients and seem to effect magic cures. They have read or heard of new treatment for chronic or fatal illnesses. They have been taught attitudes by their parents and grandparents, many of whom lived in a time when going to the hospital was a pronouncement of death, or at least a life-threatening decision.

RESISTANCE

Although preparation has been shown to reduce anxiety before, during, and after hospitalization (Petrillo and Sanger, 1980), some professionals who are in decision-making roles may not be aware of or convinced of the need to reduce psychological stress in this way. In fact, the manner in which children's stress is managed by families and hospital staffs, if it is dealt with at all, varies from no policy (which is a policy of neglect) to elaborate materials and events. Only one in three general, acute care hospitals that admit children provide preparation services (Azarnoff and Woody, 1981), so most children who are admitted receive care in hospitals that do not prepare. Since children's stress affects not only their mental health but their physical recovery as well, it would seem important to have a policy of preparation as a primary preventive.

In some hospitals, arguments of lack of money, time, staff, or space are used to prevent starting such services, even when there are a number of hospitals demonstrating that without additional resources they can prepare children for hospitalization and surgery routinely. They do this with an attitude that preparation not only assists children to cope, but also creates a more cooperative patient and a more satisfied staff.

Arguments that children are too young to think abstractly and to understand their illness or that it would be unkind to tell children of impending painful events are contrary to what is well known in learning and stress theories: that a major style of coping is to accumulate information to insure survival. In the absence of desired information, children imagine what will or did happen. They believe these fantasies and act on them. Thus a four-year-old brought in for cast removal believed her arm would be cut off and was not calmed until she placed a cast on a doll and saw it removed with a cast cutter, arm intact. And an eight-year-old believed the purpose of the arm cast was to keep the shoulder and the hand connected while the new arm grew back. Preparation therefore takes into account children's mistaken notions but assumes that even young children have concepts about the body and beliefs about what procedures will do to them. The way in which information is rapidly acquired by seriously ill and chronically ill children, in particular, forces us to look again at our beliefs about children's capabilities to learn when they are highly motivated to do so.

Some physicians in training believe that gathering physical history is time consuming enough and that any knowledge of children's perception of experiences, like most social history, is too tenuous to deal with to make rational decisions about in planning care. It is true that such information lends itself to interpretation and is not as clearly seen as measurements by instruments. But instruments are tenuous too. Blood pressure, for example, measured in the same child on the same day can differ from one cuff to another, from one placement to another, and from one physician or nurse to another. Sometimes these differences are significant to decisions about therapy. In the same way, behavioral observations of children vary from one situation to another and are not exact. Yet these are the data on which one must depend. That is why it is important to improve the instrument—oneself—so that measurements are as accurate as possible.

Some physicians who see their patients a few minutes a day may deny staff reports that their patient is in emotional turmoil, in order to maintain their own ability to function under continuous stress. Some acquire patients of families who feel reassured by the paternalistic approach that consists of telling parents that the child is safe in the doctor's hands, so that there is no need to worry or to know any further information.

Many practitioners who believe in the value of preparation but see the resistance of administrative and professional staff to begin programs, go ahead on their own and prepare children for events. Their experience shows them the anxiety-alleviating effects preparation has on children. They are not necessarily aware of others in their own hospital who are also doing this work and, in some instances, hide it so that a resistant physician does not know and therefore cannot object. This staff needs considerable support from enlightened physicians. They need a surgeon who refuses to perform open heart surgery on an unprepared child, a hematologist who requires during chemotherapy the presence of a parent or staff whose only function is supportive care, an endocrinologist who insists that children with diabetes learn about their illness and not be entirely dependent on others for care.

Preparation practices are seldom a stated policy of a hospital, except for nonrelational events such as scheduled films, preadmission tours, or coloring books sent with admission materials. Therefore, preparation services are usually random, inconsistent, informal, and insufficient. What is needed is a consistently available individual, with back-up staff, who can be counted on by children to see them through each of the more stressful stages of the hospital experience. A child should not have to cope alone because a staff person is out sick or was called to a meeting.

Many families do not thrive in situations of dependency, lack of information, and minimal support. A more outspoken and informed consumer voice is now heard from parents of rehospitalized children (Azarnoff and Hardgrove, 1981).

They want to be more actively involved in their children's care as a way of feeling less helpless. To do that, they need to be readied for the experience and to help prepare their own children, if only the staff would first give them the information and assurance they want. Parents often do not know their role prior to hospitalization, during treatments, or at home after hospitalization. Are they to continue the traditional parenting role of informing, reassuring, nurturing? Should they hold and comfort their children, or keep them lying flat in bed? Should they adjust the linens and bring toys, or stay away from a sterile field? They want answers to detailed questions, even when the need to know represents their anxiety instead of, or in addition to, a desire for the facts. When they are told the answers, assuming there are any, parents need to be told again at a later point, since they are unlikely to have heard it all the first time. Anxiety and distractions intrude into concentration. But they do hear a message on an emotional level, that their physician is interested in how they feel and can be counted on to deal with them candidly, as adults.

For those parents who wish to be more involved in their child's care, advocate that parents be encouraged to continue giving care in the hospital. If they are aware of routines and procedures, they can better help their children to become treatment ready. Parents of young diabetics, for example, would continue to give injections even in the hospital. Parents of children with hemophilia would give transfusions. Parents of children with cancer would assist with chemotherapy treatments. In that way parents can prepare their children with reassurance that the parents will be with them instead of waiting outside or in an unknown lounge. Parents also become better able to administer treatments at home. A number of hospitals have found ways to get past the legal issues and devote more energy to the humane issues.

METHODS

There are three primary ways in which children and parents can be prepared by the professional. The first is to analyze and acknowledge the context in which the child is receiving health care. Ask the family's prior relevant experiences and what benefits they anticipate from the planned surgery. This information can be obtained in the preadmission clinic visit. Since that visit is required in some hospitals before surgery can be scheduled, a preadmission preparation session can be similarly required. If it is not done then, or in addition to that session, preparation can be done as part of the admissions process. The interview in itself can help a family to feel cared about, in addition to the method of preparation that is used. The child development specialist, playroom coordinator (Azarnoff and Flegal, 1979), or family advocate on staff meets with one family group at a time. With background information, one can then help the family to better understand how the unit functions. Some children on preadmission tours want to know about equipment, where the operating and recovery room can be found, and other architectural features. Other children want to know about television, mealtime, toys, and other features that remind them of familiar, more secure times. Parents want to know relational features such as who will be caring for their children. Some will ask about participatory features such as how active they can be in visiting and caring for their children.

With both children and parents it is important to discover what assumptions are being made about the illness and treatment. The stress children experience has less relationship to the actual life risk and more to the children's perception of risk. Because children's ideas are often derived from their perception of recent events, it is important to talk with them about what has been happening in their lives. Children need to know that illness is not a punishment for bad thoughts or actions. Parents need to know they were not at fault and did not cause the illness. That is why group tours with preplanned speeches, puppet show, or media are likely to be only minimally helpful; they can reach only some of the interests and concerns of the individuals in the family, and do not usually take into account what has been happening in the family situation and the varying styles adults and children use in coping with change or stress.

A second way to prepare children and parents is to provide a support system that enhances their efforts to cope with the challenge of the unknown. For example, children develop strength in coping by steps. First they comprehend that there will be a hospitalization, sometimes learned in the doctor's office, though no one may have said that directly. Then there is the accommodation to leaving home to be cared for in a new place by strangers not under the control of the parents. Next, children realize that everything in the medical center is different: the clothes, the food, the routines, and especially the permissions. Where before parents said not to touch electrical wires, now it seems to be all right for unknown people to connect wires to children's heads for an electroencephalogram. At home, children could only void or defecate into a toilet, but now they are expected to do so into strange metal containers hidden under the bedcovers. In the next stage children acknowledge that the body will be opened and changed in an intrusive procedure. And finally, it is hoped, children believe their bodies are strong enough to regain health and not be vulnerable soon again.

That is why preparation is most effective in stages. Visits by school or youth groups prior to the time a hospitalization is needed provide information to children at a time when they can better accept it, without feeling the same degree or type of threat that children do when scheduled for admission. Many hospitals now offer such tours. Then a preadmission visit transforms fantasy into at least some reality. On admission day a renewed acquaintance with places and people begins to feel familiar. Prior to surgery, specifics of treatment procedures, according to what children want to know, help them understand how to participate in their own care and recovery. Afterwards, children can recall aloud or playact the procedure that was done, so that staff can assess what information and attitudes resulted. And a follow-up call or postdischarge interview would pick up remaining concerns or misconceptions.

Support for parents would help them to feel competent, reducing feelings of helplessness, loss of power and authority, and feelings of guilt. Prior to admission, send parents information (in their first language) about how to prepare themselves and their children for admission and hospitalization. In the hospital, encourage parents to stay with or near their babies and young children during the admission process, in the first stage of anesthesia induction, in the recovery room, intensive care unit, and the bedroom; and to be accessible to their older children on an as-needed basis. To help parents explain to and reassure their children, provide materials such as photographs of treatment procedures or figures and miniature equipment or expendable medical supplies for play sessions.

Another way to prepare children and parents is to generate a repertoire of materials and relational events from which children and parents may choose. Printed materials can include storybooks about the hospital, instructions to parents on how to prepare their children, and information on specific procedures such as cardiac catheterization. Nonprint media can include films about the hospital departments, slides about body casts, tape recordings of one child telling another what a kidney biopsy was like, photography albums showing step-by-step procedures in spinal taps. Replica or real materials can include doll-house-sized models of equipment, with stuffed animals and dolls on which to play-practice.

Relational preparation brings staff and family together to talk about feelings, to recall events that happened to cousin Joe who had the "same" illness, to wonder "iffy" questions aloud. This can be done in duscussions on a home visit, during a preadmission tour, in the playroom or lounge, or bedside. Children can then write stories or draw about their surgical experiences, express their feelings about what is happening to their bodies and their lives; then the staff helps them put together a letter or newspaper and distributes it to other staff, patients, and families. A tour of the pediatric unit by a group of children to be admitted for tonsillectomy may be followed by a crayons and paper session in which the children are asked to draw "the scariest thing you saw today," or "what part of this hospital will help me most," or "what toy I will play with when I come back."

In summary, the mental health specialist can be most helpful in preparing the pediatric family by (1) acknowledging the existing context of information and affect and (2) developing a support system that assists a child to cope with stress in manageable stages and helps parents to continue their parenting roles with feelings of competence. By building upon existing family strengths in this way and offering a repertoire of materials and relationships, the mental health specialist can offer the family benefits from hospitalization that are not only physically healing but emotionally gratifying as well.

REFERENCES

Azarnoff, P. and Flegal, S. *A Pediatric Play Program.* 2nd printing. Charles C. Thomas, Springfield (1979).

Azarnoff, P., and Hardgrove, C., eds. *The Family in Child Health Care.* Wiley-Interscience, New York (1981).

Azarnoff, P., and Woody, P.D. Preparation of children for hospitalization in acute care hospitals in the United States. *Pediatrics,* 1981 *68*(3), 361–367.

Petrillo, M., and Sanger, S. *Emotional Care of Hospitalized Children: An Environmental Approach,* 2nd ed. J.B. Lippincott, Philadelphia (1980).

5

Referral to the Mental Health
Professional

Charles E. Hollingsworth

Anyone can recognize the need for mental health intervention with a particular child or family. In the hospital setting we generally rely on physician referral. Members of the team suggest such referrals to the physician who, as the case manager, is ultimately responsible for the child's total well-being, both physical and emotional. All disciplines are becoming more assertive about suggesting or recommending referral to a mental health center when psychopathology, marital conflict, or emotional stress are recognized.

Many mental health centers for children have attempted to streamline their entry process, but most continue to require a screening interview to complete a symptom review, developmental history, family history, request for school and health reports—especially a copy of a recent physical exam—and a financial screening form to determine an appropriate and reasonable fee. Then an appointment for a diagnostic evaluation is set. This evaluation, in general, is done by a team that includes a child psychiatrist; a child psychologist; a psychiatric social worker; an educational psychologist or learning disability specialist; and, when appropriate, an audiologist, a speech therapist, or a linguistic consultant.

PSYCHIATRIC TREATMENT PROGRAM

The child's psychiatric treatment program should provide the following:

1. Individual psychotherapy
2. Family therapy
3. Marital counseling
4. Counseling focused on grief
5. Group therapy
6. Behavior therapy

7. Postdivorce counseling
8. Medication clinic
9. Relaxation techniques, hypnosis, and/or guided imagery
10. Administration

Each of these subjects is discussed below.

Individual Psychotherapy

After the diagnostic evaluation is complete, a conference is held with the parents and child to discuss recommendations. Individual psychotherapy is frequently recommended for the child. There may be conjoint family or marital therapy sessions and/or occasional meetings with the parents and therapist to discuss the child's progress.

Individual therapy may be psychoanalytic psychotherapy, play therapy (Axline, 1969), or behavior modification. The focus is on the child's particular fears, concerns, and conflicts. The therapist pays special attention to the child's perception of his world and to the defense mechanisms used in coping with his environment. Individual therapy is very useful when preparing a child for surgery or when adjustment to a recent handicap.

Family Therapy

Many centers use family therapy as their major intervention. The parents and all children in the family meet once a week for 1 to 1½ hours with one or more therapists to discuss issues that affect the entire family. Particular attention is paid to communication patterns within the family, family dynamics, and alignments and roles within the family. Minuchin's (1974) structural family therapy is a popular technique. Family therapy is very useful in families in which a child has a chronic illness.

Marital Counseling

Frequently, the child perceives stress within the parents' marriage and will develop somatic complaints as a result of internalizing his stress. In such instances, it is imperative that the parents be encouraged to seek marital counseling to allow them and the child to function in a less stressful environment.

Counseling Focused on Grief

When a child or parent is diagnosed as having a potentially fatal illness, the anticipatory grieving process begins. Referral to a mental health professional is often indicated at this time, because open communication about these fears and concerns within the family can help the family cope as the illness progresses (Hollingsworth and Pasnau, 1977). Too often, physicians wait until the family becomes dysfunctional before referring them to a mental health worker who is trained to help a family deal with their feelings. A combination of individual and family therapy is most useful for these families.

Group Therapy

Most mental health centers have some group therapy. Parents groups, support groups, and parent education classes focus on parental coping. Groups for children include activity groups, peer-interaction groups, education remediation groups, postdivorce counseling groups, chronic illness groups, and rehabilitation groups (Brandes and Gardner, 1973). These groups usually consist of five to eight individuals who meet once a week with one or more therapists to discuss their feelings.

Behavior Therapy

The therapist will design a behavior modification program for the parent and child and will meet with them once a week to discuss the progress, effectiveness, and modifications of the program. Behavior modification is frequently used for enuresis, encopresis, temper tantrums, and phobias (Task Force Report, American Psychiatric Association, 1974).

Postdivorce Counseling

There are centers that handle court-referred child custody evaluations. An interdisciplinary team with a psychiatric social worker, psychologist, child psychiatrist, and a probation officer performs an extensive 10-hour evaluation and then makes recommendations to the courts in disputed child custody cases (Sheffner and Suarez, 1975).

Children almost always need postdivorce counseling to help them deal with their feelings (e.g., the parents' marital conflict, abandonment, being pulled apart by their parents, split loyalty) and to help them adjust to their new relationships and changes in their living arrangements. Group therapy with other children who have experienced the separation of their parents is very beneficial and should be recommended early, before the child's behavior indicates maladjustment.

Medication Clinic

Most mental health clinics have a child psychiatrist on staff to evaluate children for consideration for psychotropic medication. The child should have a careful physical examination, including a detailed neurological examination, before any medication is prescribed. Each child should also have a recent complete blood count and urinalysis. The most commonly used medications are stimulants, such as amphetamines, methylphenidate, or pemoline, for attention deficit disorder; imipramine for enuresis; phenothiazines for psychotic states; and antidepressants for depression (Werry, 1977).

Any child who is on medication should be seen one week after the medication is started and then at least once a month after the child is stabilized on the medication. We do not recommend writing a prescription for more than a one-month supply of medication. This policy will encourage parents to keep appointments, so that their child can be properly followed. Parents should be warned to keep all medications out of the reach of young children. Many of these medications can be fatal if ingested in large quantity by a small child.

Relaxation Techniques, Hypnosis, and/or Guided Imagery

Relaxation techniques, hypnosis, and guided imagery are becoming widely used in pediatrics and child psychiatry. These techniques are useful in reducing anxiety, controlling pain, and affording the child a sense of being in control of his body and actions. With relaxation techniques and/or hypnosis, many children are able to undergo such procedures as bone marrow aspiration without any medication for pain control. These techniques are also used for children with functional abdominal pain, anxiety attacks, hyperventilation syndrome, and obsessive-compulsive neurosis.

Administration

Each child mental health center has an administrative organization to determine policies, provide supervision, coordinate training and teaching, and implement programs to provide services to its clients. An advisory board of community leaders is imperative to guarantee that the center serves the interests of its catchment area.

These ten components can be expanded until all the mental health needs of the children in the community are met. Such basic needs are seen in all communities.

REFERENCES

Axline, V.M. *Play Therapy*. Ballantine Books, New York (1969).
Brandes, N.S., and Gardner, M.L., *Group Therapy for the Adolescent*. Jason Aronson, New York (1973).

Hollingsworth, C.E., and Pasnau, R.O. *The Family in Mourning.* Grune & Stratton, New York (1977).
Minuchin, S. *Families and Family Therapy.* Harvard University Press, Cambridge, Mass. (1974).
Sheffner, D.J., and Suarez, J.M. The post divorce clinic. *American Journal of Psychiatry, 132;* 442–446 (1975).
Task Force Report: American Psychiatric Association. *Behavior Therapy in Psychiatry.* Jason Aronson, New York (1974).
Werry, J.S. The use of psychotropic drugs in children. *Journal of the American Academy of Child Psychiatry, 16;* 446–468 (1977).

6

Sibling Groups

Charles E. Hollingsworth

The need for group counseling sessions for siblings of children who have chronic illnesses, physical handicaps, or debiliating or disfiguring ailments has become obvious to those of us who work in the pediatric setting. Yet, very few hospitals, agencies, or foundations offer such a service.

These groups can be led by anyone with experience in conducting group therapy. Often a psychiatric social worker or psychiatric nurse is able to hold a sibling group in the late afternoon to avoid taking children out of school for their sessions. It has been our experience that these groups are well attended. We strongly encourage the mental health community to stop overlooking the tremendous psychological impact on siblings of chronically ill, handicapped, or disfigured children.

ISSUES COMMONLY DISCUSSED IN SIBLING GROUPS

Fears

Most children are afraid that the same thing might happen to them. Parents report that siblings often develop similar symptoms, have frightening nightmares or other sleep disturbances. When a child is hospitalized, the siblings develop fantasies about what has happened, what is being done, and what their brother or sister looks like. Young children can be prisoners to threatening, frightening fantasies. It is important that all siblings be allowed to visit. In their fears and fantasies they usually imagine their sibllings in worse condition than s/he may be. Also, it is an important first step in helping the sibling adjust to the impairment.

Concerns

Whenever a brother or sister is seriously ill or injured, siblings grieve for his or her incapacity and expected lifetime achievements. This grieving process goes on

---

in all members of the family, including the patient. Siblings, like parents, want to know about the condition and daily progress of the patient and should be included in periodic family informational conferences or teaching sessions.

Older siblings worry about treating their brother or sister differently. Will I become overprotective or rejecting? Can I become comfortable and accepting of the disability?

Fantasies

Young children often think that whatever happened to the brother or sister was caused by their own angry feelings toward the brother or sister. Magical thinking is common up to age eight. Sibling rivalry is present in all families, and many children feel that they are responsible for accidents or other events beyond their control because at some point, in an angry rage, they wished their brother or sister dead or injured.

Some children think that God is punishing their sibling for being bad. Children with paralysis may be accused by siblings of faking. Most children have the fantasy that a brother or sister with paralysis will some day be able to walk or use his or her extremities again.

Teasing

Children must be educated about the damaging effects of cruelly teasing handicapped or disfigured children. Group therapy is an effective arena to achieve this goal. Siblings need to be made aware that their friends or other children may tease or make inappropriate comments about their brother or sister. They will want to talk about these embarrassing situations and how to handle them. It is difficult to teach children to ignore teasing, but this is the most effective way to stop reinforcing it. Role modeling of ways to ignore teasing can be used in group therapy, as well as teaching a sibling what to say to those cruel, immature children who lack empathy for handicapped, disfigured, or chronically ill children. School teachers and counselors should give this high priority because it affects the mental health of the ill child and the siblings. Even the child who does the teasing will often later be troubled by guilt feelings for what was said or done in a group of peers.

Guilt

As mentioned earlier, siblings feel guilt for many reasons. Older siblings may have been left to supervise the young child who was severely injured in an accident. These older siblings often become depressed and withdrawn and will need psychotherapy—either group or individual—to help resolve the guilt feelings.

The need to ventilate is often overlooked, and referral is postponed by the caretakers until the older child has become symptomatic and school performance has deteriorated. We should begin to practice preventive mental health in this area.

Interference with Convalescence

Siblings may be afraid to visit their brother or sister for fear that they may in some way interfere with the nursing care of the patient. After the patient is home, siblings may be shy about interacting with the affected child for fear that in the process of play they might injure their sibling. Parents sometimes place guilt on the siblings if a child's convalescence does not go as smoothly and expediently as planned. "She would not have been rehospitalized if you had not brought that cold home from school and given it to her." "You made so much noise that he became weaker and weaker until he had to go back to the hospital." Siblings need to talk about expected and common setbacks during convalescence.

Aiding the Convalescence

From a psychological viewpoint, siblings need to be aware that brothers and sisters who are ill or injured look forward to being home with them and want to be treated as normally as their condition will permit. The staff of a pediatric rehabilitation unit should talk with siblings about how they can aid in their brother's or sister's convalescence. A positive attitude, faith, and hope are very important for all members of the family during the convalescence phase.

Being Neglected by Parents; Feeling that the Sick Sibling Is Preferred by the Parents

Many families feel overwhelmed when a child is hospitalized in critical condition. As the child's condition improves, some parents will be able to pull away to give sufficient attention to the other children at home. But there are some parents who feel that their place is at the bedside of the hospitalized child, and they relegate the household and child care responsibilities to someone else or to an older sibling of the sick child. Therefore, we frequently hear siblings talk about being neglected by their parents when a brother or sister is hospitalized. This inevitably leads the children at home to develop feelings that the parent in some way prefers or loves the ill child more than them.

We have all seen some parents who become overprotective and overinvolved in the care of the sick child during convalescence. Siblings feel left out and pushed to the periphery. The solution to this dilemma would be a family approach to the child's convalescence, with responsibilities being shared by all members of the family in an appropriate manner.

Not Understanding the Illness

Appreciation of a child's developmental cognitive level is imperative in assessing his or her ability to understand the illness or injury of a sibling. We must gear our explanation to the child's level. Explain carefully, then ask him/her to explain what you have told him/her and what s/he understands it to mean. I am constantly surprised at children's misunderstandings, even after I have been careful to explain the illness or injury at a level appropriate to age. Fantasies, fear, attention span, and readiness to accept or understand information affect the siblings' understanding, just as they affect the understanding of the ill child and/or parent. Denial and other protective defense mechanisms help the siblings cope until they are finally ready to begin to accept that their brother or sister has a serious illness or handicap.

Needing Medical Information

During sibling discussion groups, we find that most children ask for more medical information. They want to know why it happened, if it could happen to them, if it will happen to their own children. Older children will want to know if the illness is hereditary, contagious, or curable. Sometimes siblings shy away from the ill child because of an erroneous belief that the condition is contagious. This is especially prevalent among siblings of patients with cancer and cystic fibrosis. Long discussions of the curability of an ailment and what a cure or remission really means should help the sibling cope.

Coping

The process of coping, accepting, and adjusting to life with a chronically ill, injured, or disfigured sibling is one of constantly changing emotions and defense mechanisms. While not compartmentalized into distinct stages, there are some characteristics seen in almost every case—disbelief, shock, denial, anger, plea bargaining, understanding, and acceptance. I would like to stress that group therapy for siblings is an effective way to provide the education and understanding essential for acceptance and healthy coping.

7

The Comprehensive Rehabilitation Clinic

Charles E. Hollingsworth

NEED

Some children who survive devastating accidental or nonaccidental trauma with multiple residua, including neurological, orthopedic, and emotional sequelae, require intensive follow-up by various subspecialties. Parents could spend most of their time transporting their child to and from appointments to physicians and waiting in their busy offices and waiting rooms. Therefore, we recommend that each hospital outpatient clinic organize a comprehensive rehabilitation clinic, where children will meet on the same day of the week once a month and where all the disciplines involved in the child's care can be integrated to provide coordinated, consistent, optimal care for the multiply handicapped child.

PHILOSOPHY

It is felt that optimal care can be provided if communication among all the physicians, nurses, and paramedical personnel caring for a child meet once a month, or as often as needed, to discuss the patient's program, needs, and problems. If the child and parent or guardians are also present, the child can be examined by as many of the subspecialists as is indicated during one day (preferably morning only), and a summary conference can be held at the end of the clinic to discuss the child.

INTERDISCIPLINARY APPROACH

The interdisciplinary team should have a case manager clearly identified for each child. The clinic should have codirectors designated from the department of pediatrics and the division of pediatric rehabilitation. Behavioral science staff members on this team should include the psychiatric social worker, psychologist, child psychiatrist, and a coordinator of the child protection program (child abuse). In addition, other representatives on this comprehensive rehabilitation team will be occupational therapists, physical therapists, a speech pathologist, a pediatric neurologist, a pediatric orthopedist, a pediatric urologist, and an ophthalmologist. The case manager determines what other members of the team will see the child and/or family, at what times, and in what order. The case manager is ultimately responsible for the child's care and indirectly responsible for the appropriate and effective use of the other members of the team.

CONSOLIDATED TOTAL CARE

A rehabilitation program for these children and their families must integrate the physical limitations with the emotional reactions to the limitations. This clinic affords the mental health professionals an opportunity to observe the medical specialists working with the patients. The difference in style of interviewing or relating to the child may yield very different results in terms of the child's performance or cooperation. Therefore, it is useful for the medical specialists to stay in the examining room and observe the child's interaction with other members of the team. They usually find that the child displays higher functioning for members of the team who are perceived as less threatening or more familiar.

CHILDREN WITH MULTIPLE NEUROLOGICAL IMPAIRMENTS

Children develop multiple neurological impairments for many reasons. Many children are severely abused by their parents, commonly by the mother's live-in boyfriend or a stepfather. Statistics reflect an increased risk for a person who was an abused child to become an abusive parent.

Frequently the children were neglected or left unattended for only a few minutes, allowing them time to drown, fall from a high place, become electrocuted, or run into traffic.

In the follow-up, it is difficult to tell which child was abused and which was injured by accident, but one thing stands out for both: the severe degree of neurological impairment. Even with the most severe damage, we often see progress month after month; and as the child grows older, we see developmental accomplishments that delight us and the parents.

FOLLOW-UP FOR PREVIOUSLY ABUSED CHILDREN

Many emergency room physicians see children who have possibly been victims of child abuse. This is reported and investigated. Eventually, the children are released to their parents either by the hospital, the courts, or the probation department only to show up a few months later in another hospital or emergency room with serious injuries that are again difficult to explain. We recommend that these children and their families be followed closely by the Suspect Child Abuse and Neglect (SCAN) team, or Child Protection Program as it is called at some hospitals. These cases should be reviewed at periodic intervals, and the family should be provided with enough emotional support to guarantee the safety of the children. Frequent contact with these families is imperative. A child who has sustained injury resulting in any permanent residua should also be followed in the monthly comprehensive rehabilitation clinic. This optimizes the opportunity for more of the professionals involved in the child's care to discuss the child's progress and determine if the parents or guardians are providing a safe and emotionally supportive environment for the child to develop and attain his or her potential.

THE SUMMARY PLANNING CONFERENCE
AT THE CONCLUSION OF THE MONTHLY CLINIC

The comprehensive rehabilitation clinic is coordinated by a nurse who guarantees that the charts are accurate, well organized, available to the clinic, and highly confidential. These charts are periodically reviewed by a peer review committee to guarantee that the children are provided with the comprehensive scope of services that we encourage. At the end of this clinic, each health professional who works with the children meets for an interdisciplinary review of each child. Progress, care plan, and areas that need more attention or more intensive intervention are discussed.

In addition, a program has been developed to assist families in which a child has been abused. Some of these children are also followed in the comprehensive rehabilitation clinic. Our hope is that this program will prevent children from becoming so severely injured that they need to be followed in our comprehensive rehabilitation clinic.

IMPROVING PARENTING SKILLS
WITH COMPREHENSIVE FAMILY REHABILITATION

The purpose of the comprehensive family rehabilitation program is to provide emotional and psychiatric services to families that have abused, neglected, or molested their children or that are at high risk to do so. It is aimed to teach them adequate parenting skills, to involve them and their children in ongoing professional counseling, and to provide each family with a successful parental role model in the form of a friend, lay counselor, and parent aide for both parents and children. This program accepts self-referred, physician-referred, and court-referred families and provides a comprehensive approach over at least a one-year period for families involved in the program. We hope that most families can be followed for years and will remain involved in the program.

Assigning a successful parent role model to each abusing family has been proven effective in reducing the risk of repeat abusive offenses (Dr. Brandt Steele and Dr. C. Henry Kempe, National Center for the Prevention of Child Abuse and Neglect). The parent role model is called a parent aide and is carefully screened and educated about normal child development. S/he attends carefully planned in-service programs on topics of family stress, child abuse, and intervention techniques. We discourage the use of a parent aid who was an abused child, a previously abusive parent, or who has a history of serious emotional problems. While there are many emotional rewards in being a parent aide, it is a stressful, demanding role and usually involves more time than we initially expected. All parent aides are unpaid volunteers and are available by phone 24 hours a day to the family with whom they work. The parent aide will also go to the home of the family for regular visits. At any time that either parent feels the stress level building to a dangerous level, the parent aide takes the children and/or parent for an outing. The parent aide can markedly increase the quality of interaction between the parent and child and provide an excellent model for parents to improve their parenting skills.

Parent-infant and parent-toddler classes should be offered for mothers and fathers who have abused their children or who fear that they might abuse their child, and are self-referred, as well as for parents of high-risk and premature infants. These classes could teach the parents about child development and provide a supportive group therapy arena for discussion of feelings and stresses. We also recommend that each abusing parent be involved in ongoing individual or couples parent counseling at a mental health center or with a private-practice mental health professional who is willing to communicate with the parent aide. This counseling can be voluntary or court ordered.

Child abuse appears to be on the increase. More cases are coming to the attention of authorities with the increase in reporting. Obviously, more cases will be brought to the attention of the courts, and it would be beneficial if the judge in each case had a program available to improve parenting skills for these families.

In summary, a program for improving parenting skills with comprehensive family rehabilitation should include well-trained parent aides, psychiatric social workers, child psychologists, child psychiatrists, parent-infant classes, as well as group and individual counseling for the parents and the children. We must not overlook the psychological damage done to the child by an abusive parent. For children over age three, we must provide psychotherapy to help them understand their world and to help them with their fears and feelings toward the abusive parents.

REFERENCE

Kempe, C.H., Silverman, F., Steele, B., et al. The battered child syndrome. JAMA 181: 17–24 (1962).

8

Case Studies in Pediatric
Consultation-Liaison Psychiatry

Charles E. Hollingsworth

There are many reasons why the pediatrician, nursing staff, or medical social worker calls on the consultation-liaison child psychiatrist for assistance, but most frequently it is observed psychic stress in the child or family. The following case studies are typical of any pediatric hospital.*

CASE 1: ADOLESCENT DEPRESSION WITH SUICIDE ATTEMPTS

Kathy is now age 15 and in the 11th grade. She has an I.Q. of 133. Her parents separated just two months after she was conceived, because the mother felt that the husband had become insanely jealous and seemed psychotic. He reportedly would run away and spend his money foolishly, and then write bad checks. Kathy and her mother had a close relationship until Kathy began ninth grade, at which time she began to quarrel with her mother and began to stay out late at night. Kathy complained of difficulty sleeping, and her mother could not get her to go to bed at a reasonable hour. Her mother said that Kathy became quarrelsome in the ninth grade. "She was very moody. Our whole life seemed to change. She resented my telling her to do anything and resented any control." There were two episodes of strange behavior in the ninth grade: once a girl touched Kathy on the shoulder and Kathy began screaming and crying in front of the entire class for 20 minutes. In another episode, Kathy became angry at a boy and broke the window of his van. She was taken to Juvenile Hall for this, but the case was dismissed. At that point her mother insisted that she attend psychotherapy sessions with a family counselor. Her mother also felt that Kathy was taking drugs, but could never find any in her possession.

---

*In this chapter, the "we" or first person singular (I) refers to the pediatric consultation-liaison psychiatrist.

During the summer after ninth grade, while Kathy's mother was out of town at a family reunion, Kathy took her mother's new car and deliberately drove it into another car. The result was $900 in repairs. Her mother interrupted the vacation and flew home.

In 10th grade, at 14 Kathy began dating; her menstrual periods also began. She seemed to be making a good adjustment at last and continued in family counseling. When her boyfriend started dating another girl, Kathy became very distraught and made a suicidal gesture by scratching both wrists with a razor blade. She was psychiatrically hospitalized for two weeks.

In 11th grade Kathy's mood became depressed, she was not sleeping well, and her appetite was poor. She began to tell her friends unbelievable stories, and they became concerned and called her mother. Kathy told her school counselor that she had a baby named Michael, that her mother had ten children in a dirty house, and that her mother forced her to care for the children. In actuality, Kathy was an only child and her mother was very successful in business.

In the two weeks before Kathy presented to the Children's Hospital emergency room, she had become grandiose and was hyperexcited. Her style of dress had changed drastically and she was unkempt. She was brought in a state of stupor to the hospital via ambulance from the school grounds. The toxic screen revealed that she had taken an overdose of Valium and alcohol. Her mother was summoned to the emergency room and did not seem surprised about the drug usage or suicide attempt. The pediatrician managed the medical aspects of the drug overdose and placed Kathy in the intensive care unit on suicidal status. She required mechanical ventilation by respirator for eight hours. The child psychiatrist had been consulted in the emergency room and continued to follow Kathy and her mother. After Kathy was fully awake, she admitted taking the overdose and said she still wanted to die. She was transferred to the adolescent psychiatric ward, still on suicidal precautions, with a tentative diagnosis of probable manic-depressive psychosis with suicidal ideation.

In this case the pediatrician, nursing staff, social worker, and liaison child psychiatrist worked collaboratively to allow the smooth transition from a medical emergency to longer-term psychiatric inpatient care.

CASE 2: EXPLOSIVE ADOLESCENT MALE, HYSTERICAL CONVERSION REACTION

At age 15, before an all-star baseball game, Mark noticed a slight swelling of his forehead above his left eyebrow. He developed chest pain while playing as catcher during the game and was taken to an emergency room, where an EKG and other workup were normal. Now, at age 16, he feels a great deal of pressure regarding his baseball team. He feels that his coach is tough and expects him to excel more than his teammates. Mark thinks no one likes him in school and has a low self-esteem. He has had one girl friend for the past year and gets very upset if she threatens to date anyone else. She is also age 16.

When Mark's school performance deteriorated he and his parents began seeing a psychiatrist for family therapy. Mark had made low scores on school achievement tests. He was often sent to the "opportunity room" for disruptive behavior in the classroom. Recently he had been missing school two to three days per week because he did not get up in the morning for classes. In addition to attending summer school, he was working part-time and playing baseball at night.

On the evening before he was admitted to the psychiatric ward, Mark was sitting quietly in the family den when he began scratching himself. He then began hitting his father and lay on the floor as if having a seizure, with arms and legs shaking and eyes rolled back, but without losing consciousness or sphincter control. An EEG done on the morning of his admission was normal.

The child psychiatrist was consulted and filed the following report:

> Mark had been very cooperative during the evaluation with only two episodes of anger and frustration. On one occasion, he threw a chair against the floor because he did not want the nurse to take his temperature, and on another occasion he was angry because he was missing an all-star baseball game and his pediatrician would not give him a pass to leave the hospital to play in the game.
>
> Mark and Debbie have been dating for almost a year, but had known each other for several years before they started dating. Mark seems to fear that Debbie will terminate the relationship and frequently asked her if she was going to break up with him. His behavior is immature for a 16-year-old, with low frustration tolerance. He seems very unsure of himself. Debbie describes three or four breakups with Mark, always followed by Mark having some kind of attack—chest pain, pushing his fist through a door, or shaking episodes. Even if Debbie goes out with a girl friend, Mark is so jealous that he is likely to have some type of attack. Mark says that Debbie started his attacks by going to the prom with someone else the day after he had been released from Community Hospital. He had been examined in the hospital for chest pain that had occurred at school 30 minutes after an argument with Debbie and two minutes after an argument with his baseball coach. The attack occurred on the baseball field, and the coach reported that Mark stopped breathing.
>
> Because of a mild tremor of hands, arms, and legs, and his complaint of nervousness, the family therapy psychiatrist had prescribed Valium, but the tremor episodes had continued. Two nights before this admission to the hospital, Mark was asleep on the sofa beside his girl friend when he

began to shake violently. She woke him up. He was coherent and said he was having a nightmare. He reports frequent bad dreams in the past six months. The night prior to this admission he fell asleep while watching TV beside his girl friend. Five minutes later he began shaking violently, choking and gagging. This episode lasted for 30 minutes, during which he was not arousable and did not respond to cold water on his face. This frightened his girl friend and his mother. Ten minutes after he stopped shaking, he awakened with no recollection of the attack. The next morning when he awoke, he noted bilateral subconjunctival hemorrhage, for which his mother took him to see the pediatrician. The pediatrician admitted Mark to the hospital for a workup which included EEG, EMI Scan, blood glucose, a four-hour glucose tolerance test, urine for VMA, and toxic scan for drugs on serum and urine. The results of all these tests were within normal limits.

The child psychiatrist felt that Mark was very ambivalent about his relationship with Debbie. Evidence for this was their frequent arguments, his declared fear that she will leave him, and his behavior, which seems sure to drive her away.

The diagnosis was given as anxiety reaction, conversion type, with a recommendation to increase psychotherapy to twice a week and strong consideration of inpatient psychiatric treatment if symptoms persist.

CASE 3: FAMILY STRESS, PLACEMENT ISSUE, OSTEOMYELITIS

Alex is a seven-year-old second grader who had been hospitalized for 3½ weeks for antibiotic treatment for osteomyelitis in his left foot. His mother had been conferring with the pediatric ward's social worker twice a week and had been explaining that she could not cope financially or emotionally with four children under the age of 12 years. On the day the child psychiatrist was consulted, Alex's mother had told the social worker that she had been fired from her part-time job and had decided to place all four children in Synanon near San Francisco. The mother had already told this to Alex, and he was in his room crying. She had also told him that he and all the children would have their heads shaved and would live a strict and disciplined life at Synanon. She had told him that she would not see him again and someone from Synanon would come to pick him up at the hospital.

The child psychiatrist asked Alex what his plans were for the remainder of the summer.

"My Mom wants to go on a trip, but we don't have enough money. (pause) Have you ever heard about Synanon? Mom says they have a school and she wants us to go there, but if it costs too much we can't go there. I don't want to go. One of my Mom's friends at her work had a son there and she told her about it. (pause) My Dad never sent us nothing. I haven't seen him in two years. I think the County used to give my Mom some money. She has an old Datsun." He began sobbing, "I'm sorta worried that she might send me to Synanon. We went there one time so she could look it over. All the people are bald with shaved heads, even the children. (pause) I've been to surgery two times on my foot. When I was smaller I was cross-eyed and I had surgery when I was three."

"How do you get along with your brothers and sisters?" asked the child psychiatrist.

"We have some arguments at home. Mom would say, 'Knock it off' and send us to our rooms—now she says she can't take us any more; so she is giving us to Synanon."

A year earlier, Alex's mother had placed him and his siblings in a Country foster home for six weeks. She had attended some counseling sessions at a community mental health center, but had recently terminated them.

The child psychiatrist agreed to see Alex's mother again the next day, and she was more composed. She agreed to let the hospital social services investigate other alternatives for placement, but when Alex was ready for discharge his mother took him home and was again receiving welfare. Alex was very happy that he was allowed to be home with his brothers and sisters. Our child abuse intervention program provided a parent aid to Alex's mother, and she was allowed to work part-time and receive welfare. At six months post discharge, she abruptly changed her mind and placed all four of her children in Synanon in San Mateo County, and they were lost to follow-up.

CASE 4: CYSTIC FIBROSIS WITH DEPRESSION

Jackie, age 14, was from a close, middle-class family with one older brother. She had frequent colds and pneumonia, and only two months earlier had been diagnosed to have cystic fibrosis. Her reaction had been one of extreme anger. She said the doctors were wrong and that the laboratory technician had made an error. She had watched a television program about cystic fibrosis that said that most people with the disease die before age 20. Jackie was even more angry when the child psychiatrist was consulted. She would not speak to the psychiatrist at all on the first day, but on the second day she began to talk. She said she had no boy friends, but did have several girl friends. She then began to talk about how angry she was at her female pediatrician, saying, "She just lectures at me every time she comes in here." She said that the doctor tells her how she should be feeling, and she felt that no one could know how someone else feels inside, especially when you have just been told that you have something as serious as cystic fibrosis. The female physician had told Jackie that it doesn't hurt much when she takes blood gases. Jackie said she had now had gases taken ten times and she knew how much it hurts. Jackie felt that she couldn't trust anyone—nurses, doctors, or parents. The physician had told Jackie's parents that Jackie had cystic fibrosis two days before they told Jackie. Jackie had picked up the nonverbal communication that something serious was going on, yet she could not get her parents to level with her. Her mother had made the physician promise to give them a few days to find the appropriate way and time to tell Jackie.

Finding out about this delay in telling her only added to the girl's distrust and anger.

As the hospitalization progressed, Jackie's depression became evern more apparent. Her anger shifted to a quiet, withdrawn state, and she kept the curtains pulled around her bed most of the time. She began to cry and grieve appropriately about her diagnosis. She was seen daily by the child psychiatrist for two weeks and then was referred to a psychiatric social worker in the community for ongoing psychotherapy.

CASE 5: ASTHMA, REFUSAL TO TAKE MEDICATION

Sheila, age eight, has had asthma since the age of 3½ years, with frequent visits to emergency rooms at night and to her allergist's office during the day. She lives at home with her single mother and a five-year-old brother. Her physician had some concerns that Sheila was not being given her medication regularly or appropriately. The frequency of Sheila's asthmatic attacks seemed to increase at times when Sheila's mother appeared more depressed.

The child psychiatrist was consulted and asked to see Sheila on the ward, where she was refusing to take any oral medication. (She had also protested loudly when given subcutaneous injections of epinephrine in the emergency room.) She told the psychiatrist, "I don't want to take no more pills, I'm tired of being sick. I can't have any cat or dog. I don't feel good today, and the nurses wake me up and say, 'take these pills'."

Her mother reported that Sheila had been refusing to take her medication at home, and she had finally given up trying to force her. Her mother had a low self-esteem and admitted that she was tired of Sheila's frequent asthma attacks.

Sheila and her mother began outpatient psychotherapy sessions with our child psychiatry department to address the issues of chronic illness and depression.

CASE 6: SYSTEMIC LUPUS ERYTHEMATOSUS WITH HALLUCINATIONS

Martina, a ten-year old Mexican girl, was referred because of alteration in her mental status during treatment of acute systemic lupus erythematosus. Martina, the third of six children, was born and raised in Ensenada. Two months prior to admission to the pediatric ward, Martina's parents noticed that she tired more easily, became apathetic, and had a decreased appetite. At that time, she was admitted to a hospital in Mexico with a diagnosis of renal failure and anemia. On the pediatric ward she was diagnosed with nephritis due to systemic lupus erythematosus, and treatment with steroids was begun. One week prior to the psychiatric consultation, she had a sudden grand mal seizure and was put on phenobarbital, with no recurrence of the seizure. Shortly after this, she began to have periods during which she seemed confused and disoriented. Auditory and visual hallucinations were also noted. These have consisted of voices calling to her, seeing strangers in her room talking to her, and seeing actual people as if they were upside down or distorted in other ways. These episodes occurred several times per day, generally lasting a few minutes. There seemed to be no difference in occurrence between night and day.

Martina has a history of good academic progress in school and good peer and family relationships. There was no family history of mental illness.

Mental Status Exam

Martina was a friendly, attractive, petite, ten-year-old girl, who was lying in bed when interviewed. She seemed weary and spoke slowly but distinctly. She was alert but somewhat lethargic. Martina speaks basic English well and communicates well. She was oriented to place, knowing that she was in a hospital. She was oriented to time—she was correct about the date, month, and year. She described the auditory and visual hallucinations mentioned earlier. At the time of interview, her thought processes seemed intact, her language was clear, logical, and there were no loose associations.

Impression

Martina's mental deterioration is acute; her premorbid mental status was sound and age-appropriate. The waxing and waning nature of her mental symptoms, the periods of confusion that seemed delirious, and the presence of both auditory and visual hallucinations suggest a toxic organic process. Central nervous system involvement of her lupus is a good first choice as to etiology. Psychic manifestations of steroid therapy are well documented in the literature and quite variable, including frank psychosis, euphoria, depression, and more subtle personality changes. Regression in ego functioning is typically seen in illness, sometimes to the point of serious mental deterioration, as in the case of "intensive care unit psychosis." The emotional stress of this serious illness; its rather prolonged course, from her point of view; and the resulting removal from a close family, friends, and a familiar environment must also be considered.

Unfortunately, there is no way to clearly delineate etiology at this time, and all factors must be considered.

Recommendations

1. Neuroleptics and low doses of a nonsedating, antipsychotic medication may be helpful, particularly if her symptoms become more pronounced, more prolonged, and result in behavior that is potentially dangerous. I would suggest starting with Haldol (haloperidol), using 0.25 mg b.i.d. and gradually titrating upward to desired effect. The child psychiatrist will help monitor her condition if this is taken.

2. Measures that should be taken now are: increase in contact with staff; close observation to note periods of delirium and hallucinations, with help in reality testing during such periods. She will need continued reassurance that the hallucinations are not real, but in her imagination. My impression is that when lucid, she understands this idea, but will need help during periods of decompensation.

3. Periods of play activity, now begun, are helpful and should be increased if possible. It would also be helpful to introduce some teaching, more for the contact and structure it provides than for the academic advantage. Probably a Spanish-speaking teacher would be better, but if this is not possible, then perhaps some lessons in basic English.

4. The parents seem to be attentive and supportive. I would encourage their presence and also frequent visits by other relatives and friends.

5. If medically possible, removal to an open ward would be advantageous, with a view to increasing contact, particularly with other children, and reduction of her sense of isolation.

CASE 7: SEPTIC ARTHRITIS, TEMPER TANTRUMS, SULLEN AND WITHDRAWN BEHAVIOR

Jason was a 3½-year-old boy being treated for septic arthritis of the left hip. He was having extreme difficulty allowing his mother to leave the hospital, and had temper tantrums followed by sullen and withdrawn behavior.

Family history was significant in that the grandmother lived with Jason's divorced mother. One sister had died five years earlier, at age four, of chronic illness.

During this hospitalization, Jason's mother has been at his bedside almost continually. This has been in part because of his protests at her leaving, but even more because of her own reluctance to leave and her anxiety about his condition when she is absent. Recently she has begun to leave his room for brief periods, which he has tolerated fairly well even when no one else was present. His mother has also left twice for extended periods (up to about seven hours), but felt compelled to call the hospital and check on his condition while away. This is a pattern that has existed since Jason's birth. His mother states that she is "paranoid" about something happening to Jason while she is away. She denies that she reacted to her first three children like this and thinks that she relates to Jason in this way largely because of the loss of her third child five years ago.

Jason also has been demanding while in the hospital, has temper tantrums if he does not get what he wants from mother, and generally has had a sullen, withdrawn demeanor. Mother states she has always had difficulty setting limits for him, does not discipline consistently, and thinks he is "spoiled rotten."

Growth and Development

Mother's pregnancy with Jason was wanted, but occurred in the midst of marital distress toward the end of the marriage. During the pregnancy she was under considerable emotional stress. Physically, the pregnancy and delivery were unremarkable, and Jason's major developmental milestones have been grossly normal.

Interview with Jason

Jason appeared to be tired, irritated, and depressed when I first met him. He was in a cast that immobilized his left hip, was having some discomfort, and would occasionally point to the left hip and try to get mother's attention. He responded only briefly to me, telling me his name and that he did not like the hospital. While I talked with mother, Jason occupied himself fairly well with toys, but occasionally would demand attention from his mother and was visibly annoyed if she did not respond immediately.

Mental Status

Jason is an alert, well-developed 3½-year-old boy, who appeared depressed and withdrawn. His speech was age-appropriate and he could use simple sentences. There was no indication of psychosis, autism, or organicity.

Psychiatric Diagnosis

The following psychiatric diagnosis was made: (1) psychological regression due to acute illness and hospitalization; (2) capacity for separation, impulse control, and frustration tolerance less than normal for age. This probably represents a developmental deviation in response to environmental factors.

Recommendation

Jason's behavior in the hospital has improved somewhat and probably will continue to do so as he feels better. This will be facilitated by helping mother to separate and set limits more comfortably.

The important concerns here are the questions raised concerning Jason's development. His mother has created a very close relationship with Jason, has difficulty allowing him to separate, probably over-gratifies and over-stimulates him, and has unreasonable fears concerning his health and well-being. His mother has indicated that she is interested in outpatient psychotherapy. The child psychiatrist has arranged for further evaluation as an outpatient, will continue to follow the case while in the hospital, and will assist with any psychiatric interventions that may be necessary.

CASE 8: DIABETES MELLITUS WITH BEHAVIOR PROBLEM

Penny is a 13-year-old half-Mexican-half-Indian female diabetic who was admitted to the pediatric ward in a diabetic coma. She has a long history of insulin-dependent diabetes mellitus, which has led to multiple hospitalizations in the past. The circumstances preceding the last hospitalization are roughly as follows: The day prior to hospitalization, Penny was very active, riding her bike until late in the evening. She then stayed up until about 11:00 doing the dishes. The next day she woke up feeling unwell and told her mother she planned to stay home from school. Her mother agreed and expressed some concern about her daughter's condition. During the day, Penny became progressively lethargic and withdrawn, and her mother expressed some concern over this. Neither mother nor Penny checked her urine or thought to call the physician at this time. Later in the day, her mother became increasingly alarmed and finally took Penny's temperature. On finding a fever of 103 degrees, the mother brought Penny to the hospital in an apparently comatose state. The mother notes that Penny has had total responsibility for her diabetes for some time now, giving herself her own injections and checking her own urine when she remembers. The mother is uncertain of what precipitated this recent attack, but feels it might be related to some interest that she showed approximately a week ago in returning to work. Though Penny overtly agreed with this, her mother doubts that she would support this change. Penny has been living with her mother for the past year. She spent the previous year with her father in Fresno. The mother has very little insight into Penny's emotional difficulties. During the year that she was away, her mother visited her at most two to three times. Since Penny returned to her mother, her mother says that things have been going fairly well for her. The mother feels that Penny has some friends now, whereas before she was more socially isolated, that she has been more physically active, and that she is even involved in some social groups, such as a group on "Indian consciousness." Penny is currently in the eighth grade in regular classes and doing fairly well, according to her mother. Her mother says that Penny has always been a quiet youngster, has little contact with other people, and shows little initiative. She is especially quiet around nonfamily members. Her mother notes that Penny complains a lot about "almost anything." The mother denies any other difficulties with her daughter.

Penny has two older siblings, living with her father, and one younger sister also living with her mother. The mother denies any significant family difficulties, with the exception of the two older boys, who were placed on probation briefly for vandalism. She also denies any family history of psychiatric illness, alcohol, or drug use. The parents were separated when Penny was four years old, and the mother says, "The children didn't seem to mind."

Mental Status Examination

Penny is a somewhat thin, lethargic, apathetic youngster who has very poor eye contact and shows little interest in the examiner and, in general, has tremendous difficulty in relating. She answered questions put to her with grunts, nods, or one-word answers. She essentially denies any difficulties or worries and professes little concern over her medical problems. She seems to have very little insight into her recent hospitalization and family conflicts that might have contributed to it. Any kind of formal intellectual testing was impossible due to a lack of cooperation.

Impression: (1) Depression secondary to chronic illness; (2) probably passive-aggressive, passive-dependent personality.

Assessment

Penny has suffered a number of stresses, including a lack of maternal interest, multiple deprivations and losses, and chronic illness. These have combined to lead to an extraordinary ambivalence about dependency needs and an essentially maladaptive solution to these problems. These have begun to coalesce into fairly rigid character traits, which are likely to be difficult to modify. The assessment is superficial and difficult to make, given the lack of cooperation on the child's part and given the mother's obvious denial. Nonetheless, it is clear that an attempt at intervention is warranted and may be lifesaving. Effectiveness with intervention would have to hinge on the mother at this time. She must be convinced of the seriousness of her daughter's difficulties and of the need for finding more adaptive solutions. If the mother sees psychiatric help as a vital component of management of her daughter's difficulties, she might be able to follow through on referral. This could probably most helpfully be placed in terms of "you must help your daughter help herself." Mother and daughter should at least initially be seen together, as it is unlikely that Penny would be able to attach to anyone at this time and that even if she did, the mother would probably be unable to continue to get her to appointments if she were not directly involved. I have taken the first step in strongly suggesting the need for treatment to her mother, and she has at least overtly agreed. Given pressure from all quarters, it is hoped that she will follow through with outpatient psychotherapy for Penny and herself.

Follow-Up

Two years after the above report, at age 15, Penny was readmitted in diabetic ketoacidosis. She had persistent depression and poor cooperation with treatment. She and her mother had not followed the pediatric liaison psychiatrist's recommendation for outpatient psychotherapy. She now had proteinuria secondary to diabetic nephropathy. After the patient was stabilized medically, she was transferred to the adolescent psychiatric inpatient unit of the hospital, where she had individual and group psychotherapy for six weeks before being discharged home to her mother.

CASE 9: DIABETES MELLITUS, ANXIETY, FEAR OF DEATH

Valerie is a nine-year-old girl who celebrated her birthday just a few weeks ago. She lives with her natural mother, who is employed out of the home, and with her father, who currently works two jobs as a truck driver. There is also a brother who is six years old and in first grade. There are no other persons in the home at the present time.

Valerie was admitted to the pediatric ward six weeks prior to psychiatric consultation with newly diagnosed diabetes mellitus and a glucose level of 500. Consultation to our service was requested because the child seemed anxious and was reluctant to eat, and the mother was expressing apparently excessive anxiety, making frequent phone calls and verbalizing some worries that her daughter would die soon.

History of the Present Illness

For the last couple of months, the mother has noted that Valerie has been eating and drinking more frequently, but that she has been losing weight. The mother thought the diagnosis would probably be "worms," and so she was shocked when she went to the pediatrician's office and learned that Valerie has diabetes and would require hospitalization for insulin titration. The mother said she cried after they left the pediatrician's office, but she did not explain to Valerie what the crying was about.

Valerie has been basically a healthy child, the one major exception being a problem with ureteral reflux. The mother says, "Valerie has half of one kidney that is nonfunctional," a chronic problem of considerable distress to the mother. The only time Valerie had been previously hospitalized was for one night, when she was about five years old, for an uneventful tonsillectomy with no major sequelae and no apparent major behavioral or emotional regression by the child.

To the best of the mother's knowledge, there is no diabetes mellitus on either side of the family. The genetic history is incomplete because the father was adopted.

Development History

Valerie was described as an "excellent baby," with the only infant problem being that she was a picky eater. She was very close to her mother and the mother felt that her child was "sensitive." Her father thinks that since toddlerhood she has been a "pleaser" and that she is a child who "holds in" her feelings. The mother agrees that as a toddler she would cry even with a little "no no" from the mother. But she had significant developmental milestones on time, started kindergarten with no significant separation anxieties, and her mother thinks that, despite the sensitivity, Valerie has always been a "very independent child."

Stresses within the family during the past year include a series of four accidents at work in his truck for the father between one and two years ago. This year Valerie was diagnosed has having ureteral reflux, with apparently some nonfunctional renal tissue. Also, in the spring of 1978, her younger brother was hospitalized for about six weeks with a fractured femur after being struck by a car. The significance of this may be that Valerie had been told to be "responsible" for this brother and watch out for him along the street. She was often told this, and on that particular day she apparently remained anxious all day long, until she found the opportunity to tell her mother how scared and how guilty she felt that her bother had been hit and was injured.

This past summer Valerie began to gain weight and developed a "pot belly." The mother would tell her from time to time that she really ought to go on a diet, and about once a week Valerie would announce that today she was starting her diet. Otherwise, the past few years have been relatively unremarkable ones for the family. The family is described by the mother as one that is close and that verbalizes its concerns, but there are indications from the father that the mother worries a great deal out loud and that, although concerns may be expressed verbally, affect may not be shared with any sense of support.

Hospital Course

One day after admission, Valerie was tearful about the frequent blood tests and injections, but she was taking a somewhat active part in her care, testing her own urines. Three days after admission she was described in the chart as alert and playful. But after dinner there was an episode of nausea and vomiting that went on into the evening. Stabilizing this child on insulin has been difficult because of episodes of nausea and vomiting, and because she has been rather inactive, staying in her room, and has been a picky eater. However, according to the chart, her affect waxes and wanes; at times she is very active in learning about her own care, whereas at other times she mopes a bit.

Interviews with the Child

When the liaison psychiatrist met with Valerie she was eager to talk about her worries. She requested that the psychiatrist close the door and draw the curtains around her bed. We talked immediately and quite directly about her concerns. She told me that she believes she caused her diabetes by eating so much this summer, particularly candy. Secondarily, she believes that "it was kind of a bad thing to give herself this diabetes," and what is going to happen now is that she will have to stay in this hospital "forever." She became a little tearful as she described that staying here forever would mean never seeing her friends and only having intermittent contact with her family. Then she told me that she is afraid that after staying here forever, she will die here. She describes fear of what the process of dying might be like.

In summary, this is a little girl who considers that her illness is due to something she did wrong, and that the consequences will be separation from family and friends, and death. She has apparently been resistant to getting up and getting dressed in the morning, and has been staying in bed, which seems to be playing out the role of a little girl who might die. She seemed to accept my clarification on these points.

She willingly drew for me a picture of her family, which showed everybody else smiling and happy. She started by drawing a big smile on her face and changed it to a substantial frown. We talked about the fact that sometimes you are expected to keep a stiff upper lip and might go around smiling when you really feel very sad and unhappy. One other interesting aspect of the drawing was her attention to sexual detail, with a penis for the father and brother, muscles for the father, breasts for the mother, and nipples for herself. She expressed some delight in including these details in her drawings.

Interview with the Parents

The child psychiatrist met with the parents once together, then with the mother alone, and then with the mother and Valerie together. It was clear to me that the frequent telephone calls by the parents while Valerie has been in the hospital were a result of the mother feeling that she is out of control and that a good mother stays in control of the parenting of the child. She is worried about giving up the parenting aspect of life to the hospital staff. She expressed fears "that Valerie might develop an insulin reaction in her sleep" and the staff might just think she was sleeping normally, and that Valerie might go downhill and die in her sleep. It seems that the father gets up at home at 2 A.M. to go to work, and the mother awakens with him. They both feel anxious; so the father calls the hospital to make sure that Valerie is OK. Only then can the mother turn over and go back to sleep, while the father can go off to work. The frequent phone calls and demands to know what is going on seem to stem from an anxiety that has something to do with being a mother who remains in adequate control. I am really not clear on the details of what is causing this, but I think that the mother's own personality organization will probably stabilize after she gets substantial clarification and teaching on the subject of diabetes and gains experience caring for her daughter as a diabetic child. Until then I think the phone calls will continue.

Diagnostic Impression and Recommendations

My impression of Valerie is that she is experiencing what may be a normal reaction of childhood in the face of a major emotional stress. The situation bears close observation to see if she moves into a somewhat longer period manifesting an actual reactive disorder of childhood. I do not think that there is major psychological pathology evident in the parents or in this child, but that we are seeing a response to stress. We can conceptualize the response to the diagnosis of a major illness much in the same way we can conceptualize the response to death. It is, after all, partly a grief reaction, with denial, anger, and frustration. I think the family may be helped to get through this grieving and readjustment time. In order to minimize emotional problems that could result from the faulty response to stress, I am going to suggest to the mother later today that they continue to meet with me at least a few more times, and perhaps longer in the out-patient psychiatric clinic. They must also maintain the important pediatric and diabetic teaching contacts with the physicians and other staff at the hospital.

In terms of ward management right now, I think that, bearing in mind that this child will continue to fear that she might be dying, it will help if the people dealing directly with her let her know that she is not in the hospital to die. I think she is now beginning to understand why she is in the hospital, and may be somewhat easier to help with this problem now than she was. I think that as she is convinced that she is going to continue to live, it will be easier to encourage her to take an active involvement in her diet and exercise, as well as in her testing of urine and injections.

CASE 10: SICKLE-CELL DISEASE WITH DEPRESSION

This psychiatric consultation was requested by the pediatrician because Diane had become depressed, withdrawn, and infantile.

Diane is a 16-year-old black female who has been known to have sickle-cell disease since the age of two years. She has had sickle-cell crisis with severe pain approximately two to three times per year. She is fortunate that she has not had any serious complications of sickle-cell disease, such as kidney disease, liver disease, or cerebrovascular accident.

Academically, she has been an average student in the 11th grade. She worked during the summer giving out sample cigarettes, and was still employed part-time when the present sickle-cell crisis began.

She lives at home with her mother, who works for the U.S. Post Office, her father, who has been retired from the U.S. Post Office for three years, and an older sister, age 19, who shares a bedroom with Diane. Diane has an unmarried brother, age 35, who lives in San Francisco, and a sister who lives in New Mexico, but was visiting Diane when the present sickle-cell crisis began. Diane is the youngest child and has always been treated as the baby of the family. Diane and her sister have both been dating occasionally, but neither has a steady boyfriend. Diane describes herself as a quiet, shy girl, who keeps everything to herself and never talks to anyone about her feelings—not even to her mother or sister. She also describes her sister as very quiet. Diane told me that her family is Catholic, but has not attended church in three years. She told me that she has been depressed about her disease since she read a pamphlet this summer that said that sickle-cell disease patients die by age 20 (and she is 16). She has had difficulty sleeping at night and has been staying up watching late movies until 2 or 3 A.M. because she could not sleep. On weekends she has been sleeping until 11 A.M. She also stated that she does not have much of an appetite, but blamed this on hospital food. She was in pain during my first interview and said that the pain in her side made her depressed. She was not in pain on my second and third interviews, and was somewhat more talkative.

She has a limited understanding of sickle-cell disease. She was able to draw pictures of normal red blood cells and sickle-shaped cells. She knew that she should avoid very high altitudes, which might precipitate a sickle-cell crisis, and told me that she had tolerated a plane ride to Mexico City and Acapulco because the plane was pressurized. She also tolerated the high altitude of Mexico City without going into crisis. She stated that she did not know that sickle-cell disease is hereditary, and she did not have any understanding of genetic probabilities. She mentioned that she had not thought much about getting married, but probably would some day, and wants two children—a boy and a girl. She mentioned that a cousin in Alabama has sickle-cell disease with more frequent episodes of crisis than Diane has.

She said that her mother takes care of her at home when she is in pain and that the only medicine she has ever had at home for pain is aspirin.

My impression is that Diane suffers from depressive neurosis secondary to physical illness: sickle-cell disease.

I feel that Diane should be referred to a psychiatrist who can see her regularly. It would also be helpful if someone could explain heredity and the genetic aspects of sickle-cell disease to Diane and her family. I will continue to follow her throughout this hospitalization on a daily basis.

CASE 11: SEIZURE DISORDER, DEPRESSION, BEHAVIOR PROBLEM

Bob, age 13, had been hospitalized on the pediatric ward for petit mal seizure disorder. His pediatrician had requested child psychiatry consultation because he had been refusing food, drink, and medication in the hospital and was a behavior problem on the ward.

Bob's petit mal seizure disorder had been poorly controlled on Zarontin (ethosuximide) for several weeks, the apparent reason being poor compliance in taking his medication.

There has been a struggle between mother and son for some time on the issue of taking the medication, and his mother confided in me that she often used physical force to get her son to swallow the medication. Three months prior to this admission, Bob discontinued his Zarontin (ethosuximide), ostensibly because his father told him he really didn't need to take it any longer. A few days later, he apparently had a staring spell while crossing the street, and was struck by a car. He was hospitalized at Community Hospital for two weeks. Rehospitalization began here six weeks ago for surgical repair of at least one and perhaps both knees.

There is a long history of personal and family problems. Four years earlier, at age nine, he was evaluated in the psychiatric outpatient clinic for hyperactivity, with shoplifting and fire setting. Apparently, the boy never got into treatment in the psychiatric outpatient clinic following the evaluation there.

Key points from that evaluation include that Bob is the youngest of six children, but the product of the tenth pregnancy to a mother who was 26 years old at his birth. There were severe medical problems during the pregnancy and beginnings of life. The mother reports herself as "sick" throughout the pregnancy. Bob was born by an induced breech delivery, weighing six pounds, one ounce. The mother had a cardiac arrest during the birth and told the psychiatric social worker that she was "clinically dead" at the time of his birth. The baby had an intestinal infection early in life and was placed on a special diet at the age of six weeks. He had pneumonia twice during the first year. There have been two prior surgeries, one for a tonsillectomy at the age of three, and the second at the age of five to remove an undescended testicle and insert a prosthetic testicle.

Bob has been in classes for the educationally handicapped because of multiple behavior problems. History from the hospital chart indicates chaos in the home over many years. The mother has been married four times. Bob's natural father left the home when Bob was six months old, and his mother subsequently remarried three times. The natural father, who is allegedly an alcoholic, abruptly returned to the family home three years ago and moved in. The mother says that Bob and his father have never gotten along well and that Bob was difficult to manage during the summer when things were particularly tense at home. She adds that Bob has been much easier to manage and no real problem since his father left a few months ago.

The noncompliance with the Zarontin (ethosuximide) medication has been a chronic problem. The mother herself says that Zarontin (ethosuximide) makes Bob nauseated.

Hospital Course

Bob was admitted to the pediatric ward for a knee repair six weeks prior to this consultation, which was accomplished one week after admission. The nursing staff feel that his behavior is immature. He has often refused food and drink from some nurses, while taking it from others. The same has been true with medication. The hospital chart shows three episodes of emesis (vomiting). The first episode contained pill fragments. The nursing staff report that when Bob was told to turn off his TV and go to sleep last Saturday evening, he refused and responded to the staff person with a raised fist. His mother told me that two days prior to his surgery, while she was visiting, Bob began crying and asked that she take him home.

Examination of the Child

I first met with Bob on the day prior to his surgery. He was lying in bed with the covers pulled up to his chin, and when I entered the room he was not occupied in any activity. He is a well-developed, well-nourished male who looks his stated age of 13, except for a rather babyish face. During the time that we talked, he remained in bed with the covers pulled up to his chin. I did not observe any staring spells or any obvious seizure activity, but I did notice several episodes where for 10-20 seconds the right corner of his mouth twitched. There were no bizzare behaviors. His affect was a bit silly. He was not really cooperative with the exam and said that I was correct when I surmised that he did not particularly want to be talking with me. His speech was a bit hesitant. When he did talk, in brief sentences, the rate and rhythm were normal. This thought process showed no signs of psychotic disorganization. There was a paucity of thoughts that were shared with me. His thoughts were neither loose nor tangential.

He was oriented to person, place, and time. Insight and judgment were difficult to assess. He did seem to know that he required surgery for his leg injuries. He would not really talk much about taking Zarontin (ethosuximide), so it was difficult to assess his feelings regarding this issue.

Bob did indicate that he felt somewhat sad about the surgery. He let me know that it really did not hurt too much when his father left the house this summer, but he would not talk about this to any great extent. I let him know there were several reasons I thought he might be feeling depressed now: (1) his school year has started and he misses his classmates and other school activities, which he has enjoyed in the past; (2) he cannot go out and be active now; (3) he cannot ride his new dirtbike because of his recent leg injuries; and (4) his father left the family again last summer.

Meeting with the Mother

I met for an hour with his mother on the day of Bob's surgery. She is a well-nourished woman, who was appropriately dressed and groomed. She made good eye contact. Her thought content revealed that she perceives people as either good or bad. She said that she makes instant judgments when she first meets a person, and she sees Bob as being just like herself. She also told me that she and Bob have not been having any fistfights lately, but that threats of physical blows are common in the home.

Assessment

I think that this is a boy who is quite immature for his age, and who is living in a home with a mother who probably has a borderline personality organization. Both mother and child are easily overwhelmed, and are easily frightened when relating to other people. I think there is such a close mother and child bond that too many attempts to change this boy would lead to anger on the part of the mother, who would feel threatened. While the boy is in the hospital, some basic suggestions for dealing with him would include the following:

1. Decide what things absolutely have to be done (essential medication, such as any antibiotics he might require) and limit struggles with him to those absolutely essential areas. For instance, I would not get involved in struggles over what or how much he eats.

2. I do not think this boy is able to relate with all members on a shift. He deals in instant good or bad judgments. It might be in the staff's as

well as the patient's, interest not to insist that he relate with all staff members equally.

3. I would keep the same basic ideas in mind for the mother, who is very close to her son and seems to function in a rather disorganized style.

4. If a system of rewards or punishment is necessary to get him to do the essential things, I would deal in rewards rather than punishment. Find out what he wants—like the use of his radio—and encourage it as a reward for good behavior.

5. I think the staff may need to talk about how frustrating this boy is as a patient. This is one of those times when the staff can really support each other in getting through a difficult convalescence with a patient.

6. I will be glad to talk with the staff to see if we can pool our ideas in ways to keep things as peaceful as possible in caring for this boy.

7. Antiseizure medications are to be decided by the pediatric neurologist. I am not very hopeful that this boy will comply with anticonvulsant medications outside the hospital.

8. I have reminded his mother about the helping agencies available to her if she needs assistance with Bob's behavior. She denies that any such help is needed right now, but apparently she has recently utilized one agency when in crisis, and perhaps would do so again if things got bad enough.

CASE 12: RAPID DETERIORATION WITH BRAIN TUMOR

The pediatric neurologist requested child psychiatry consultation for Tom, an 11-year-old boy, and his family in anticipation of a possible severe emotional crisis. The diagnosis of inoperable brain stem tumor (glioma) was made just one week after the onset of his first symptoms of deviated eye movement and slight slurred speech. The pediatric neurologist had been a tower of strength to this emotionally close family, but had also been honest about the possibility of rapid deterioration because of the size and location of the tumor. Tom and his parents knew that this was probably a terminal illness and that chemotherapy or irradiation were not likely to be helpful. Tom's parents are young, in their early thirties, with two younger children. Tom had been the star pitcher of his baseball team and had won a trophy for being the best goalie in his division of soccer.

Tom and his parents decided to try chemotherapy and radiation treatment as their "last hope." His parents had been having some marital problems before his diagnosis was made, but this crisis brought them closer together, and they seemed to be a strong emotional support for each other. Initially, the pediatric neurologist was worried "that they were taking this tragic news too well," but the stress soon began to show up; the mother began to complain about the nursing care, insisting that she would not leave Tom's bedside as long as he was in the hospital.

Interview and Mental Status Examination

Tom is an appealing, bright, articulate boy who seems overly mature for his age. His physical appearance is commensurate with his serious illness. He relates to adults in a fairly open and responsive manner. His use of language, vocabulary, the types of questions he asks, his awareness of his surroundings, and his hospital experiences indicate a sophistication and intelligence chronologically advanced, with no gross deterioration of thought process. He is fully oriented.

Tom explained to me that he has a brain stem tumor, that he would be treated with both radiation and chemotherapy, that his doctors hope the tumor will go away, but that they are not sure it will. He did not directly broach the subject of his death, but did comment once that it would be good to raise the railing on his bed because "you could commit suicide by falling off the bed." On another occasion he had arranged blankets around him in bed and told his mother that it was his coffin.

Impression

Tom's premorbid development has been good in most areas, with the exception of some age-inappropriate social development with peers. That is, Tom experiences difficulty in peer relationships, while relating to adults in a somewhat pseudomature manner. This is related to an overly close relationship between mother and son, considerable investment in him, and perhaps a somewhat distant husband-wife relationship.

Tom is currently exhibiting an increasingly dependent clinging relationship to mother, which is in part a normal reaction to his illness and, in part, encouraged by the preexisting closeness. The family system as a whole is coping with this crisis in an appropriate manner.

Recommendations

Supportive psychiatric counseling is indicated for both Tom and his parents and can be provided by either the liaison psychiatrist or the psychiatric social worker assigned to the service. The mother is bearing the brunt of this crisis and will probably require increasing support to continue to function adequately.

Tom has found significant relationships with some staff, which are useful to him supportively. I would caution that as his condition deteriorates, there may be a tendency to pull away from him. Hopefully, awareness of these issues will minimize this reaction.

In addition to the usual interaction with nurses and doctors, which is very important to Tom, I would encourage the continuation of occupational therapy, educational tutoring, and other activities to the extent that he is capable of participating in them.

Follow-Up

Tom was discharged from the hospital one month after his first admission.

The physical examination at the time of discharge showed Tom to be nonambulatory. If brought to a standing position he could stay in one place, but he was too weak and ataxic to walk without support. His left arm was weak, and he seemed to have a left facial paresis. A closer evaluation revealed a gaze paresis. He can close his eyes, but the right eye is unable to resist active opening force. His left lip droops slightly, and there is a hint of his tongue deviating to the left when extended. His speech is good, and his articulation is also good. Swallowing is difficult both with liquids and solids. Sometimes the liquid would come back out through his nose. The air exchange in his lungs is good, but he is unable to cough. His lungs were clear on auscultation. The abdomen was soft and there was no organomegaly. During the last weeks of hospitalization there have been no problems with urinary incontinence. There is clonus in the left foot and an upgoing left toe.

Tom was made as comfortable as possible at home. There were frequent home visits by his pediatrician, pediatric neurologist, and pediatric oncologist, as well as a psychiatric social worker. Tom died quietly in his sleep six weeks after going home from the hospital. His parents continued in outpatient counseling for three months after his death.

CASE 13: TRANSVERSE MYELITIS AND DEPRESSION

Hector is a 13-year-old boy who developed transverse myelitis one month prior to request for psychiatric consultation. His illness had caused lower-limb paralysis and loss of bladder function. His physical medicine and rehabilitation physician requested the psychiatric intervention because of "possible developmental problems and depression which are suggested by Hector's behavior in the hospital, which has at times been uncooperative, demanding, passive, and dependent." He also frequently withdraws from social contact and has brief outbursts of temper.

During the several days prior to this consultation, Hector regained bladder control and partial use of his legs. It is important to note that his mood and attitude also improved during this time, no doubt not coincidentally.

Hector lives with his mother and his 15-year-old sister, Debbie.

Past History

I interviewed Hector on one occasion, and his mother and sister together on another. It was noted by the staff that the mother had visited infrequently and, in fact, some of the staff who have been working closely with Hector had not seen her. I found it difficult to contact her, although she was cooperative once reached. Hector's mother is a rather attractive, but weary and depressed woman who conveys a sense of detachment, which raises the question of the quality of her involvement with her family. During the interview, in fact, Hector's sister supplied more pertinent information and conveyed a more accurate understanding of Hector than did his mother. In all fairness, it should be noted that his mother is currently attending the trial of the people accused of murdering her brother this past year. This may be decreasing her capacity to be involved with Hector at this time.

The only problem that the mother could identify as genuinely concerning her, other than the present illness, was Hector's difficulty in school during the past year. He had entered seventh grade following a move to a new district, had left behind old friends, and encountered a new environment and many new people. Hector ditched school for a while, felt that his teacher was overly critical and did not give him enough help, and had some difficulty with his school work and with making new friends. He began to receive special instruction in math, and by the end of the year seemed to have made a reasonable adjustment to the new school, at least from the mother's viewpoint. The mother was not able to recall his specific report card evaluation and, even though she stated she was concerned about Hector's school problem, she made no move to address this problem either through the school or other agencies. She states that, in general, Hector has progressed satisfactorily in school and has not been retained in any grade.

Other problems that the mother identifies are Hector's moodiness, his tendency to lose his temper easily, to become hurt and hide in his room sulking, and his frequent arguments with his sister. However, she does not see these as problems impeding his development, does not see any need for professional help for Hector, and comments, "That's just the way he is." There apparently is no history of delinquency, other serious behavioral problems, or symptoms of serious psychiatric illness.

Hector does have a number of friends, both older and younger, and is active in play outside the home with them. He has recently started a newspaper route and experienced some difficulty organizing it. He and his sister have apparently worked out an arrangement whereby they will share the tasks involved, and she is cooperating by taking over the route while Hector is in the hospital.

Interview with Hector

I found Hector working on a model car and apparently enjoying this task. Other staff members later commented that he seemed to prefer solitary activities and does not like group activities. He was cooperative and spoke to me for nearly an hour. Hector talked about how frightening it was to lose the use of his legs and about how at first his mother did not believe his complaints. He was optimistic about recovery of full function and was pleased at the progress he had made already.

Hector was able to identify his current illness and problems at school last year as his only problems. He blamed the school difficulty on going to a new school, where he felt "like an outsider," and on his teacher, who picked on him, was critical, and at times made fun of him. He stated that math was the most difficult subject and asked me if he could have someone help him in math while in the hospital.

I was impressed by Hector's not knowing what kind of work his mother did, by his telling me that he often made his own meals, and by his statement that his mother had not visited him for several days. He was vague and rather evasive when asked more questions about his mother.

Hector also talked at length about his friends, about playing in the park frequently, and about how much he enjoyed tennis and basketball.

Mental Status Examination

Hector is a somewhat chubby, young adolescent who was cooperative, but somewhat guarded in the interview. He remained seated in a wheelchair, but was able to use it actively and effectively without help. His speech was relatively normal but suggestive of a culturally deprived environment. Hector's thinking was clear, with no indication of psychosis or organic brain syndrome. He was able to express himself well and had no difficulty understanding me. He had a somewhat blunted affect, but occasionally there were flashes of humor, and more often he had spontaneous speech. No formal assessment of knowledge or cognition was attempted, but he seems of approximately normal intelligence.

Psychiatric Diagnosis

(1) Hector suffers from reactive depression secondary to acute illness, with regressive features such as easy loss of temper, withdrawal, and overdependency; (2) developmental deviation in a number of areas, particularly cognitive development and social relationships. Other significant personality traits are low frustration tolerance, tendency to emotional lability, difficulty with self-assertion, low

self-esteem, and a chronic, mild depression. These traits are compatible with Hector's development in a fatherless family with a mother who seems somewhat distant and vague.

In summary, Hector has areas where he does not function optimally, but is making progress that is considered satisfactory by his family and immediate cultural environment.

Recommendations

I would encourage Hector to talk about his present disability, how frightening it was initially, and how encouraging it must be for him to be making progress now. It is important to be sensitive here to possible misunderstanding by Hector of the significance of his illness, whether or not he is concerned about possible future consequences, and how quickly he expects recovery. Hector's tendency to isolate himself from group activity is indicative of his difficulty in relating to others and the feelings he has about himself. I expect he will resist participation in group activities, but it would be good to encourage him to do so. In view of his present stage of development (young adolescence), his past history in a fatherless family, and his current need to separate from his mother, it may be that he will respond more positively toward male staff.

Educational difficulty is the only area which both Hector and his mother recognize as being a problem for his development. It does not appear that he has had testing for learning disability. This could be done now (psychoeducational evaluation) and would be made available to his school. This testing would indicate specific academic strengths and weaknesses and would be helpful to the school in planning an effective educational program for Hector.

The other issues of Hector's development—depression, poor control of temper, some difficulty with peer relationships—could be dealt with in therapy in an outpatient clinic setting. However, it would require the mother's awareness of these issues and appropriate motivation on her part in order to develop a continuing treatment plan. Neither of these criteria appear to be met at this time. His mother stated that she would prefer to wait until Hector had recovered from his present illness before considering the question of assistance in other areas.

CASE 14: PARAPLEGIA, ADJUSTMENT TO IMMOBILITY

Psychiatric consultation was requested for this 9½-year-old female to suggest an acute intervention for her reactive depression, to help her family understand and accept her neurological disabilities, and to assist in an educational assessment of the child's remaining capabilities.

History of Present Illness

Annie is the eldest of two female children in a single-parent family. She was physically healthy and appeared to be adjusting satisfactorily to the separation of her parents and to her reading disability. One month prior to the consultation, she was severely injured when a vehicle hit her as she crossed the street to follow her mother into a store against her mother's instructions. She sustained multiple injuries, including a cervical spinal injury with resultant paraplegia distal to the T-1 level, a fracture of the left humerus in its distal third (Annie is left-handed), and multiple intrathoracic and intraabdominal injuries necessitating chest tube suction, tracheostomy, and splenectomy. In addition, there were two documented cardiac arrests with cardiopulmonary resuscitation, two previous hospital transfers before the patient was admitted here, and a cervical spinal fusion at the previous hospital, with postoperative immobilization, a body cast, halo splinting, and a hanging left arm cast. Annie was apparently comatose for an indeterminate length of time, with fluctuating neurological status, as described in reports from the two previous hospitals.

According to her mother, Annie was unconscious and not breathing when the mother arrived at the accident scene moments after it occurred. She received CPR from a passerby who apparently happened to be associated with the respiratory therapy unit at a nearby hospital. The mother noted that she was able to communicate with Annie six to seven days after the accident and, because she has been particularly concerned about her daughter's mental ability, has given her different tasks and tests along the way. Annie was able, through visual cues, and hand grasps for "yes" and "no," to recognize her mother, father, and an aunt; to remember people from the past; and a few days later, with her mother working with her, was able to count to ten. She was able to hold a card for the game of Candyland that the family played with her, and she was verbally able to identify the colors that each family member had: red, green, and blue. She was able to laugh appropriately with her sister, Donna, and a nephew, Tony. She was able to show anger by saying that she was tired of listening and telling members of her family to "shut up, I don't want to hear any more." She was able to ask for and see her nephew, Tony, to whom she is quite attached.

In addition, her mother relates how Annie was able to talk and relate well to the social worker, who used a hand puppet of Kermit the Frog to express some anger and scary feelings that she was probably having from her very stressful ordeal. Since the accident, the mother notes that when Annie is angry or wants to assert some control, she actively will not listen or will not talk.

Developmental History

Her mother indicated that she and Annie have been very close and that Annie has only been away from her one other time, and that was for one week at age six when she visited a maternal grandmother. This is where she became great pals with six-year-old nephew, Tony.

Hospital Course

Since admission to the pediatric rehabilitation ward, Annie has apparently been withdrawn and so quiet on the inpatient rehab unit as to raise the question of whether she could, in fact, speak at all, or whether she might be silent because of psychological response to her injuries, her multiple moves from the different hospitals, and her present new surroundings here at the rehab unit. This is what prompted the consultation.

Interviews with the Child

I met with Annie briefly on the day the consultation was requested. She acknowledged my presence visually with good eye contact and verbally agreed that her Mom and I could leave the room and talk for half an hour and come back. In the process she asked to have a book that her mother was reading to her to be left at the bedside to comfort her while her mother was gone.

Mental Status

In the interviews the following mental status was gathered from rather limited observation.

Appearance: Annie is an attractive, dark-eyed, dark-haired girl with a very expressive face.

Affect: She appeared apprehensive initially, then willingly made eye contact and was able to understand questions about how she signals the nursing staff and other caretakers here on the rehab unit when she is scared or lonely. She was quite animated and explained that she does not have a way to signal or show others when she is in distress, especially at night. She showed considerable relief that someone had asked her such a question, understood her plight, and apparently would look into it. Speech was infrequent, soft, whispered in phrases and short sentences. She would speak more to her mother than she would to the examiner.

Sensorium: The child recognized her mother, that I was someone new, and appeared to understand that we would be away for about half an hour talking and then we would return. She was not alarmed by this, but made arrangements for her own comfort while her mother was gone.

Thought Processes: She appeared to understand her mother and me and spoke coherently in phrases and short sentences.

Judgment: She understood that her mother and I would be gone for awhile and asked to hold a book that mother was reading to her.

Insight: Apparently Annie has demonstrated sufficient insight with the social worker through her discussions about internal feelings through the use of the puppet Kermit.

Assessment

This is the case of a young, left-handed girl with preexisting reading disabilities, from a single-parent family, who appears at present to be in a subacute response phase to massive physical and psychological injury and loss, including the accident itself, the multiple surgical and medical procedures that followed, the repeated neurosensory examinations to determine the level of neurological function, the confinement of her dominant hand, her head, and body in casts, and the vocal insult secondary to the tracheostomy. Also, she has loss of control of nearly everything, except whether or not she would engage others visually with eye contact or verbally with speech.

Her retreat to more infantile behavior, her attempt to isolate or deny massive overload of negative feelings, and her use of visual/verbal communications as a way to control others can—and in this instance probably do—represent a normal response at this phase of her grief reaction and reorientation to her significantly altered new self.

Diagnostic Impression

1. Adjustment reactions, early phase
2. Suggestion of delayed separation individuation phase in psychological development.

Recommendations

1. An increase and extension of her sense of control through a bedside light switch or buzzer control. Use of her free hand in self-feeding or attempts at self-feeding, reading, kneading clay, drawing, and other activities that she would have been capable of doing with her dominant hand.

2. An increase in her awareness of her retained abilities by pointing out to her repeatedly through action (this might be done through occupational therapy) those things that she is still capable of doing.

3. Helping her to absorb and accommodate in small steps to the massive emotional overload that she has recently had. This could be done through play and puppet therapy dealing with the appropriate themes of grief and guilt.

4. An increased sense of belonging to and relating to others. This can be facilitated through a hand-held family album, which helps to reattach her visually to her family. Use of family and support staff interactions for nonmedical relationships, for example, occupational therapist visits by volunteers or other children. Eventually Annie will go to the activity room to observe and participate in some of the activities as well as she can with her left hand so that she will begin to feel more involved in activities with other children from the rehab unit.

CASE 15: PARAPLEGIA, DIFFICULTY IN ADJUSTMENT

History of Present Illness

Kim, age 16, was driving a friend to a party at Kim's boyfriend's (age 20) apartment when the car went off the road and down the embankment. While Kim's friend had no significant injury, Kim suffered a spinal cord transection. Kim awoke in the ambulance en route to Community Hospital.

She was noted not be able to move her legs and to have decreased sensation below T-8. When stabilized, she was transferred to the pediatric rehab unit, where she underwent a bone graft and the placement of a Herrington rod. In the hospital, she also developed a urinary tract infection. She was in considerable pain from her injuries and from the infection. She spent several weeks in the intensive care unit, where, according to her mother, she acted in many ways like a martyr—so much so that everyone got involved with her and would give her their addresses. When she was in the intensive care unit, she was, according to her mother, by far the healthiest patient there. She was transferred to the rehabilitation ward, where she was the oldest child, and also the sickest. There the mother felt she became depressed and moody; this usually manifested itself by her talking back to her mother.

Prior to the transfer to the rehab ward, the mother had spent two weeks at Community Hospital camping out on the hospital grounds in a Winnebago trailer with Kim's boyfriend and a stepsister. When she came to our hospital, the mother spent a lot of time with Kim. When Kim left the rehabilitation ward and became angry with her mother, her mother became aware that she had been treating Kim in a different way since the accident. She resolved after that to go back to treating her as she had previously, encouraging Kim to be her own person, speaking very frankly to her about her condition, and expecting Kim to continue to work hard and use the talents that she had.

Kim and her mother both felt that of all the people in the family, Kim was the one who could best bear the blow of an accident of this sort. Both she and her mother are confident that Kim will be able to deal with the stresses that will follow. Both feel certain of the boyfriend's fidelity. He has expressed the desire to Kim to "be her legs." The mother says that from time to time Kim tests him by bringing up the issue of being a burden.

Currently the mother is having the house made suitable for a wheelchair by having ramps installed and big bathtubs put in the house.

Kim is beginning a rehabilitation program, learning transfers, and will begin to learn to dress herself in the next few weeks. It is estimated that she will be in the hospital for two months.

One of the incidents that focused staff attention in Kim's handling of her injuries was an incident in the radiology suite, where she was asked to swallow some barium. At the time, Kim said that she was in severe pain. According to the notes, she was very upset in the suite. Kim explains this by saying that she felt very bad that day.

Two weeks after admission to the hospital, there was a staff conference in which Kim was told the extent of her injuries and that she would never walk again. She became upset at this conference. However, when interviewed afterward, she said that she had known these facts all along, but had not wanted to hear them.

Currently, many high school friends visit and call. In addition, her biological father has visited, and Kim feels that they have become closer as a result of her injuries.

Developmental History

Kim was a nine-pound, six-ounce baby who smiled almost at birth, who talked from six months, and did not walk until 12 or 13 months. She showed no visible anxiety to strangers and did not have noticeable oppositional behavior. The mother did note, though, that around the age of two she suddenly became afraid of water, even though she had been swimming in it since several months old. The mother felt that, since childhood, Kim always had a jealousy of her older sister, despite the fact that the mother spent equal time with both of them. The mother feels that Kim would never admit such jealousy, however. There was considerable marital strife during Kim's childhood, and her father became an abuser of alcohol. When Kim was ten, her parents divorced, and at that time the father allegedly told Kim that she was to blame for the marital breakup. After this, for six months, Kim had difficulty in school, with some behavior problems at home. Her mother felt that after that time she began to treat the sister and Kim differently and began to encourage Kim to "be her own person." Her mother said that Kim had no other problems in school. Kim began menstruating when she was 12, and her mother discussed the facts of life with Kim and her other daughter in a frank manner. The mother remarried a year ago and said that Kim has been very pleased with her new stepfather. Kim confirms this and says that although the house at first seemed like a railroad terminal, it was really quite nice. Kim describes herself as getting her best school grades this year, and her mother said that she is also developing an interest in working with young children.

Examination of the Child

Kim was interviewed on one occasion, a day after the rehabilitation conference in which she was told her prognosis. She was interviewed while lying on a stretcher; during the course of the interview, she received two telephone calls— one from her maternal grandfather and one from a friend. She spoke of the accident, saying that she was very happy that her friend had not been injured in the accident. She said the first thing she remembered about the accident was waking up in the ambulance and being in great pain, and the attendant not being able to give her anything for it. She described her background in some detail, speaking of the arguments between her mother and father. It was her opinion that the family stayed together in part so that she would have time to grow up. She spoke of having some difficulties in the sixth and seventh grades, about the time that the divorce took place. She said that this enabled her to get those things out of her system, so that she was much more reliable in junior high school. She described herself as very much interested in social events, and that that was her major activity. She spoke of her boyfriend and the things that they used to do together. She spoke of her mother's remarriage and expressed a great deal of liking for her new environment. She spoke of her mother, saying that her mother would often think of the things that she, Kim, had in mind, and would verbalize them. She felt that the mother had been very supportive and helpful in the hospitalization. She spoke of her recent injury, her determination to deal with it, and go on in her pursuits. She had not made any specific plans, however. In general, she was very open and friendly.

Mental Status Exam

Appearance: Attractive, 16-year-old girl lying on a stretcher; somewhat nervous; good eye contact, and quickly engaged the interviewer in discussion.

Mood: Mood was labile during interview; she seemed happy, but admitted fluctuating moods.

Affect: Full range.

Speech: No observable abnormality, except for slight pressure of speech, at times, when talking about her injuries and future plans.

Thought: There were no delusions or hallucinations, no paranoid ideation, no ideas of reference, no vegetative signs of depression, no suicidal or homicidal ideation. She exhibited some denial, but appeared to see things realistically.

Orientation: She knew the date, month, year, and where she was hospitalized.

Digit Span: She numbered six digits forward and four backward. She knew three out of three objects in two minutes.

Abstractions: "A bird in the hand means if you do something good it is worth something."

Similarities: "An apple and a pear are fruit; a dog and a cat are animals."

Judgment: What would you do if you found a letter lying in the street? "I would probably read it." What would you do if you found a fire in a theater? "I'd get out." Insight was fair.

Assessment

Kim, for all her labile moods, appears to be grappling with the issue of her injury in a very constructive manner. As an adolescent, there are two major concerns for her—her body image and her identity. Currently, she is being given support in these two areas by the many friends who call, by her boyfriend, and by her family.

She has some sense of denial in dealing with her injuries. However, some amount of denial seems necessary in patients with this type of injury in dealing with their lives. So long as it does not interfere with her treatment or her development, it may be constructive.

Although at this time Kim does not appear to need ongoing psychotherapy, I think that it was important for us to have made an initial contact. I have told Kim and her mother that should the occasion arise when Kim feels the need of talking, that such services are available here. I have also indicated to the mother that I would be willing to talk with the father or stepfather if they desired, or to talk with her in the event that a crisis arises.

Recommendations

It is important to continue to deal directly with Kim and to inform her of any plans for her future, because this fosters her independence.

CASE 16: BRAIN CONTUSION, EXPRESSIVE APHASIA, HYPERACTIVE BEHAVIOR

The reason for the psychiatric consultation was (1) to help define the psychiatric components of the patient's expressive aphasia, since he was noted to make no attempt to form words while on the rehab unit in speech therapy; and (2) to facilitate nonverbal expressions of his reactions to the stress of his recent massive injury.

History of Present Illness

Charlie is the fourth of five children and lives with his mother, maternal grandfather, and his two youngest siblings, ages seven and five. There is a long history of chronic family stress: a psychotic episode in the mother, the children being court dependents, placement of the two older children with relatives, and working with a protective services counselor as recently as a year ago.

On the day of the accident, Charlie ran out in the street to retrieve his new puppy and was struck by a car's side mirror, causing a left parietal depressed skull fracture and reported exposure of brain tissue. He received emergency care and cerebral decompression at Community Hospital. His mother remembers that although he was somewhat delirious, he still was able to call out her name, "Mama, Mama." He was stabilized there and transferred to our pediatric rehabilitation unit, where the speech therapist noted his lack of effort to form words. This raised the question of the psychological components of his inability to speak.

Developmental History

Apparently, the pregnancy and developmental history are normal. According to his mother, Charlie had no trouble learning to speak and was using short sentences by age two. Prior to the head injury, there was already a pattern of using or not using speech in response to certain situations. His mother remembers that Charlie would be quiet, withdrawn, and frequently would not speak for varying periods of time; or he would behave as if he did not hear his mother and point to things. This usually occurred when he was angry; frustrated; told he could not do something, such as watch TV; or when he had been corrected or criticized. His mother was so concerned about this that at one time she thought he might have difficulty with his hearing. Coincidentally, after Charlie's accident, his five-year-old brother apparently withdrew behaviorally and began rocking and not speaking. According to my conversation with the mother, that brother is now seeing a psychiatrist because of this. His mother also stated that she feels that she may be a "problem," that she has ignored Charlie, that he was one of her "left-out children," that she would "take things out on him." She also had worried about the fact that he was very slow in school. He has attended preschool and apparently got along fairly well with the other children. His first year of kindergarten was a trauma, however, and he wanted to play all the time. He is presently in his second year of kindergarten, and the mother states now that he is more interested in what the teacher has to say. He was said to be hyperactive in kindergarten.

The mother also feels that Charlie's personality may, in effect, have changed since the accident and be better since his head injury. He is smiling more and is more affectionate.

Interviews with the Child

Charlie had recently begun moving the previously paralyzed right arm and leg, and his mother claimed that he had said the word "Mama" at her coaxing. The mother dates the onset of his not speaking to the time after the brain surgery and appears to ascribe a causal connection. Charlie, on first meeting, was a frightened, sad, angry-looking child, with half his head shaved. He sat in a wheelchair, head down, lips in a frown. There was no verbal response, but he seemed to understand what I said and would point appropriately. After he warmed up a bit to my presence, he wrote his name for me with his left hand. Later, in the playroom, he was noted to be lashing out at nearby objects, either by hitting them or knocking them over. I redirected this behavior to throwing bean bags at a wooden clown box. During this activity he used both arms, the left being stronger than the right. Another modification of the activity was "bombing" the clown box with the bean bags, while with each hit I would say the word "boom" loudly. When he became quite excited, obviously enjoying this activity, he said, with a medium-volume voice and quite clearly, "boom." Later, outside in the play yard, he pointed to the slide and, after being unable to get me to see what he was pointing at, said, "crat," apparently meaning the word "that."

On subsequent visits, he remembered me on sight, smiled and wanted to play or race in his wheelchair.

During the interview with his mother, while she was visiting Charlie one evening, she was trying to get him to say "Mama." He was voicing the sounds "puh puh." I suggested that she ask him to make the very sounds that he was already making. When she did this, Charlie shifted to a different set of sounds. This was repeated for three different sounds. Each time the mother repeated the sound he was saying and asked him to repeat it, he would shift to a new set of sounds. She also told me that on the past weekend with Charlie while he was home on a pass, his puppy ran out of the back yard again. He became quite excited, ran out to the back yard, closing the gates, and called "Droop, Droop," for the dog's name, Droopy.

Summary

In summary, we have a right-handed six-year-old boy from a disruptive and occasionally chaotic family, with a history of slow learning in school and a pre-injury behavioral pattern of using or withholding speech and behaving as if deaf as an anger reaction to frustration, criticism and/or deprivation. This boy then sustained a severe head injury to his dominant hemisphere language centers and left upper motor control centers. He is presently in an early psychological adjustment phase to this massive trauma and appears to be using some of his old behavior patterns of speech withholding and opposition, overlaid on the more profound organic speech impairment secondary to the brain injury. With this combination of deficits, he can sometimes muster appropriate monosyllables at times of high emotional charge, reminiscent of some stroke patients.

Diagnosis

1. Profound neurological impairment involving speech centers in the dominant hemisphere.
2. Preexisting behavioral pattern of the use and nonuse of speech in response to anger-provoking situations.
3. Increased dependent behavior and anger about injury, with the added problem of a limited mode of expressing his feelings.

Recommendations

1. Continued programs of speech therapy, physical therapy, and occupational therapy for this child.
2. Encouragement of nonverbal expressions of his reactions to the injury and loss appropriate to the hospital setting.
3. Charlie will probably need long-term, specialized help in schooling, with eventual learning disability evaluation, language reacquisition, and ongoing verbal and nonverbal psychotherapy to process the recent trauma and to cope with his long-term handicaps. The use of play therapy is indicated, and certainly his mother should be in ongoing counseling.

CASE 17: DROWNING VICTIM, PSYCHIATRIC CONSULTATION FOR PATIENT'S MOTHER

Kirk was an 11-year-old athletically talented boy who lived near the beach. His mother had just this summer began to allow him to go to the beach for surfing and "boogie boarding" alone. Kirk's parents are divorced. His father is a dentist on the east coast.

Kirk had drowned in salt water and was rescued by the lifeguard, but he had remained in a deep coma, with flat-line EEG tracings. He had continued breathing on his own when his mother and his physician had made the long and agonizing decision to disconnect the respirator four weeks after he was admitted to the intensive care unit.

Psychiatric consultation was requested for the mother because she was having difficulty coping with his condition and had begun angrily lashing out at the nurses and doctors. During Kirk's entire hospitalization his mother had been rather guarded about herself and her background. She would allude to her family and personal problems, but refused to talk about them. She was somewhat apprehensive about meeting with a psychiatrist, but was willing to do so, and was basically cooperative. She had difficulty in leaving her son's bedside and feared that if she left the nurses would make some mistake that would result in Kirk's death.

During the second interview with the psychiatrist, she was able to talk about her guilt feelings for allowing her son to surf at such a young age unattended by an adult. She expressed hope that there would be some improvement in his condition, and she felt frustrated because the hospital staff had not been more encouraging. She agreed to see the psychiatrist three times per week while Kirk was hospitalized. After six more weeks, he was transferred to a skilled nursing care facility. One week after admission, he expired with aspiration pneumonia. His mother then began seeing the same liaison psychiatrist once a week as an outpatient.

CASE 18: JAPANESE-AMERICAN BOY
WITH APHONIA FOLLOWING ENCEPHALITIS

The reason for child psychiatry consultation was to evaluate the psychological components of this youngster's aphonia following encephalitis with left-leg paralysis and to make appropriate psychological management recommendations.

History of Present Illness

Kyto is a nine-year-old Japanese-American boy, the third of five children, living with his biological parents, three brothers, and one sister. They came to the United States from Tokyo 18 months prior to his hospitalization. Kyto, according to his parents, is a rather shy boy. He had successfully completed kindergarten this past June and spoke English with his brothers and sister. He developed a viral-like encephalitis, leaving him aphonic and with left-leg paralysis. Since admission one week ago, he has made no sound or any effort to do so. I observed him with his parents for about 15 minutes. He was eating a peanut butter-and-cracker snack and focused his attention on this activity to the almost total exclusion of interaction with his parents. He responded nonverbally with opposition and/or withdrawal behavior to parental chatter, cajoling, and physical contact. The next day, after a short, nonverbal peekaboo game with him, I learned that he had made some sounds that appeared to be foreign words. This was confirmed through an interpreter in an interview with the parents. The father stated that Kyto spoke a few short but coherent and appropriately pronounced phrases in Japanese to him and his mother over the phone on Wednesday and each day since. Occupational therapy notes indicate that his withdrawn and inhibited behavior had alternated with rather nonspecific aggressive behavior at about the same time.

Developmental History

Kyto was a full-term infant with uncomplicated delivery. He had a severe febrile illness at about one month of age and, though his parents felt that he had returned to a normal developmental pattern, he was the slowest of all of their children to begin speaking, beginning at the age of two rather than at one and one-half, like the other siblings.

He has been fairly healthy since that time, and his developmental maturation appeared to be on target. He has also related well to his parents, siblings, peers, and in school during the past year. The parents indicate that his favorite activities are riding a tricycle and playing soccer. He also enjoys watching television cartoons, especially Superman, and likes going to school and drawing with crayons. His favorite foods are beef, chicken, apples, grapes, and small tomatoes. His parents note that when he is angry he becomes quiet and wants to be left alone for about ten minutes, which is the cultural norm for Japanese children. His parents also feel that Kyto is quite shy; his hiding behind hands and frequent turning away are evidence of this.

Interview with the Child

In an interview with Kyto and in interaction with him today, he was being isolated for enteric pathogens, in a crib with the sides up, scribbling with a yellow marker in a coloring book. I verbalized each of his actions in English and then I began doing, on a separate piece of paper, what he was doing in his coloring book. He gave me a long look and then hid his actions from my view. I next drew a picture like the one he had been coloring. He looked at it and compared it to his coloring book. He then curled up and closed his eyes, periodically checking to see if I was still in the room. I drew a picture of a boy riding a scooter, pointing to the boy and saying, "Kyto." When he saw this he closed his eyes for even longer periods. I placed the drawing inside his crib. Hearing the noise of the paper rustle, he opened his eyes and saw the picture. He began hitting it with his yellow marker and then began to tear it up. At this point, I reached in and did some mirror behavior by tearing it up with him. Again he withdrew and closed his eyes.

Summary

This is the case of a nine-year-old Japanese boy, with a history of slightly delayed speech development and recent American enculturation, who developed aphonia and left-leg paralysis after a viral-like encephalitis and intubation. Aphonia in a child who makes no attempt to speak or make any sound, but appears capable of nonverbal communication and maintains motor control of tongue, lip, and vocal cords is compatible with the diagnosis of hysterical or conversion mutism. Postencephalitis depression and/or emotional retreat to an earlier behavioral level secondary to severe stress can still be significant factors.

Diagnostic Impression: Probably hysterical mutism. Postencephalitic depression.

Recommendations

Increase Kyto's sense of security with a picture of the family at his bedside (this has been discussed with the family, and they will bring one in), phone conversations with parents and siblings; tape recording of family voices; and use of some Japanese words by nursing staff.

Increase Kyto's sense of enjoyment by using his favorite foods: beef, chicken, apples, grapes, etc.—even food brought from home (although this needs to be cooked according to hospital regulations)—and favorite activities, like tricycle riding and playing soccer on the patio (also drawing with crayons and paper and watching cartoons and Superman on TV).

Increase his play activity opportunities, as is already being done in occupational therapy. The child psychiatrist will follow the patient while he is on the pediatric rehab unit.

CASE 19: CEREBRAL PALSY, DAY SURGERY FOR WOUND DEBRIDEMENT AND UNEXPECTED PROLONGED STAY IN HOSPITAL

Tammie is a bright eight-year-old who has mild cerebral palsy due to a traumatic premature double-breach delivery. She came into the day surgery program of the hospital for an inguinal wound debridement and dressing change. She had been promised by her parents that she would be home in time to watch afternoon cartoons on TV and would be able to leave with the family the next morning for an Easter vacation to her grandparents' home in Honolulu.

When she was brought back from the operating room, both her legs were in casts, with a wooden separator between her legs. The surgeon explained to the parents that this had become necessary because the wound was not healing.

He added that Tammie would be required to stay in the hospital for about two weeks. The mother became quite upset—the nurses used the word hysterical to describe her reaction—and the liaison child psychiatrist was called.

When Tammie was completely awake, the surgeon, liaison child psychiatrist, and her parents explained the reason for the leg casts and for the hospitalization. Tammie cried and said that she had been tricked. She was very distrustful of everyone for several days and would begin screaming if any nursing personnel came into her room. Her mother kept a vigil at her bedside night and day. The liaison child psychiatrist talked with Tammie and her parents daily and helped Tammie begin to trust again. An agreement was reached with the physicians and nurses that every procedure, regardless of how minor, would be explained to Tammie before she was touched. Tammie regained self-control and was able to cooperate with dressing changes, blood drawing, and intravenous-injection site changes throughout the remainder of her hospitalization. Her parents began seeing a family counselor to talk about parenting a child who has cerebral palsy, because they had gained insight into the distrustful aspect of their constantly pampering Tammie and did not want to further damage her ego development.

CASE 20: CHRONIC IMMUNODEFICIENCY DISEASE WITH DEPRESSION

The child psychiatrist was asked to do this consultation by the pediatric immunologist because this patient with dysgammaglobulinemia has been chronically depressed for the past several months.

History

Ted is in the fourth grade. He has had dysgammaglobulinemia since birth, diagnosed at the age of two years by a family physician in Oregon. He has been worked up at several medical centers, including the recent workup in Seattle. He has had many admissions for this problem. He is currently admitted to the pediatric ward for central line placement for hyperalimentation. He has been losing weight over the last several months, and his appetite has decreased. He has not been able to take adequate amounts of nutrition by mouth because of stomach pain and because of stomatitis and blistering in the mouth. The blisters in his mouth have improved, and the stomatitis is much improved. Recently he began having severe stomach pain, which has made it impossible for him to eat. His mother works as an advertising executive in Los Angeles and has been curtailing her hours of work because of Ted's illness. She has been staying home to care for him and has limited work to one day per week. She is very understanding of Ted and has tried to help him with his depression. She reports that their social life consists of a few friends, primarily her friends. Ted has only one friend who visits—an eleven year old boy named Tony. Ted has been able to leave home occasionally to go to the beach for a short period and occasionally to go to a movie. However, he has been rather weak during the past six months and has not had sufficient exercise tolerance to be out of the house for very long periods. Last year he missed two to three days per week from school for much of the year. Toward the end of the school year, he was missing up to four days per week. His mother estimated he missed two to three months of school during the year. Two years ago he had a home tutor and this program worked very well. His mother is hoping that he will be able to have a home tutor for this school year as well.

Ted's mother reports that he has lost 13 pounds in the past year, having weighed 73 pounds in June and currently weighing 60 pounds. Ted states that the stomach pain has lasted for at least a month and that he literally cannot eat. There has been no vomiting, but a lot of gas, cramps, and pain. In describing his liver illness to me, the mother said that Ted had some form of hepatitis for several years. He has had three liver biopsies as well as several liver scans.

Personality Assessment

I asked Ted's mother to describe his temperament now. She said that when he is well he is in good spirits and is easy to get along with, but when sick he becomes easily frightened and very pain conscious. His depression seems to make his convalescence much more difficult. She said that he is frightened of receiving the long line for hyperalimentation, but at the same time he feels some relief. He hates IVs with a passion; he has had so many. She also reports that he is afraid of anesthetics. He hates intensive care units because of the noise and tubes and IVs and needles. She says that he has a fear of being unconscious and out of control.

The mother became tearful when describing medical students and other academicians who come to see Ted because of their interest in his dysgammaglobulinemia. She reports that while he was hospitalized in Seattle, many medical students came by to see Ted. She said that they had been prepared for that and they had actually gone to Seattle to let the physicians there have a look at him. She states that during other hospitalizations, however, when Ted was sick, a long parade of people came to see Ted because of his unusual illness. Ted frequently resents this and feels that he should be asked before people are invited to have a look at him. He feels that it is unfair to have him on display. She feels that anyone who comes into Ted's room should introduce himself. She said that Ted usually does not express displeasure at people barging into his room without introduction or explanation of why they are there, but that when they leave he cries and becomes angry and hostile. He wonders why the people came into the room and would like to be told exactly why. He feels that his privacy is frequently invaded. He is a modest boy. He feels that in the hospital he has a lack of privacy and that people should respect his privacy more. She says that at home he is not particularly modest. He does not like people doing things without his mental permission.

His mother's impression of his illness is that, in general, he does not catch things from other people. Usually when he becomes sick, it is because of his own bacterial flora or viral flora, and that it is his own body becoming weak that causes him to become sick. She said that he has never asked her, "Why do I have this illness?" or "Why can I not be healthy?" She says that recently his mouth was disfigured with large blisters and large swollen lips. His teeth have been pushed out of alignment because of the blistering in his mouth. She is very pleased that he now looks much more natural and that the blisters have resolved on his lips and mouth. She says that he is extremely affectionate and loving toward her and looks to her for protection. She says that initially he did not feel sick during this hospitalization, but after just a few days she has noticed that his mood was deteriorating and his depression increasing.

Mental Status Examination

I noted Ted to be slender and poorly nourished. He was lying quietly in bed. On several occasions he became tearful. He whined and fretted. He seemed to have very little energy. At various moments, he seemed to have intense abdominal pain, and then became even more tearful. His mother was able to comfort him and to help have him do relaxation techniques to block our the pain.

Ted's affect is appropriate. His mood certainly is depressed. He does not talk much voluntarily. He frequently gives the response "I don't know," without even listening to the question. He blocks people out by pretending to be watching TV or hiding behind a book. I am not sure that he is always reading the book. He uses a magazine to hide behind when people are talking to him. Ted does not want to talk about his depressed feelings, his fears about his illness, or his fear of being in the hospital. He generally talks only about his mother and answers questions more calmly from her than from me.

His thought content is difficult to assess at this point, because he does not talk freely of his fears and concerns. There is no evidence of any thought disorder, no evidence of hallucinations, delusions, or memory deficit. There is no evidence of any organic brain syndrome.

Ted's intelligence is difficult to assess because of his lack of cooperation and unwillingness to participate in any games or simulated school activities. However, he did tell me that he can read at a sixth-grade level. He seems to be intelligent. Insight is considered good and his judgment is also considered good.

Diagnostic Impression: Chronic depression with chronic illness: dysgamma-globulinemia.

Recommendations

I recommend that Ted have a large clock in his room so that he can tell time. I also recommend that he have a daily calendar with designation of time when different procedures are scheduled (e.g., bandage changes; appointments with people such as myself and people from the Child Activity Program; and nurses, who might be able to play cards or backgammon with him).

I believe that he also needs a picture of himself and his mother, so that when the mother is not here, he will have symbolic representation of her. Other things can be brought from home, such as posters, to make him feel more at home. We will have a goal of working toward him allowing his mother to be away for work during the day while he is hospitalized.

I will be coming by to see the patient each day to talk with him. I will advise the nurses to announce their reason for coming into his room and to introduce anyone they bring with them. I will discourage any academicians or students from coming and I will urge other members of the staff to do the same. I will encourage the staff to respect Ted's privacy.

I will also work to help him with his chronic depression. After he has had hyperalimentation for a few days and begins to regain his strength, I will push for him to become involved in activities on a schedule that would allow some environmental control. This should help with his depression.

CASE 21: CEREBRAL CONCUSSION AND
OPPOSITIONAL BEHAVIOR

Carolyn, age eight, was admitted to the pediatric ward after a fall from a ladder with subsequent nausea and vomiting and evidence of increased intracranial pressure. The liaison child psychiatrist was asked to see Carolyn because of her oppositional behavior and in order to evaluate her mental status.

History of Present Illness

Carolyn was in her usual state of good health until the morning of her accident, when she was climbing a ladder to dive into a pool and fell backwards, sustaining a head injury. She was unconscious for a short period of time. On awakening, she was exceedingly combative and aggressive. She was taken to her private physician's office, where she began to vomit. She was then admitted to our pediatric ward. Numerous studies have been done, including a normal EMI scan near the time of admission, and a normal spinal tap.

Carolyn's behavior in the hospital was combative, and she was apparently disoriented. On the second day after admission, she fought all attempts to put in IVs and required five people to restrain her in order for them to be placed. She asked for her IV to be taken out; since she was not eating well, the IV was no longer needed, and her request was granted. Her physician at the time had made the observation that after that incident, Carolyn was somewhat more cooperative. The next morning, however, she was found wandering down the hallway, continually wanting to leave the hospital. She spoke very little, except for making continual moaning noises and repeating the words, "I want to go." She did not know specifically where she wished to go.

She showed an ability to walk and seemed to recognize where her room was. She was able to perform simple tasks, such as putting on her slippers. She was also able to eat. She did this without the use of implements. After the meal she threw her bowl in the sink, something that she does at home because she washes the dishes after meals. The mother noted that the child also had picking behaviors, where she would spend lots of time picking her nose or picking at her face.

On the third day she was not very responsive to the staff. When her mother was present, she would hug her briefly, or hug her father, and ask to leave, but would not elaborate further. She was given some of her favorite toys, which she hugged. She also displayed an interest in watching Bugs Bunny on TV. However, she would often fall asleep during these programs and tended to be quite sleepy in the day.

An EEG done on the afternoon of the third day showed diffuse frontal slowing.

Developmental History

Carolyn was the first child in this family. There were no problems with pregnancy, and the mother had a normal delivery under spinal anesthetic. Carolyn weighed seven pounds, four ounces at birth. There was no neonatal jaundice. She cried a lot when she was first born, but there were no problems.

Carolyn was breast fed for three to four months and then bottle fed. She was weaned without difficulty from breast to cup because she had no fondness for the bottle. The mother does not remember at what age the child smiled and sat, but she walked at 11 months. She began to talk at about one year; her first words were "Dada" and "Mama." She also exhibited anxiety in the presence of strangers around the age of eight months.

The negativism present during the second year of life was noticeable with this child, although not as much as with the second child in the family. She was toilet trained without difficulty, by the use of a reward system, toward the end of the second and beginning the third year of life. The toilet training took six months or so to accomplish. The mother is not exactly sure of the dates.

The mother remembers that the child showed no special interest in sexual matters, nor was there any particular identification with the mother or father. The child had no phobias, but had periodic nightmares. On one or two occasions she awakened screaming, very frightened, and apparently had had a night terror, but there has been none of this in the past year or so. The mother is not sure of the content of the nightmares, but feels that they may have concerned bugs. Since that time, the child has wanted to sleep with the door open. The first school experiences were with preschool at the age of three. The child initially clung to the mother, but then accommodated well to school.

Carolyn has been an average student in public school. She did well in reading and social studies and seemed to enjoy going to school. She has lots of friends that she plays with. This summer there was no summer school, so she participated in a swimming program, did lots of swimming and ice skating, and also went to a day camp. She seemed to have no problem with children and was doing well in the swimming pool—so well that she often had to be told by the teachers to swim instead of talking with her friends. There were no outstanding emotional conflicts or disagreements at the time of Carolyn's fall.

Examination of the Child

Carolyn was seen on two occasions. On the first occasion, she was lying in bed watching TV. Attempts to communicate with her were followed by her pulling the sheets over her head, looking away, and uttering a moaning sound. The interview was conducted with her mother in the room. During this interview, Carolyn covered her eyes and went to sleep. She uttered no words during that time.

The second interview was the following morning. She was met when she was wandering down the hall moaning, "I want to go." She had wandered as far as the exit door. When asked where she wanted to go, she was not able to say. She managed to find her way back to her room. When her father came to visit, she seemed to recognize him and allowed to be hugged by him, but as soon as he set her down she wandered off to the end of the hall again. Familiar items were brought to her, including familiar games. She had no interest in the games. She accepted her stuffed animals when she was given them, and clung to them. She did not seem to respond to the staff in any individual way at the time I was present, and kept up a diffuse moaning sound, alternating with periods of silence.

Mental Status Exam

Appearance: Carolyn is a thin, pretty, eight-year-old-child who maintains very transient eye contact.

Mood: She has a highly labile mood.

Affect: Her affect is also labile and seems to be of full range.

Speech: Carolyn uses very few words, speaks little—without connecting the sentences—and resorts often to moaning. Her speech has no discernible vocal abnormality.

Thought: There is no evidence of hallucinations or delusions. The speech seems to be concrete. There is not much evidence of any purposeful opposition in her thoughts, which seem to be reactive to stresses and are an avoidance mechanism.

Sensorium: Carolyn appears to be disoriented, sometimes not knowing where she is. She is not able to participate in any form of formal psychological or mental status evaluation. She is noted to be picking at her nose and her face, and appears to cling to familiar things as a way of organizing her environment. Her memory cannot be formally assessed, but there is some question of how well she retains the memory of her experiences. Her judgment and insight are impaired.

Diagnosis

This child exhibits a posttraumatic organic brain syndrome, which could be considered a delirium or a posttraumatic amnesic state. This is manifested by a labile sensorium as well as labile moods, and also by the picking behaviors that she engages in.

Recommendations

In treating these states, it is best to keep familiar items from home around the child, as well as calendars and newspapers, in order to orient her and to keep her in a comfortable environment. It is advisable to limit the stimuli in these cases, but to remind her continually where she is. When she asks where she is going, for example, it is important to tell her that she is on the pediatric ward of the hospital. If her behavior becomes difficult to manage with reassurances, restraints may be necessary. Major tranquilizers are sometimes advised, such as Trilafon (perphenazine), 2-4 mg, for sedation (the dose depends on the child's weight). As to outcome, it is variable in these cases. Full recovery may occur, of course, but when cannot be predicted.

I have spoken with Carolyn's parents and will be available to them for any sort of supportive therapy they feel is indicated. Also, I believe that psychological testing is indicated at such time as her sensorium is sufficiently clear to help us better understand the degree of her cognitive limitations and strengths.

CASE 22: ASTHMA, IMMATURE OPPOSITIONAL AND
MANIPULATIVE BEHAVIOR

Child psychiatry consultation was requested to (1) determine if Joan's immature oppositional and manipulative behavior on the ward could be related to the communication style between mother and child and (2) offer guidance in improving communication at home with Joan.

History of Present Illness

Joan is a four-year-old female child. She has no siblings. This is her second admission for asthma, which she has had for 1½ years. Her behavior appeared to be immature, oppositional, and manipulative, especially in relationship to her mother. For example, she often refused to eat for her mother or to answer questions. Because the mother showed apparent increased sensitivity to this childhood illness, having herself developed diabetes at age 18, the staff believed that the mother was having difficulty in setting limits for Joan. Because of the child's anticipated short-term hospitalization, an initial interview was held in Joan's room. I spoke to Joan and her mother and observed their interaction for about 45 minutes, then set up an appointment with the parents for the following evening. Joan, however, was discharged the next day, having improved more rapidly than expected, and the appointment was appropriately cancelled by the parents. They left word that they would contact me via the liaison psychiatry service if they felt the need to do so.

Developmental History

The developmental history focused primarily on Joan's separations from her mother. The mother states that for the first 1½ years she and Joan were extremely close, to the near exclusion—and disgruntlement—of her husband. Joan began attending nursery school before age two, and has continued to do so because of the mother's need to work. Joan has no neighborhood playmates and is an only child. The father is gone much of the time because of his job. The family situation reveals that when the family is home together there is a tendency toward diadic interactions, while the third person has to wait. Joan, of course, has the most difficulty waiting. The mother admits to being more lenient with Joan than her father. They try hard to talk, explain, clarify, and verbally control their daughter. However, after the "umpteenth time" of repeating a request or a correction, Joan may get a spanking and be sent to bed. The parents strenuously try to avoid this maneuver.

Observations of Joan, Her Mother, and Interactions

Joan appeared to be an attractive, intelligent little girl who seemed to be having difficulty deciding whether she was sad, angry, or lonely. This was accompanied by fearfulness and a complaining, clinging attitude toward her mother upon the arrival of the interviewer and, later, the respiratory therapist. The mother was a pleasant woman who was concerned and candid about her problems with Joan.

Joan would interact with me only grudgingly, and she repeatedly engaged mother's attention with some question or activity, only to appear to tire of the interaction and become absorbed in the program on the TV screen in the room. At these times, her mother and I would continue our conversation, which Joan would interrupt again with complaints or requests, only to lose interest again to the TV.

The mother's interactions with Joan were mostly of a helpful but corrective nature, putting Joan off just a little bit longer so that she could finish her sentence. I do not remember any spontaneous praising of Joan, although there was frequent touching and comforting.

Recommendations

The child psychiatrist indicated to the mother that many children of Joan's age may think they have done something bad to bring about the illness. This tends to cause an increased desire to be close to mother. The long hours that Joan spends away from both parents may also contribute to this desire for closeness, especially when she is not feeling well.

Positive reinforcement of Joan with praise or her mother's visible pleasure in her activities would probably help Joan to feel closer to her mother and better about herself while she is in the hospital. This might lessen some of the clinging. It was recommended that both parents discuss their limit-setting policies and try to agree more closely as to what is allowed and what is not.

CASE 23: CLEFT LIP REPAIR, HYPOSPADIAS REPAIR, SHORT STATURE

History of Present Illness

Gordon, age 14, lives in a foster home and was being seen once a week by a psychologist because of a history of delinquent behavior. The psychologist had also been collaborating with the pediatric urologist in order to prepare Gordon for an operation for further correction of his severe hypospadias. He had one previous operation at age three for hypospadias. He is also followed in the endocrine clinic because his height is below the first percentile, caused by delayed bone age. Results of a recent 24-hour suppression test for growth hormone were pending. Gordon also has a history of petit mal seizures earlier in life, but is not on medication for them at the present time. He has had severe dental caries with poor mandibular and maxillary development. He also is said to have a cataract of his right eye. In the past, he was noted to have a speech impairment with poor articulation and hypernasality, but at age 11 surgeons constructed a pharyngeal flap with good result. His speech is now clear and easily intelligible, with no resonance problems, although I do detect some hypernasality with certain words. He also has a mild conductive bilateral hearing loss.

Past History

Gordon had been in trouble between the sixth and seventh grades and had been sent to juvenile hall for three months while the court decided what to do with him. Gordon would not talk to me about the incident that caused him to be sent to juvenile hall. He said that it was private and did not need to be discussed at this time. The biological father died when Gordon was six years of age. He told me that his father was killed in an industrial accident. The parents had lived together until that time without separations or any previous divorces. Gordon's mother remarried when Gordon was 11 or 12 years of age.

Gordon was placed in a foster home at age 13. He had had to repeat kindergarten at age five, but made Bs and Cs from first through sixth grades, except for reading, in which he made Ds and Fs. Since moving to the foster home, Gordon's grades have improved to As and Bs, except for reading, in which he continues to make Ds. Gordon reports that he is cruelly teased by classmates because of his short stature and because of the scar from the cleft lip repair. We discussed the surgery that was planned for correction of hypospadias, and he seems well prepared emotionally and educationally for this procedure.

Mental Status Examination

Gordon is an attractive, blond boy who appears quite short and underweight for his age. His mood is cheerful, he has a full range of affect, his thought processes are intact. There is no evidence of delusions or hallucinations. His thought content is age-appropriate. His intelligence seems to be average or above average, although his ability to do calculations is poor. He can do addition and subtraction. He has difficulty with multiplication. He can do multiplications by twos, threes, fives and tens, but not the other numbers. He cannot do division. He does not read at grade level. His reading is probably at fourth- or fifth-grade level. His insight into his circumstances seems to be appropriate. His judgment is appropriate. He reports that if he saw a fire in the waiting room of a theater he would try to put it out or call for help. He seems to have no real worries about the operation. He says that the operation has been explained to him and that he understands that he will have anesthesia.

Impression

I believe that this is a boy with a specific learning disability who will need special educational assistance to complete his education. He seems to be a well-adjusted young man emotionally, and I found no evidence of thought disorder or any glaring abnormalities on the mental status examination. I think that he is well prepared for the surgical procedure that is to be done tomorrow, and that there are no contraindications to going ahead with the correction of hypospadias.

Recommendations

I would strongly recommend that Gordon have an educational assessment while he is here on the pediatric ward, to determine if we could suggest some special assistance at his school.

CASE 24: FUNCTIONAL ABDOMINAL PAIN

Reason for Consultation

The consultation to Child Psychiatry was requested because Shelly, age 10, has a long history of abdominal pain of unknown etiology. An extensive medical workup has already been done and is negative. Psychiatric consultation is obtained at this point for additional evaluation of a possible psychological component to the pain.

Chief Complaint

Shelly tells me her worry is that nobody has figured out why she gets stomach aches. The mother voices a similar concern, coupled with the awareness of a possibly psychological component.

Present Illness

Shelly has approximately a two-year history of mild, intermittent, generalized abdominal pain. Two months prior to admission there was an acute exacerbation of the pain. Shelly had had the flu, and was apparently given Bicillin. She had a generalized skin eruption of hives, apparently in reaction to the Bicillin. The itching hives were treated with an oral cortisone preparation. According to the mother, about 12 hours after taking the cortisone, there was the onset of severe abdominal pain, which has long outlasted the episode of flu, hives, or cortisone. The pain has persisted for two months, and the child has been out of school all this time. She recently tried going to school, apparently on two different days, but her mother describes her as coming home "white as a sheet" and in pain, and the family has not sent her back to school again. The mother says Shelly keeps up with her lessons at home and does the homework on her own, and that other children sometimes visit her at home. Shelly showed me the workbook that she has been doing at home, which does show a number of As and Bs and very careful school work.

On the initial meeting with the mother, she discussed marital relationship problems that were occurring around the time of the onset of Shelly's severe pain.

Developmental History

Shelly is the only live birth to this mother, who had a total of six pregnancies. After a difficult pregnancy, Shelly was born premature, weighing three pounds. The mother describes with some emotion that this child is understandably "very precious" and that she thinks she probably has been "a bit overprotective." Five other pregnancies resulted in either premature delivery or full-term still births caused by severe rh blood type incompatibility.

In-Hospital Course

The hospital documented a weight of 85 pounds twice during the hospitalization. This careful documentation was done because there was a report that Shelly had lost several pounds in the past two months. On multiple examinations in the hospital, it was noted that Shelly complained of pain but did not give the expected physical responses to palpation of the abdomen. She also showed some affect that was inappropriate to the experience of pain. She just looked too happy.

Diagnostic Interviews

I met with the mother, who seemed quite anxious about her daughter and eager to find a reason for the stomach aches. She brought up the two-month absence from school and said that she herself had taken a two-month leave of absence from her job as a bank teller. She hoped to return to work soon, but felt somewhat uneasy about leaving home when her daughter was undergoing such a stressful time. The mother appears to be a woman of average intelligence, who is quite involved in her daughter's growth and development. She warned me that she did not think Shelly was going to be very pleased to see a psychiatrist, as the child had expressed anger that anyone could suggest that her pain might be psychological in origin.

When I met Shelly, who is an attractive child of average height and weight, she was wearing a neat dressing gown and furry, pink slippers. She came willingly with me to her room, and together we drew the curtains around her bed, as she requested this for privacy. She asked why I was here to see her. When I told her who I was—that my consultation was requested because of the difficulty figuring out what was causing her pain—she responded, "Now, that's a real doctor." She went on to say that she was glad I did not make an automatic assumption that her pain must be imaginary. She discussed her likes and dislikes, showing me some projects of "things she likes to do with her hands." She was also willing to draw a picture of herself. She started out drawing a small figure of a girl with a smiling face, and arms that came together so that the hands were over the abdomen. She then said she could draw "another me." She drew basically the same picture with minor differences in detail. When I asked her the difference between the two she pointed out specific differences in the shoes versus slippers, etc. Then she looked straight at me and said that she could draw a picture of "the real me." I said I would be interested in this, and she drew a somewhat larger picture of a girl with an enormous frown, dressed in a long dressing gown similar to the one she was actually wearing. She added a caption of the girl saying, "I hurt!" Shelly willingly wrote her name neatly above her picture. She then drew a football player who is saying, "We won." (This is what she had originally told me she was going to draw before I asked her to draw a picture of herself.) She gave me the picture to keep. She told me she had seen a psychologist when she was much younger, when the decision was being made as to what grade she was going to enter, and she was annoyed at him and the blocks and tasks that he gave her.

Shelly talked with me about her pain, saying that she has it all the time. She showed a rather blandly smiling face as she told me this. However, when I talked with her rather seriously about the subject, she got an expression of real distress on her face as she told me that she was very upset that nobody had yet figured out why she has the pain. She hid her face in the pillow for a while as she talked about being upset about receiving no answers.

Mental Status Examination

Shelly is a child of average appearance and behavior, except for a somewhat bland affect when initially talking about her pain. Her speech and thought were appropriate for a child of 10 of at least average intelligence. Her insight and

judgment included an awareness that being out of school was an associated problem in its own right. Her sensorium was not formally tested but, grossly, showed
no major deficiencies. Her affect had the brief time of inappropriateness noted,
but other than that was neutral in its resting tone and ran the range of sadness
through annoyance, all of which seemed appropriate to the stream of talk.

Diagnostic Impression: Functional abdominal pain.

Recommendation: Outpatient psychotherapy for both child and mother.

CASE 25: COHEN'S SYNDROME, DIFFICULTY IN SWALLOWING

Reason for Child Psychiatry Consultation Request

Joshua, age 14, has had difficulty swallowing for two months. Medical workup has been normal and the pediatricians were concerned about an emotional
component to the patient's dysphagia.

History of Present Illness

The patient has carried a diagnosis of Cohen's syndrome, which includes
hypotonia, obesity, prominent incisors, and mental deficiency. The patient had
been doing very well until one year prior to admission, when he fractured his
ankle and required a cast for several weeks. At that time he began to gain weight.
He gained several pounds during the next few months, and his mother decided
to have him go on a restrictive diet, eating as balanced a diet as possible, but
smaller amounts. The mother also went on the diet, and during the past 4½
months she went from 167 pounds to 132 pounds.

Approximately two months ago, the patient began complaining of difficulty
swallowing solid foods. The mother does not know of any psychological stress
occurring in the family shortly before or during this period of difficulty with
swallowing solid foods. The patient is able to swallow liquid foods without
much difficulty. The mother had noted, however, that in the past two months
he has eaten at a much slower rate and seems to keep the food in his mouth
longer. The patient has not had episodes of vomiting or diarrhea, but has complained during the past two months of substernal chest pain, which he says is
mild. He also has pain in the lateral right rib cage. His mother took him to a
physician for evaluation of this problem. An EKG and chest X-rays were said
to be normal. His mother has not seen any episodes of hyperventilation in this
patient. She reports she has seen him short of breath and exhausted after riding
his bicycle at fast speed.

There is a strong family history of cancer, and this was one of the mother's
concerns when she was told that there were swollen lymph nodes in Joshua's

neck. Joshua's father died of lymphoma when Joshua was three years old, and Joshua rarely talks about his father's death. Three paternal uncles have also died of cancer. The patient's mother states that the patient has never verbalized a fear of cancer or of death. She feels that the difficulty with swallowing is caused by swollen nodes in the patient's neck and that perhaps the penicillin that was given prior to his coming to the pediatric ward caused the lymph nodes to reduce in size.

During the hospital course the patient has continued to have difficulty swallowing solid foods. When asked if there has been any episodes when the patient could not swallow at all, the patient's mother reported none. On one occasion, while eating in a restaurant, the patient was not able to swallow bits of hamburger, whereas he could swallow his milk shake.

Hospital Course

During the five days of hospitalization Joshua continued to have difficulty in swallowing. When the esophagram was done, the impression was that it was a probable-normal study; however, the patient only swallowed very small boluses of barium, and was reluctant to do so. It was felt that there might be slight impairment of the peristalsis of the esophagus but that that was probably a result of the small boluses of barium.

Development

Joshua was one year old before his parents noticed any abnormality in his development. He did not walk until he was 1½-2 years of age, although he had been crawling since ten months. His talking was also delayed, and his mother reports that he never learned to talk fluently. He understands quite a bit, but there is much that he does not understand for his chronological age of 14 years. However, Joshua is very observant. He sometimes tells his mother if she runs a red light or if she is going up a one way street in the wrong direction. His mother reports that he also tends to be bossy and occasionally tells her how to run the household. Joshua has been in special education classes in school and is currently in such a class.

Social History

Joshua has very few friends except for those in his classroom. He does not bring friends to his home, and the family does not socialize with other people in the community. His brother occasionally brings friends, who talk to Joshua but do not play with him. Because of Joshua's mental retardation, his family is not able to leave him at home for long periods of time. They usually try to leave him alone no longer than one-half to one hour. He also is not able to go into stores to make purchases by himself. When accompanied by his mother, however, he can do simple shopping and help to find items that are on his mother's shopping list. He cannot count change or tell time. Joshua enjoys watching TV and seems to have a fair attention span. Although he does not seem to understand much of what is happening on TV, he does laugh at cartoons. He usually watches detective stories. Joshua enjoys riding his bicycle. This seems to be one of his best activities. He will ride the bicycle at fast speeds for up to an hour and come home exhausted and short of breath. His mother feels that he is better coordinated when riding the bicycle than when he is walking. Joshua also enjoys throwing darts at a target. He is very curious and likes to try to build models. Joshua frequently paints pictures of houses and trees and the sun, and will spend a great deal of time drawing these same pictures over and over.

School History

Teachers in Joshua's special education class report that Joshua is very well liked in the class by both students and the teacher, that he is "a little gentleman at school and well behaved."

Mental Status Examination

During my interview, Joshua was continuing to eat his breakfast, although it was rather late in the morning. He was chewing very slowly and had food in his mouth during the entire time that he was talking to me. He seemed to understand most of my questions and had difficulty giving answers. His answers were short and his articulation was poor. His intellectual level seemed to be somewhere near first grade. His I.Q. is probably around 60 and does not equal that of normal first graders. There was no evidence of psychotic behavior.

Thought Content

The patient did not seem overly concerned with the physical aspects of his illness. He was not very spontaneous in terms of his mood during the interview; however, his mother reports that he is usually more spontaneous and cheerful than he has been during this hospitalization. He did not discuss fears of dying or of having serious illness. When I discussed his memories of his father, he did not mention any worries about his father's terminal illness.

Dynamic Formulation

This is a 14-year-old male with Cohen's syndrome who had done reasonably well until fracturing his ankle one year ago, after which he began to gain weight.

He responds very well to his mother. After his mother urged him to lose weight, the patient became very conscientious in his effort and took great pride in bringing the scale in each day to stand and show his mother that he was continuing to lose weight. Then, approximately two months ago, he began having difficulty swallowing, especially solid foods. He secured a great deal of attention from his mother because of this problem. At this point, I am not totally convinced that there is not some medical problem either causing or contributing in some way to this dysphagia. Even though the esophagram appears to be relatively normal, I would be interested in the esophageal motility studies, if they could be done. These studies need not be done at this time, but if the problem continues for several months, I think this should be considered. The serious malocclusion is also a possible contributing problem. My evaluation did not disclose any serious psychological stress or problems that could be directly related to the dysphagia. It is certain, however, that the patient is getting a great deal of secondary gain from his mother for this problem.

Recommendations

1. Strong positive suggestion to the patient that his swallowing will improve and that within a short time his swallowing of solid foods will again be possible.
2. Continued follow-up of the patient in the pediatric outpatient clinic.
3. If the swallowing problem continues, we would see the patient at the child psychiatry clinic for a behavior modification program for him and the mother.
4. If the swallowing problem continues for several months, I would strongly urge that esophageal motility studies be done.

In summary, I do not feel that this patient has anorexia nervosa or hyperventilation syndrome. There is a possibility that his swallowing difficulty may be related to secondary gain. It will be necessary to follow him for several weeks to determine the nature of his problem.

CASE 26: FRIGHTENING VISUAL EXPERIENCES

Reason for Consultation Request

This five-year-old boy had some very frightening visual experiences during the past week. The interview with him and his mother was conducted for one hour in the afternoon and for 30 minutes that evening.

History of Present Illness

Conrad is a five-year-old boy who lives with his divorced mother and his seven-year-old brother. Conrad attends kindergarten. He has an almost perfect attendance record, having missed only one day during the school year.

Conrad suddenly awoke from his sleep approximately five nights ago, screaming in terror but fully awake, saying that it seemed that he could see something, but he could not tell what it was, and that it seemed that it was far away from him. He also related having dreams about his maternal grandfather who had died two months ago. Conrad talks about speaking to a man who is in heaven. Conrad says he has had several dreams about the man, but that those dreams are not frightening and he enjoys talking with the man.

Approximately two days ago, Conrad, in the daytime while awake, experienced a visual phenomenon in which his mother, who was standing very close to him, seemed to be far away and her head seemed to be very small. This lasted for approximately 15 minutes and then went away. One day prior to admission, this same experience reoccurred. This was very frightening to the child.

The mother reports that Conrad has been a nervous child and is afraid of loud noises, such as sonic booms or thunder. Last summer, whenever there was an electrical storm Conrad and his seven-year-old brother would get in bed with the mother and sleep for the night.

Conrad's parents were divorced when he was 2½ years old. The mother had an ongoing relationship with a boyfriend for the past two years. The relationship was terminated by the mother two weeks ago, and she thinks this could be affecting Conrad. When asked if the mother had any boyfriends, Conrad said no, and that she had not been dating. The mother was surprised that Conrad was denying the fact that she had been dating for the past two years.

Conrad has not had any other visual disturbances or hallucinatory experiences. The mother reports that he is vindictive. If she disciplines him or he becomes angry at her, he will go into her bedroom and pull all the covers off her bed. Also, if his brother makes him angry, he will go into the brother's bedroom and write on the walls with crayons. She says that on several occasions Conrad has put things in his mouth that she considered dangerous. As recently as one month ago he ingested a large quantity of blue food coloring. She reports that approximately six months ago he began to use swear words such as the "F" word. On two occasions she washed his mouth out with soap. Since then he has not used swear words, and she has not washed his mouth with soap.

I asked her how she disciplines him. She says that she sends him to his room for ten minutes, that he screams and leaves the door open. She has spanked him on occasion and she also takes the bicycle away from him.

He and his brother each have a bedroom. They leave a light on in the hallway at night and do not have a night light in the room. Recently, Conrad was given a picture of a spaceman floating around the moon, but it had to be taken down because he was so frightened of the picture. He is especially afraid at night and frequently comes to the mother's bedroom stating that he is afraid. The mother says that he picks up some of his nervousness from her and that he is also frightened of loud noises. There is no family history of psychiatric illness.

Environmental Assessment

The mother states that the house is in a rural area, with farm land within three blocks of their house. Planes occasionally spray cotton and lettuce fields. She states that recently she bought some new clothes for Conrad at a discount store and that she did not wash the pants before he wore them, although she washed the shirts. She does not know for sure if his first visual disturbance occurred on the day that he wore the new clothes for the first time. She insists that there are no medications in the house that he could have been exposed to, except for Allergy Relief Medicine (A.R.M.)®, and she does not think that he ingested any of this. He has no history of convulsions. He was adopted at the age of ten months and had been with one foster family for this entire period. She states that his developmental milestones were all normal, that he was walking by 14 months, and talking at a normal time.

Mental Status Examination

Conrad's mother reports that he is either very happy or very sad. He gets upset easily. He is vindictive when he is angry. In my interview with the child, he talked somewhat hesitatingly. He did not appear to be hallucinating at the time of the interview; he did not appear to be frightened. His mood was slightly sad. He answered all questions appropriately. He did not seem to be preoccupied with any bizzare ideation. He seemed of average intelligence. He could count to 100. He knew his ABCs. He knew his colors. There were no loose associations to his thoughts, and his judgment was considered good. I felt that there was no evidence of a thought disorder.

Impression

My impression of this child is that he has an adjustment reaction of childhood, adjusting to the mother's termination of her relationship with her boyfriend and to the death of his grandfather two months ago. I believe that his visual experiences are illusory phenomena and not hallucinations. I do not believe that there is a serious emotional disorder in this child. I would strongly recommend that if this problem does not clear up in a short time, Conrad's mother should consider having him in psychiatric counseling.

Recommendations

My recommendation to the mother would be that she observe Conrad; if the visual phenomena continue, she should contact me or his pediatrician. Also, I would recommend a toxic screen and careful neurological examination for this child.

CASE 27: CHRONIC PAIN, PARAPLEGIA, SLEEP PROBLEMS, HALLUCINATIONS

History of Present Illness

Six months prior to this hospital admission, Becky, who is now ten years old was at home alone with a younger brother. He walked into the bedroom and pointed a real, loaded revolver at her and said "bang." She knew that it was a real gun and attempted to grab it from him. The gun discharged, striking Becky in the spine, resulting in paraplegia, with the bullet left embedded in her right scapular area. Becky and her brother had been placed in foster care after that incident because her father could not afford a baby-sitter or caretaker for them. Becky's mother had been hospitalized in a state psychiatric hospital for ten months with "chronic undifferentiated schizophrenia."

Becky was admitted to the pediatric rehab ward because of severe complaints of pain in her right scapula in which the bullet was lodged. Her physician felt that there was no reason for this pain and that it probably represented a somatic delusion. Her foster mother said that Becky had not slept well for two weeks, had frequent nightmares, and complained of hearing people talking about her and calling her name two days ago when no one was around. Becky had been placed on an antibiotic for a kidney infection two weeks earlier, and her foster mother wondered if this medication might have caused the deterioration in Becky's mental status.

Observations and Assessment

Becky was seen individually. She presented as a very attractive, neatly cared for ten-year-old girl. She was able to wheel herself into my office and began talking quite readily. Throughout my entire time with her, there was an obvious intense, underlying anxiety accompanying all of her speech. Her speech was extreme in its amount and suggested an almost run-on quality. Her intelligence was considered to be very high for her age, as evidenced by the vocabulary she used and her ability to communicate her needs.

Her primary emotional preoccupations were of fearfulness as she described the frightening auditory and visual experiences. The image of a man in black coming at her with a gun was particularly frightening, and she mentioned it quite often in the interview. When asked whether she thought the man was really there, she explained that she realized that he was not actually in the room, yet she believes quite strongly that she had this vision and heard voices of people who were claiming to come to get her. Throughout much of this description, there was also the preoccupation with the safety of her sister. Much dream and fantasy experience was described throughout my 45 minutes with her.

Her affect seemed slightly inappropriate, as she related these events in a very consistent and somewhat smiling manner. Only once in the interview did she fail to respond in the usual, rapid-fire quality that I have already described. I asked her, "What will happen to you in the future?" After a long pause, she looked visibly upset and then continued to relate how she hoped things would work out for her. The overwhelming suggestion from her response was that she was concerned and unclear about the most basic type of fear, that for her own life and safety.

Projective testing will be very valuable in clarifying the underlying nature of Becky's mental status. The experiences that she has described certainly constitute paranormal occurrences of excessive fearfulness, yet there is an element of reality contact throughout all of the description. Projective testing, particularly with the Rorschach method, would clarify the extent to which her reality contact is impaired.

Summary and Recommendations

While there are clear disturbances in ego functioning suggestive of some thought and affective disturbance, a diagnosis of psychosis is not made, since Becky's reality testing and object relationships appear to be strong. Her reactions should be considered serious and require a high priority for care. This girl may very well be close to an acute psychotic break. She is laboring under tremendous fear for her safety. Some of the issues surrounding these feelings no doubt include: (1) the confusion and emotional binding that she is experiencing around family ties; (2) the after effects of her paralysis, which can be assumed to have been only superficially worked through; (3) the perceived rejection by her father, who has had no contact with her since she was placed in foster care.

Some immediate and specific recommendations are as follows: (1) coordinate these impressions with the prescribing physician in order to rule out the possibility of toxic side effects from the medication Becky is taking for a kidney infection; (2) begin ongoing psychotherapy; (3) there should be continued observation to determine if Becky needs antipsychotic medication for hallucinations; (4) begin projective personality testing to clarify the extent and nature of ego functioning.

9

SCAN: A Hospital-Based Program for Identifying Suspected Child Abuse and Neglect

Morris J. Paulson, Susan Edelstein, Mary Spencer

The term SCAN (suspected child abuse and neglect) has been used interchangeably with the concept of the child protection team (CPT). Prior to the pioneer paper of Kempe et al. (1962), the medical profession and social services were involved only minimally in any formal, interdisciplinary health team approach to understanding that phenomenon of family violence now identified as child abuse and neglect. Two decades of clinical collaboration and research studies have clearly established the need for and importance of a child protection team within every medical facility, large or small.

The medical health of the pediatric patient cannot be separated from concern for the emotional and social welfare of the child. Therefore, any combined team approach bringing together the disciplines of medicine, nursing, social service, mental health, law enforcement, and the juvenile court will maximize the identification, diagnosis, treatment, and rehabilitation of abused children and their families. No single discipline can provide all the necessary techniques and knowledge bases that will assure maximum care of the pediatric patient. Multiple disciplines working together provide a dynamic gestalt, which, like group psychotherapy, becomes more powerful and more healing than the resource of any single individual, agency, or discipline (Paulson et al., 1974).

SCAN: A VEHICLE FOR IN-HOUSE EDUCATION AND COMMUNITY CONSULTATION

As early as 1970, Rowe et al. described a hospital program for the detection and registration of abused and neglected children at the Yale University Medical Center. A team with representation from pediatrics, child psychiatry, and social services created a registry for the detection, admission, reporting, and treatment (DART) of child abuse, and also provided consultation and education to all house staff interested in or involved in cases of suspected or identified abuse. Detection included a detailed history taking, medical examination, home visits, and consultation with family physician, community agencies, and school authorities. Over an 18-month period, there were 183 referrals, attesting not only to the incidence of ongoing child maltreatment, but to heightened medical management and responsibility in identifying over 10 cases a month—cases that may have escaped identification were it not for the intervention of such an early protection team of pediatric health specialists.

Additional functions of an intervention and protection team have been formulated by Schmitt (1978), who, along with his collaborators, defined the purposes of the child protection team and delineated its structure both within a hospital setting and as an adjunct to community consultation. As a guideline for implementing such a combined team approach for the better identification of abuse and neglect, Schmitt et al. (1980) provide policies and procedures that were found highly effective in Colorado, procedures that, with modification, can become a model for establishing similar programs throughout the nation.

With an increased number of abused children being referred to the UCLA Hospital and Clinics for diagnosis and treatment of child abuse, there developed a need for implementing a similar child abuse intervention team within the hospital. Representatives from medicine, nursing, social service, the Neuropsychiatric Institute, and campus police became a nucleus of professionals from which has now developed a SCAN team, a team consisting of over 20 members who meet weekly to consult on every case referred to the UCLA Hospital and Clinics where there exists either suspicion of abuse and neglect or injury to a child of unknown and undefined cause. From a modest number of referrals per year, the present SCAN team now evaluates 25–30 cases per month. An "on-call" consultant is available 24 hours a day, seven days a week, to facilitate the identification and diagnosis of child maltreatment. He/she provides immediate consultation to those staff members on the wards and in the emergency room who, faced with such a crisis and perhaps lacking an expertise in child abuse evaluation, can have available an immediate resource person knowledgeable about the medical, social, and legal issues of child abuse and neglect.

The SCAN team meets weekly reviewing all ongoing cases of child physical abuse and neglect, emotional deprivation, emotional abuse, substance abuse, and sexual abuse and molestation. Medical treatment, crisis intervention for the family, psychosocial assessment of the home, review of suggested treatment plans, and follow-up—all are topics for discussion by the interdisciplinary team. Resources within the hospital and Neuropsychiatric Institute are used to provide psychosocial treatment for the parents and for the child. Where that is not feasible, there is extensive community consultation to facilitate a community referral closer to the residence of the family. In addition to weekly meetings oriented specifically to the diagnosis and treatment of child abuse, the SCAN team also meets monthly to discuss policy and procedures specific to the improvement of services to children and to hospital house staff education.

The UCLA SCAN team differs in several ways from Schmitt's child protection team. While Schmitt's program consults on approximately 100 cases per year, the UCLA team reviews and consults on 300–350 cases per year. Schmitt recommends a maximum team size of 10 professionals, while the UCLA SCAN team is more than double that number. Schmitt describes a "nuclear team" of three people who see very few of the families directly, but who, having a background and training in child abuse, are an available and immediate consultation resource for the house staff. At UCLA the entire team, meeting as a body, provides an available interdisciplinary consultation resource for those professionals and services involved in the identification and diagnosis of suspected child abuse. In order to enhance consultation with the Los Angeles County Department of Public Social Services (DPSS), a permanent member of the DPSS supervising staff attends each weekly SCAN meeting, bringing her knowledge and expertise, especially in those areas related to placement, temporary custody, and juvenile court proceedings.

In California, all cases of suspected child abuse must be reported to both the local law enforcement agency and the Department of Public Social Services. To facilitate this liaison, a member of the UCLA campus police department attends weekly as a permanent member of the team. In those cases where a child is at "high risk" and must be detained either for medical reasons or because of a continued threat to the child's welfare, the campus police are immediately available to place a "police hold" and to take the child into protective custody. In those situations involving an outside law enforcement agency, the campus police again become the liaison with that agency, expediting the filing of complaints and assuring that the outside agency "follows through" on the investigation of suspected abuse or neglect. In those cases where the severity of the injury and the nature of the evidence requires the arresting of the parents, this is also done by the campus police, in consultation with the SCAN team.

Schmitt feels that since police involvement frequently jeopardizes therapy, it should be used only in emergencies or when parents do not cooperate with child protective services intervention. The experience at UCLA and with the Los Angeles Police Department and Los Angeles County Sheriff's Department indicates otherwise. Developing a close liaison with law enforcement in general, and with law enforcement agencies having specialty teams trained in the investigation of child abuse and neglect, is essential. Such liaison between the UCLA SCAN team and the local police departments has been very positive. Prior to the detaining of a child or the arresting of a parent, there will always be ongoing discussion between all parties concerned and the parents. While there is often angry denial and hostility from parents, the SCAN team approach has been found supportive, reassuring, and helpful in facilitating referral of the family for further medical and psychological treatment, even after police involvement.

An additionally important link in community networking is the relationship of the SCAN team to neighborhood drug treatment programs and Methadone clinics. Because of an increasing number of substance-abusing mothers delivering addicted newborns, there is a need for close linkage between the hospitals and the community. Initially, there may exist resistance toward SCAN involvement, as it often means that mothers delivering children manifesting withdrawal are automatically reported. Such reporting is seen as a breaking up of the family, depriving the newborn of its rightful biological mother, and substituting even more inadequate foster homes as a temporary placement. However, through consistent efforts to clarify goals, by inviting an exchange of staffs, and by regular case conferences on specific families, a closer and more therapeutic liaison can be developed. The community drug clinics will see the SCAN team's goals as protecting the child while making every effort to preserve the integrity of the family (Newberger and Bourne, 1978).

SCAN members must also participate in the founding and operation of local child trauma councils. Such councils represent the interfacing of disciplines, agencies, and educational institutions involved in the identification and treatment of child abuse. Because of the recognized expertise of SCAN members, they are often elected to leadership roles—developing programs, conducting educational workshops, and providing the lay community with parent training classes and infant-mother clinics. On a countywide level, SCAN members can provide similar leadership roles on community health department task forces, which focus on planning of child abuse policies and services and coordinating of interagency treatment, research, and training programs. Such community education and consultation therefore become vital responsibilities for the SCAN team, over and beyond those rendered within the hospital and affiliated outpatient clinics (Paulson, 1978).

GUIDELINES FOR THE MEDICAL MANAGEMENT
OF CHILD ABUSE AND NEGLECT

A recent publication by the Office of Human Development Services, HEW, provides a comprehensive set of guidelines for the hospital and clinical management of child abuse and neglect (Schmitt et al., 1980). Integrating the knowledge of seven nationally known experts in child abuse intervention and treatment, this manual is comprehensive, descriptive, and will be a valuable resource for any medical facility, large or small, wishing to organize a child abuse intervention team of professionals. The following five management objectives provide the foundation stones for organizing such a team:

1. Identification of abused and neglected children;
2. Providing necessary medical care;
3. Carrying out all legal mandates regarding reporting;
4. Collection of all specimens and evidence necessary to document the diagnosis of child abuse;
5. Providing a supportive and therapeutic milieu to parents in order to promote maximum motivation for intervention, treatment, rehabilitation, or placement of the child when necessary.

In order to implement these objectives, the authors describe in detail nine important topical areas about which the SCAN staff should be fully informed and knowledgeable in order to maximize the management of a referred case of suspected abuse. These nine topical areas are:

1. Management objectives specific to personnel and laboratory facilities;
2. Responsibilities of all medical and nonmedical personnel;
3. Defining legal policies and reporting procedures;
4. Triaging emergency room procedures and protocol;
5. Physician guidelines for managing physical child abuse and neglect;
6. Physician guidelines for managing sexual abuse and incest;
7. Physician guidelines for managing nonorganic failure-to-thrive;
8. Newborn nursery: identification of and intervention with high-risk families;
9. Child protection team protocol.

Recognizing the variability of resources and personnel within each community, the guideline manual establishes standardized procedures for physicians, nurses, and hospital and clinic administrators. Health care facilities are divided into three types of settings, with policies and procedures specified for each:

1. Type I health care facility, such as a pediatrician's office, a clinic, or an emergency room, that sees children but has no pediatric ward;
2. Type II health facility, such as a hospital with a small to medium pediatric ward, that sees less than 30 child abuse cases per year;
3. Type III facility, such as a children's hospital evaluating more than 30 cases of child abuse per year, a university medical center, or a large county hospital.

By describing the resources and policies needed for each of these three facilities, by documenting the personnel requirements, laboratory and X-ray facilities necessary, and by prescribing the legal policies and procedures to be carried out, any medical care facility within each of the three types above can implement a responsible SCAN program.

CASE HISTORIES AND THE ROLE OF SCAN

Physical Abuse

A five-year-old male child was brought to the UCLA emergency room with a chief complaint of pain and swelling of the inner lining of the mouth. He was well until the evening before admission. During the physical examination, bruises and lacerations were noted on the back, hands, and right arm. The child was withdrawn and depressed, showing a blank facial expression and unusual compliance during the physical exam. Full-body X-rays disclosed a healing fracture of the radius and ulna of the left arm. The dental SCAN consultant felt the oral lesions were typical of a caustic burn and not mouthwash, as claimed by the mother.

Following SCAN consultation with the pediatrician, a diagnosis of suspected child abuse was made. The campus police were informed, and a police hold was placed on the hospitalized child. The findings were discussed with the parents, who were then informed of the legal mandate for reporting and the probable role of law enforcement. The parents were subsequently arrested for child abuse, the child was declared a dependent ward of the court, and, following discharge from the hospital, was placed in foster care.

Past medical history of the child and family was very important, reflecting how, in the earlier absence of a SCAN team, a high-risk child and an equally high-risk mother were not identified previously as living in what was probably an "at risk" home. The child was born prematurely, eight months after his sibling, remaining five weeks in the neonatal intensive care unit. At four months of age, he had a feeding problem and was followed in a high-risk infant clinic. When the child was nine months old, his mother was admitted to a psychiatric facility with auditory hallucinations, hearing voices telling her to kill the infant. At that time, the infant was hospitalized for failure to thrive and was subsequently placed voluntarily by the mother in a foster home. Following two years' placement in the foster home and concomitant psychiatric treatment for both parents, the child was returned to the biological home, where he stayed until the present admission to UCLA with fractures and caustic burns in the mouth.

In retrospect, it was evident that there had been an earlier failure in the management of this high-risk child and family. Had a SCAN team existed previously, all of these stresses would have been evaluated in terms of an unwanted child in a home with an overwhelmed, emotionally distraught mother who never had an opportunity to develop a meaningful emotional bond with her child. The mother had been giving many messages, consciously and unconsciously, indicating her own failures as a mother and her inability to provide for the emotional and physical health of her child. The present SCAN intervention provided the necessary pediatric consultation to prevent further life-threatening abuse of a child. Through collaboration with child protective services and the juvenile court, SCAN helped provide a home environment that will hopefully allow for the positive development of this boy—mentally, emotionally, and physically.

Sexual Abuse

A 14-year-old female, one of four siblings, was brought to the pediatric outpatient department clinic by her mother because the daughter allegedly had sexual intercourse with her boyfriend. The mother was concerned about venereal disease and the possibility of pregnancy. During the interview, the girl revealed that when she came home from a date with her boyfriend two nights earlier, the father flew into a rage, forced her at knife point to go to a motel, and then had intercourse with her. The patient reported a history of intermittent vaginal discharge since age 10 years; but sexual intercourse had never been considered by the family pediatrician. The 13-year-old sister also revealed that the father had been fondling her for over two years and had also been physically abusive. During the initial history, the mother denied any knowledge of these facts and seemed not to know what had been occurring in the family. Both girls said they could not go to their mother and tell her of the molestation by the father, saying that she would not understand and that she never seemed able to protect them from the physical abuse that she continually witnessed.

The examining pediatrician immediately talked with the SCAN consultant. Because of the incest and sexual molestation of the two girls, the campus police were notified, and the children were taken into protective custody. Unfortunately, the children were separated, two going to MacLaren Hall (a county shelter for children) and two placed in a temporary foster home. In the meantime, the mother contacted a battered-women's shelter, which, acting on behalf of the mother, successfully petitioned the dependency court to grant temporary custody of the four children to the shelter home, where all five were then housed. Two weeks later, just prior to a disposition hearing, the mother disappeared, along with the three youngest children and the husband.

Several important issues were dealt with by the SCAN team. Even though sexual molestation had been occurring for years, no physician had ever inquired as to possible incest or molestation. It was the examining pediatrian who, with sensitive yet direct questioning, was able to emotionally support the girl and enable her to share the secret and guilt of incest, something the girl was not able to do with her family doctor. The SCAN consultant provided information on reporting to the house staff and, in addition, provided support for the two girls following their revelation of the ongoing molestations. While the consequences of reporting and intervention in this case led to a negative outcome, the steps taken by SCAN were professionally sound and legally correct. In retrospect, the four children should have been kept together in a suitable foster home or in some other supervised "out-of-home" placement. Because the legal system allows such perpetrators to post a small bond and then remain free to return to the family and again threaten the children, the children of necessity were the ones who had to be placed and who, unfortunately, were made to feel that they were the incarcerated and guilty persons, not the molesting father. While there were mixed feelings within the house staff regarding the consequences of reporting the two cases of molestation, the SCAN team felt that the appropriate and necessary legal and professional steps had been taken. The consequent failure of the "system" to properly protect the welfare of the children in no way detracts from the legal responsibilities of reporting molestation and sexual abuse of two children (Paulson, 1978).

The Substance-Addicted Newborn

An infant delivered at UCLA went into withdrawal shortly after birth, with a subsequent toxic screen showing evidence of heroin. The unwed, 27-year-old mother had previously placed two other children in foster care, stating that she did not want them, but she did want this newborn child and would be able to take good care of it. The mother had been in a number of drug treatment programs for the past seven years and had been briefly incarcerated several times for drug trafficking. The present infant was conceived while the mother was prostituting, and she was not sure who the father was. She was raised by an alcoholic mother, was molested at age 14 by a boyfriend of her mother, and ran away from home at age 16, supporting herself by selling drugs and prostitution.

It is standard UCLA hospital policy that any newborn child showing evidence of withdrawal due to the mother's earlier ingestion of drugs is automatically taken into protective custody, with a "police hold" providing the necessary time for the staff to undertake an evaluation in cooperation with law enforcement, protective services, and public health. In smaller hospitals, where no SCAN team exists, such a child would often go unreported. The mother and newborn would be assisted through the withdrawal, but then perhaps discharged to the community with little if any follow-up or postnatal care.

In the case of this mother and newborn, the authorities were notified, and, following termination of withdrawal, the newborn was placed in a licensed foster home pending a preadjudication hearing. The SCAN team worked with the mother and the local drug treatment center to implement greater supervision over the mother and to monitor her post delivery behavior. Although somewhat reluctant, the mother accepted a referral to a day treatment center, where she could also learn basic elements of child care and child growth and development. While in the hospital, the obstetrics and pediatric nursing staff had carefully observed mother and child, noting the gradual development of bonding. They also provided much reinforcement to the mother in terms of developing a greater emotional attachment to her baby. A SCAN member presented these ward observations at the dependency hearing and assured the court that the infant would be followed regularly in the child development clinic while the mother would be obtaining outpatient psychotherapy at the Neuropsychiatric Institute. Recognizing the medical and educational supports being provided by the hospital and noting the mother's apparently genuine wish to stay in therapy and to keep her child, the dependency court returned the child to the mother. The County Department of Public Social Services maintained a close supervision over the child. Both the drug treatment center and the Neuropsychiatric Institute provided regular follow-up information to the dependency court. Hopefully, with such professional monitoring and close SCAN consultation, the child will be provided a positive home environment in the care of its biological mother.

The Premature Infant

A two-month premature girl was delivered to a 21-year-old mother and a 32-year-old father; spending the first nine weeks of life in intensive neonatal and postnatal care. The mother had a drug history, the marriage was chaotic, and both parents were acutely angry at the medical staff and hospital over the infant's lengthy hospitalization and several postponements in discharge dates. Because of the prior drug history and evident marital discord, the SCAN team consultant was called in to provide recommendations. The parents were further infuriated, feeling that this was a reflection of their incompetence as parents.

Within the SCAN team there were divergent feelings over the possible reporting of the family to protective services for post-hospital follow-up and supervision. The mother was off drugs, and certain positive bonding experiences were noted by the inpatient pediatric staff. However, because of the angry, volatile nature of the husband-wife relationship and because there was no extended family to support the mother, the father, and the medically delicate newborn, SCAN did recommend a referral to protective services and to public health. One of the house staff physicians, along with the pediatric social worker, made a number of home visits for medical and psychosocial follow-up. At six months after discharge from the hospital, the child was progressing relatively well, the marriage appeared more stable, and the parents were accepting the visiting public health nurse and protective services worker with a more positive show of appreciation. Without such an initial SCAN consultation and continued social networking with other hospital resources and community agencies, this premature child may well have become a victim of at least parental neglect, and possibly family violence and abuse.

Other High-Risk Children

High-risk children are those children born to unwed, adolescent mothers; those who have congenital defects; those born in an emotionally unstable, chaotic household; those having mentally retarded parents; those who are premature, or of the wrong sex, or who remind parents of an unwanted pregnancy. High-risk parents include those mothers having no prenatal care; who did not want the pregnancy; who initially wanted to abort the pregnancy; or who initially wanted to give up the child for adoption, but later, because of family pressures, decided to keep the infant. High-risk home environments include those homes where the unemployed father temporarily or permanently takes over child care responsibilities, or where crowded home conditions do not provide privacy for the parents and sufficient free space for the children. Large families, with children born in close succession and where the mother lacks support from an extended family, are families at risk. Other high-risk environments include mothers with an abnormal pregnancy or abnormal delivery, or with neonatal separation secondary to illness or prematurity. Prolonged illness of the mother or child in the child's first year of life or separation of the mother and child during the first six months of life, when bonding and attachment experiences are so vital, are other kinds of family stresses that should be recognized as contributing to a high-risk environment for both infant and parent.

In such situations as those above, what can the SCAN team do? Health professionals from all disciplines must be alert to the indices of stress, especially when the young mother is presenting for the first time in the prenatal clinic. A high-risk parent may show behaviorally, verbally, and nonverbally many indications of ambivalence with regard to the expected or newborn child. Rejection statements relative to the fetus or newborn should be immediately recognized as indications of potential bonding failure. Recognizing such prenatal responses, both parents should be counseled and referred to prenatal parenting classes— classes that include not only basic facts with regard to growth and development of the child, but that allow the parents to verbalize negative and ambivalent feelings in a therapeutic milieu that fosters emotional growth and development. In terms of primary prevention, it is here that the combined resources and network of SCAN team members within a hospital setting can provide the necessary intervention and education referrals for those parents facing overwhelming postdelivery responsibilities.

PROFESSIONAL ISSUES IN THE FUNCTIONING OF A SCAN TEAM

A SCAN team, to be effective, must be fully informed as to existing laws within the state that mandate required action by professionals when neglect, abuse, or maltreatment of a child is suspected. SCAN, in a consultant relationship with the hospital and the community, serves therefore to advise, to recommend, and even at times to require the implementation of specific actions by concerned professionals. Although child protection laws vary among the states, there is general consensus that mandatory reporting is essential, even though it initially received considerable professional resistance.

Since 1974, when all 50 states enacted mandatory reporting laws, there has appeared the concept of the child protection team, representing an interdisciplinary body of health-related professionals networking within the hospital and with the community. With an increasing use of the acronym *SCAN*, mainly within health service centers, ambivalent feelings have developed with regard to a possible "labeling effect" when the letters *SCAN* are placed on or in a medical chart. For some physicians, the stamping of these letters implies a judgment by medical peers of inappropriate pediatric management. In the family, there is often engendered anger, resistance, hostility, and frequently lack of cooperation, especially when a SCAN team member is introduced to the parents or when, subsequent to a SCAN consultation, there is a report made of suspected abuse of a child, or at times even the temporary "out-of-home" placement of a child. Schmitt's recent text, entitled *The Child Protection Team Handbook*, has given some impetus to the use of the letters *CPT*, but, in general, there is a more widespread use of *SCAN* to signify the team of professionals involved in the management of children at risk of parental abuse and neglect.

A recent publication by the Education Commission of the States (1980) reviews most recent state statutes with regard to child protection laws. Thirteen important issues are discussed:

1. What element(s) of child abuse must be reported?
2. Who must report suspected cases of child abuse?
3. When must a report be made?
4. To whom must a report be made?
5. Immunity for good-faith reporting.
6. Penalty for not making a mandated report.
7. Abrogation of privileged communication.
8. Color photography and X-ray evidence.
9. Temporary protective custody and emergency placement of a child.
10. Central registry.
11. Child protection teams.
12. Guardian *ad litem* counsel for the child.
13. Public education.

These issues and questions should be clearly understood by any SCAN team. In summary, the identified trends in child protection laws are as follows. Every state requires the reporting of nonaccidental physical injury and neglect. While 46 states also require the reporting of sexual abuse and molestation, physicians, nurses, and social workers in all 50 states are mandated to report. Almost all states require both an oral and written report within 36-72 hours from the time of suspicion of maltreatment. In 28 states, reporting is made to the local department of social services; while an additional 19 states require reporting either to social services or to a law enforcement agency. In only two states is reporting to law enforcement alone. Reporting in good faith assures immunity from liability in all states. Therefore, those who so report cannot later be found in jeopardy even though subsequent proceedings may not substantiate the suspicion of abuse. It is in this area that the SCAN team can provide reassurance to those practitioners who fear involvement by reporting and who otherwise are apprehensive about reporting potentially litiginous parents even though a high index of suspicion of abuse exists.

Almost two-thirds of all states provide criminal and/or civil penalties for nonreporting. Yet to date, no criminal penalties for nonreporting have been rendered. However, two civil cases in California—both against nonreporting physicians—have resulted in civil liabilities being levied, one to the amount of over $400,000. Privileged communication in numerous civil and criminal hearings has heretofore protected the alleged perpetrator. However, with respect to child abuse, 19 states have rescinded the status of privileged communication between husband and wife; 22 abrogate this status between doctor and patient, and 20 abrogate all privileged communication except that between attorney and client.

In the related area of medical documentation of physical and sexual abuse, health professionals are often hesitant to pursue the gathering of medical specimens or evidence of trauma and/or assault. Almost half of the states now permit health agencies and physicians to take necessary color photographs and radiographs of an abused child, even without parental permission. For those major medical centers to whom suspected abuse is most frequently referred, it is imperative that the SCAN team in such diagnostic centers be fully informed as to the hospital and state limitation of privileges specific to the gathering of information necessary for both correct diagnosis and treatment of inflicted abuse, and for information necessary for later civil and/or criminal prosecution of the perpetrators.

On the basis of severe jeopardy to a child, protective services or law enforcement may act to protect the child through emergency removal and/or placing the child in temporary protective custody pending later dependency court hearings, which then prescribe for varying periods of time temporary or permanent custody and care of the child in question. Frequently, it is one of the SCAN members who may in a court of law be required to present medical and social findings, plus SCAN consultation reports and recommendations, in order that a wise judicial opinion be rendered regarding the child's best present and future well-being and custody.

Recognizing the phenomenon of repetitive abuse and "hospital shopping," and acting to identify as early as possible probable abuse of a child, more than 80 percent of the states have created statewide central registries, which become the repository for all reported cases of suspected and substantiated neglect and abuse. Such a pool of information becomes an available data bank for any agency or professional evaluating suspected abuse. By making such information available to the appropriate authorities, a central registry can be instrumental in tracking abusive parents, many whom are transient both within a county and within a state.

It thus becomes evident that the diagnosis and treatment of abused children is not within the realm of any one specific health or social agency. A child protection team can be the cornerstone of effective diagnosis and subsequent treatment. Consultation liaison within the network of medicine, law, social service, law enforcement, and mental health is enhanced and maximized by the establishment of such a SCAN consultation team within every hospital—urban, suburban, or rural. The size of a medical facility and community catchment area will dictate the extent and breadth of participating professionals in such an ongoing, constantly available consultation team. However, in even the smaller hospitals and emergency receiving centers, there should be a team consisting of a physician and nurse specialist, each trained in the identification of child abuse and knowledgeable about the social-psychological concomitants of violence to children. Liaison with the community public health nurse and public social services can therefore provide maximum cross-disciplinary referral and collaboration.

When identification of nonaccidental, inflicted injury results in judicial prosecution, maximum protection for the child can be assured through a child advocacy program employing the concept of guardian *ad litem* (guardian appointed by the court) for the minor. Theoretically, while the department of social service in the dependency court represents the child's best welfare, in practice such an agency serves multiple roles, some of which may not always be to maximize the child's best interests. Therefore, a court-appointed guardian for the child, now existing in 46 of the 50 states, can provide maximum legal representation for the minor.

In Los Angeles County, for example, the dependency court is conducting a multiyear research study comparing the effectiveness of specially trained, non-lawyer guardians *ad litem* with that of guardians *ad litem* holding a law degree. If, in fact, equally effective representation can be provided by nonlawyer representation for the child, then many more children now unrepresented in courts of law can more effectively be represented. It is evident that child abuse is not an acute problem only for health and welfare professionals; it is an acute problem for the community and the nation. Through public education of the lay community and professionals and technical education of educators and scientists, through the medium of SCAN and the child protection team, society can assure the highest level of proficiency in the adequate diagnosis and treatment of child abuse.

PHYSICIAN RESISTANCE TO REPORTING SUSPECTED CHILD ABUSE

Privileged communication between physician and patient has been the cornerstone of medical practice since the Hippocratic oath was postulated. Today however, 22 of the 50 states have conscientiously examined this concept of confidentiality, specifically as it applies to the reporting of suspected abuse and/or neglect; and have in fact waived the right of the physician to remain silent. For many, this has caused great resistance and resentment, insofar as the courts are seen as legislating specific aspects of medical practice. From a practical viewpoint, there is a large gray area between parenting behavior that is appropriate discipline and that which constitutes undue corporal punishment or physical assault upon a child. Even more, standards of discipline and punishment have strong cultural and ethnic roots that in many ways determine not only judicial opinion in both juvenile and adult criminal court, but determine also the way in which parents and educational institutions exercise punishment of children. It is because of this vast gray area in differentiating abuse from punishment that many physicians, especially pediatricians, are reluctant to become involved in the reporting of suspected abuse. This lack of clarity in determining what constitutes abuse is shared equally by allied health specialists who, many times looking to the physician for leadership, are reluctant to make an affirmative statement about any suspicion of abuse that would appear to challenge the non-egalitarian authority relationship between the physician and nonphysician health specialist.

The acutely ill, brutalized infant presenting in a county hospital emergency room rarely is a diagnostic problem for the examining physician. Nor does the physician have any reluctance to report such a case to the appropriate authorities. However, the middle-upper-economic WASP child presenting in a major medical setting and referred by an outside colleague for diagnosis of undetermined injuries becomes a source of great professional and medical concern. For example, a 2½-year-old girl was brought to a pediatric clinic by the paternal aunt who reported the child as saying that the maternal grandfather had burned her on the vagina with a cigarette. What the examining physician saw was an abrasion resembling impetigo. The child was unable to indicate verbally or through diagnostic play therapy whether she had been burned. The physician, when charting his findings and history, said with great humility and anguish,

"I just can't stand these cases. They're so frustrating. You just never seem to know whether it's abuse or not."

Compounding the problems of diagnosis are many reality factors inherent in any major emergency room setting, such as inadequate and incomplete information, limited time available for detailed examination and history taking, and lack of staff trained in the recognition and identification of suspected abuse (Friedman et al., 1979). Many physicians are poorly trained to do a social history or social-psychological assessment of a child and family. Even more, they feel acutely uncomfortable in asking very specific and necessary questions regarding the actual physical or sexual abuse of a child. Professionals must here realize that the law requires only reporting of suspicion of abuse; the law does not require *that* specific professional to prove the fact of abuse. That responsibility lies in the hands of others, once the reporting of suspicion is made. Remembering this, physicians and other allied specialists will hopefully be able to maintain greater objectivity in interviewing and feel less inhibited in asking important but necessarily personal questions.

Many physicians are reluctant to report less severe cases of abuse and/or neglect, saying, "The system won't do anything anyway, so why become involved?" While the great majority of professionals are responsible in the performance of their duties, there are those occasional persons who, because of "burnout," emotional exhaustion and overwork, lack of training, or indifference to the job, refuse to adequately follow through on a referral. The family is not helped; instead, they are made angry and resentful at being reported. The physician is frustrated because he is blamed by the parents for reporting, and is at times even subjected to all forms of intimidation and threats of legal action. Compounding the physician's frustration even more is the experience of being subpoenaed to testify in either a dependency hearing for the child or in the superior court where criminal charges against the perpetrator are being heard. Not only does courtroom testimony and trial preparation require a great deal of time, effort, and loss of income, but, even more, the opposing attorney will frequently attempt to "downgrade" professional testimony by verbal assault, innuendo, and demeaning of the physician's responses or testimony. This assault upon the dignity of the physician as a trial or expert witness is all too common in many courts of law. It therefore behooves the physician to prepare well before testifying, to have all evidence in a well-ordered and documented form, and, above all, not to let the courtroom behavior of an opposing trial attorney be a source of personal or professional threat or intimidation. For example, on the basis of all the data available from a lengthy medical-social-psychological examination of a neglected child, a physician testified in a dependency hearing recommending that inadequate as the home and parents were, it was better to keep the child with its siblings and biological parents rather than induce great separation anxiety and fear in the child by having it placed in a licensed foster home. There was a calculated risk that the severe discipline and physical and emotional neglect might again occur. However, with court-ordered supervision of the family by protective services and counseling for the child and its parent, both the physician and the judge wisely agreed to return the child to the parents. Such a decision, though, is a heavy, burdensome responsibility, one that is emotionally draining for the professionals involved in these important decisions regarding the health and life of a child.

An additional reason for physicians being reluctant to report is their lack of adequate training and education in the medical-legal-social-psychological aspects of child abuse. Taking the medical history on the possible etiology of a peptic ulcer involves much less emotional strain than taking a detailed history on a gravely and viciously battered or burned child, or on a seven-year-old child raped and sodomized by its biological father. It is the rare medical school or residency education program that provides the necessary training and experience in doing a thorough, sensitive interview of an abused child and an abusing parent. Lacking this kind of formal, well-supervised clinical training, many physicians, nurses, and other health professionals are therefore acutely anxious when confronted with the responsibility of interviewing, evaluating, and diagnosing a child-abusing family.

Helfer (1975) in his article "Why Most Physicians Don't Get Involved in Child Abuse Cases and What to Do About It" details eight reasons for such minimal involvement. These are:

1. Medical school training was insufficient.
2. Physicians are not trained in interpersonal skills.
3. Doctors have great difficulty working with members of other disciplines as peers.
4. The drain on time, finances, and emotions for the physician in private practice is truly extensive.
5. Physicians have a fear of testifying in court.
6. There is minimal personal reward, and these rewards are hard to identify.
7. When one does get involved, he or she is often confronted with a community system that is less than helpful.
8. Physicians have rarely been trained to see themselves or to act as agents for change.

If these eight conditions exist within health delivery systems, it is understandable that child abuse is underdiagnosed and underreported. It is incumbent upon those professionals on the SCAN team, expert in understanding the etiology of child abuse and neglect to provide the necessary educational and training opportunities to counteract these resistances. Working within a school of medicine and residency education department, the interdisciplinary team of SCAN can provide a positive learning and consultation experience that will contribute significantly to the primary prevention, and more effective secondary and tertiary intervention with abused children and their families.

Equally essential is an awareness and acceptance of the fact that working with abused children and abusing parents can often be an unrewarding, thankless, and an emotionally painful experience. Society teaches that parents should love their children and protect them from all harm. As professionals in the field, we profess that the great majority of parents are supposedly well intentioned and well meaning in the rearing and disciplining of their children. But we also see a significant number who are viciously cruel, inhuman, and purposefully and violently assaultive to children. The nonpsychotic mother who placed a lighted cigarette upon the eyeball of her infant; the enraged but nonpsychotic father who seized a child by the foot and smashed its head against the wall; the parent who purposefully scalded a child's penis because he was occasionally enuretic— all these are examples of acutely painful human tragedy that give the diagnosing and treating physician no sense of personal reward or professional fulfillment.

From the beginning of diagnosis to the end of treatment of such children, the physician must be considerate, thoughtful, controlling of his emotions, and able to render maximum medical care to the child. However, the anguish within may in part contribute to the high rate of suicide, substance abuse, and addiction reported among physicians. The doctor, the nurse, and all the allied professionals joined together to provide medical care for the abused child and abusing parents suffer an inner pain of great magnitude. SCAN, representing a combined group of understanding, caring, thoroughly trained colleagues, can nonetheless be a major element in the healing process of abused children. As a consulting resource for both the hospital and the community, SCAN and the child protection team play a significant role in the prevention, identification, and treatment of child maltreatment.

THE DENTIST AS A SCAN CONSULTANT

Considering that 50-60 percent of all physical child abuse occurs to the head and neck areas, it is essential that a pediatric dentist be a member of the SCAN team. Head trauma may involve short-term or long-term dental consultation, especially when trauma to the mouth area requires extensive orthodontic repair. Dental testimony also plays a significant role in the determination of inflicted trauma versus accidental injury. For example, a nine-year-old boy was brought to a dentist by his mother because of damage to his teeth supposedly caused by being hit by a ball. The dentist immediately observed marked dental neglect and acute apprehension on the part of the young child. Further examination of the broken teeth and damaged jawbone convinced the dentist that such damage could not be caused by a child throwing a ball. Talking supportively to the boy, the dentist elicited information that the father had in fact punched the boy in the mouth for talking back. The poor dental hygiene was also evidence of medical neglect on the part of the parents. From a legal point of view, severe dental neglect can be the basis for filing neglect charges in a dependency court. When the dental neglect occurs in conjunction with other evidence of medical and physical neglect, the dentist becomes an important member of the SCAN consultation team.

In terms of felony child abuse, dentistry has also been called into court to provide expert witness evidence that bite marks on a child's body were in fact purposefully inflicted by a parent. By matching the bite marks on the arms and legs with a dental mold made from the father, a dental professor was able to provide confirming evidence as to the identity of the abuser and the nature of the inflicted bodily trauma. It is evident that the dentist can and must fulfill several important roles as a SCAN team member. First, as an expect in orodental trauma, he can testify as to the nature of mouth and head trauma in terms of diagnosing nonaccidental injury to a child. Secondly, in terms of treatment intervention, the dentist can be a part of the rehabilitation planning. Like all permanent members of a SCAN team, the dentist also accepts the responsibility of "on-call" SCAN consultant, providing knowledge and expertise not only to the medical emergency room and pediatric house staff, but to other members of the dental school and dental community.

In those centers for the health sciences where schools of medicine, dentistry, nursing, and public health comprise a unified health service, the dentist plays a major educational and teaching role. Dental students and others can learn first-hand about the relationships between dental neglect, medical neglect, and failure on the part of parents to provide the necessary oral care for a child. At the UCLA School of Dentistry, a protocol for evaluation and referral of suspected child abuse and neglect has been developed and is a basic part of the education of all dental students (Blain, 1979). For the private practitioner, the SCAN team and the pedodontist are valuable educational resources not only for specific case discussion, but in terms of providing continuing education programs on the relationship between child abuse and dentistry. The dentist, like all other health professionals, is required by law to report suspected child abuse and neglect. Yet, such reports are rarely made—often because the busy dental practitioner is unaware of his legal obligations, and sometimes because the dentist does not want to become involved in the emotionally charged (and at times legal) complications forthcoming from reporting suspected abuse or severe dental neglect. Graduate courses can provide an opportunity to develop skills for interviewing victims of abuse as well as the suspected perpetrators. In any case, while dentistry in the past has been only minimally involved in the identification and reporting of suspected child maltreatment, there is an increasing awareness of the responsibilities of the dentist to protect the child who is a potential victim of neglect, as well as to identify the victim of abuse and neglect when such a child presents itself in a dental office.

BURNOUT: A PROFESSIONAL RISK

Burnout of professionals working in the field of child abuse and neglect happens frequently and for many reasons. The nature of the violent acts; the frequent resistance, anger, and defensiveness of the abusing parents; and the frustrations in working within a less than perfect health delivery system provoke ambivalent and at times intense and unpleasant emotional and physical responses. Even the concept of mandatory reporting creates intraprofessional strife and disharmony. The bipolar concepts of "compassion versus control" (Rosenfeld and Newberger, 1977) characterize the strong professional differences of opinion with regard to the so-called "labeling" of a family and the reporting of an incident of suspected abuse or neglect. For example, even the hospital policy of reporting an infant to Protective Services if a toxic substance is found in the newborn's toxic screen can be highly controversial within a hospital. On the one hand, reporting is mandatory by law specifically for the protection of the infant. On the other hand, many health professionals and child development specialists feel that separation of a child from its mother at birth is justified only under the most extreme conditions within the home or in the mother. Those professionals who report such a case are at times viewed as punitive, judgmental, and more oriented toward a judicial and law enforcement approach to child abuse intervention, while those who are more lenient with respect to reporting are seen as more oriented toward a social service and rehabilitation point of view.

Opposition to mandatory and automatic reporting of all cases of suspected abuse is based on a lack of available diagnostic and treatment services once a report has been filed. In many health centers, large and small, once one accomplishes the necessary awareness raising and training in child abuse (Davoren), the volume of identified and reported cases often becomes overwhelming, with few centers or agencies having sufficient numbers of trained staff to work effectively and sensitively with the referred and reported abusing families. The families themselves provide minimal gratification for the professional, especially in the identification and early management stages—the stages where hospital personnel and SCAN members are most involved. The parents are often lonely, isolated, frightened, and angry. Although on one level they may be relieved that the abuse has been discovered and help is available, outwardly they often withdraw into rage, denial, and threatening and verbally assaultive behavior. The children are usually troubed and frightened and deeply loyal to their parents, rarely realizing the life saving interventions being made on their behalf by the professionals.

Such clinical aspects of child abuse intervention contribute significantly to burnout in hospital and agency professionals. SCAN teams can be most helpful in lessening these stresses and providing team support for those members and hospital staff under special pressures specific to a particularly difficult and administratively controversial case of reported child abuse. One of the major steps toward the prevention of burnout is the dividing and sharing of responsibility in "working up" a case. Such responsibility and decisionmaking must not rest solely on the shoulders of one individual. In health service centers, the SCAN team must be a consulting body. This consultation must be available in person, by phone, and in regularly or specially scheduled conferences. While the actual management of child abuse is done by the professionals coming into contact with the family members on a particular service, the SCAN members must be constantly available. By having the professionals directly involved in case management and the SCAN team as consultant members, the volume of child abuse cases can be divided, burnout can be minimized, and the families can be provided with maximum care and treatment.

While shared responsibilities are an effective antidote to burnout, it is also essential that all SCAN team members and hospital staff be provided maximum training opportunities, so that every individual feels more confident in basic skills, more aware of resources, and can use such educational programs as a momentary and rewarding diversion from the daily responsibilities of child abuse intervention.

While there may be many differences in approach and opinion among SCAN team members, they value the individual opinion of each other and their own contributions to SCAN decisions. Requests for frequent consultation are seen as recognized strengths of the team and not as a sign of ignorance on the part of the information seeker. Since gratification does not readily come from the families themselves, and at times does not come from senior hospital staff and administrators involved in a difficult case, team support is especially crucial and rewarding. The multidisciplinary nature of the SCAN team is intellectually broadening and stimulating for its members and provides opportunities for a free and open interchange of feelings.

SCAN teams can do much to lessen the burnout of hospital staff by being available for consultation; by lessening the anxiety of staff through sensitive listening and support; by providing basic and essential information on procedures and policy; and by lending a guiding hand to those professionals unfamiliar with the ambiguities of child abuse systems, services, and regulations. The SCAN team helps the hospital professional find an answer to the difficult question "What is child abuse?" As is known by all who work within this field, there is still much ambiguity as to what is or is not child abuse and neglect (Giovanni and Becerra, 1979).

PRESENT AND FUTURE DIRECTIONS FOR SCAN

SCAN is now recognized as a necessary and valuable aspect of interdisciplinary child abuse intervention. Whether within a hospital setting or in a community treatment agency, there must be a cadre of specially trained, knowledgeable and available professionals who can be used in a consultant and evaluation role when a case of suspected or identified child abuse is referred for evaluation, diagnosis, and treatment. What are the steps to be implemented to maximize the functioning of SCAN so that it can make a meaningful contribution of progressive change within the community?

1. There must be a continuing education of lay citizens and professionals with regard to the nature of child abuse and how society must intervene in both a preventive and remedial manner.
2. There must be increased governmental support for primary and secondary intervention programs in order to provide expanded consultation, service, education, and research into child abuse.
3. On a community level, there should be organized child trauma councils that will bring together all those health and welfare professionals who, united, can provide an integrated approach to the prevention and treatment of child abuse.
4. On a statewide level, there must be a consortium of child trauma councils, bringing together the combined resources of all the local trauma councils. Information can be shared, new ideas can be promulgated, and a united approach can characterize a statewide, coordinated approach to improving the family life of its citizens.
5. Outreach to the rural communities has been minimal. To date, the greatest amount of money and manpower has been directed to the urban population. We cannot generalize from urban social conflict to rural social conflict. Each community has its own special needs. Each must be offered an opportunity to participate in and reap the benefits of an active child abuse intervention team.
6. Community consultation is an antidote to institutional and agency abuse of children and families. Community consultation is an antidote to professional burnout. The SCAN team must take an active role in the operation and implementation of programs of community consultation and agency sharing.
7. There must be a recognition that "alternative lifestyles" and changing patterns of family life have in many ways created a threat to the stability of the family and the role of parents in the disciplining and rearing of their children. Professionals must be aware of these societal changes and variations in social structure. Professionals must be trained to

understand such social conflict and metamorphosis in order to provide the necessary supports to families in need and families in transition.

8. There must be a greater recognition of the importance of clinical research in primary prevention and secondary intervention. Social-economic-political-emotional-family concomitants of domestic violence must be studied, and the findings of successful intervention must be shared with all those agencies and professionals working in the area of child abuse and violence within the home. The long-term needs for secondary intervention must be recognized. However, the immediate needs for primary intervention must not be shelved in order to deal effectively with the crisis conditions within the home today.

9. Interagency collaboration can bring together the resources of medicine, nursing, education, mental health, law enforcement, and the judiciary. Combined in effort, such collaboration can provide guidelines and approaches to child abuse prevention that will ultimately eradicate the great epidemic of child violence experienced today.

SCAN, as a team of such interdisciplinary experts, can provide a leadership role in the implementing of the nine points noted above. This is the challenge.

This paper was supported by Catholics of Motion Picture, TV, and Radio and Recording Industry.

REFERENCES

Blain, S. *A University Based, Multidisciplinary Program for the Detection and Early Management of the Abused Child, with Emphasis on Community Agency Referral and Case Follow-Up.* National Child Abuse Conference, Los Angeles (October, 1979).

Davoren, E. On being self-aware. Personal communication.

Education Commission of the States. *Trends in Child Protection Laws—1979,* Report No. 128. Denver (1980).

Friedman, A., Cardiff, M., Sandler, A., and Friedman, D. Coping with the dilemmas of child abuse. In *Working for Children: Ethical Issues Beyond Professional Guidelines,* J. Mearig, ed. Jossey-Bass, San Francisco (1979).

Giovannoni, J., and Becerra, R. *Defining Child Abuse.* The Free Press, New York (1979).

Helfer, R. Why most physicians don't get involved in child abuse cases and what to do about it. *Children Today, 4,* 28-32 (1975).

Kempe, C., Silverman, F., Steele, B., Droegmueller, W., and Silver, H. The battered child syndrome. *Journal of the American Medical Association, 181,* 105-112 (1962).

Newberger, E., and Bourne, R. The medicalization and legalization of child abuse. *American Journal of Orthopsychiatry, 48,* 593-606 (1978).

Paulson, M. Early intervention and treatment of child abuse: Our nation's mandate. *Psychiatric Opinion, 15,* 34–38 (1978a).

———. Incest and sexual molestation: Clinical and legal issues. *Journal of Clinical Child Psychology, 7,* 177–180 (1978b).

Paulson, M., Savino, A., Chaleff, A., Sanders, R., Frisch, F., and Dunn, R. Parents of the battered child: A multidisciplinary group therapy approach to life-threatening behavior. *Life Threatening Behavior, 4,* 18–31 (1974).

Rosenfeld, A., and Newberger, E. Compassion vs control. *Journal of the American Medical Association, 237,* 2086–2088 (1977).

Rowe, D., Leonard, M., Seashore, M., Lewiston, N., and Anderson, F. A hospital program for the detection and registration of abused and neglected children. *New England Journal of Medicine, 282,* 950–952 (1970).

Schmitt, B. *The Child Protection Team Handbook: A Multidisciplinary Approach to Managing Child Abuse and Neglect.* Garland STPM Press, New York (1978).

Schmitt, B., Broso, D., Carroll, C., Gray, J., Grosz, C., Kempe, C., and Lenherr, M. *Guidelines for the Hospital and Clinic Management of Child Abuse and Neglect.* Children's Bureau, Department of Health, Education and Welfare Publication No. (OHDS) 80-30167 (1980).

10

Physical and Emotional Abuse of Children: Prevention and Intervention Strategies

Morris J. Paulson

PRIMARY PREVENTION

If society is to provide fully for the emotional health of the pediatric patient, it must look to the multiple factors within the child and within the family that contribute to impairment. This is especially true for families in which physical, emotional, and sexual abuse of children occur (Paulson, 1978b). Often abuse is unnoticed and undiagnosed until that tragic moment when ultimate parental indifference, frustration, anger, or purposeful violence explode, resulting in severe injury or even death to a child (Caffey, 1972). It is therefore vital that all professionals and agencies responsible for providing pediatric care be fully informed as to the multiple causality of child abuse and neglect, and be equally knowledgeable about prevention and intervention strategies helpful in the care of pediatric patients and their parents (Green, Gaines, and Sandgrund, 1974).

It is becoming increasingly evident that abuse of children is not an isolated phenomenon, but is a manifestation of domestic stress and family violence, where the infant-child becomes a life-threatening, conscious and/or unconscious scapegoat for parental frustration (Lystad, 1975; Green, 1979). Many definitions of child abuse exist, each reflecting the medical, legal, sociological, or psychological orientation of the writer. Conceptual definitions of child abuse in the early 1960s focused primarily upon physical signs and symptoms of abuse and neglect. Kempe et al. (1962, p. 17) in part defined the battered-child syndrome as "evidence of possible trauma or neglect (fracture of any bone, subdural hematoma, multiple soft tissue injuries, poor skin hygiene or malnutrition) or where there is marked discrepancy between the clinical findings and historical data supplied by the parents." Gil (1970, p. 50), in describing the Brandeis study on child abuse, provided a further definition of child abuse as "when an adult physically injures a child, not by accident, but in anger or deliberately."

Throughout the two decades since the battered-child syndrome was first described, revisions of earlier definitions have been made, each reflecting the

Table 10-1

Referrals to the California State Child Protective Services Bureau
for the Calendar Year January–December, 1978,
Prorated to the USA Census

Reason for Referral	California Population ($N = 22,000,000$)		USA Population ($N = 220,000,000$)	
	N	%	N	%
Total Family Cases	80,333	100	803,330	100
General neglect	47,249	59	472,490	59
Physical abuse	16,575	21	165,750	21
Intentional deprivation	4,862	6	48,620	6
Sexual abuse	4,006	5	40,060	5
Other	7,641	9	76,140	9

broadened understanding and conceptualization of the multiple factors contributing to emotional, physical, and sexual assault of children by adult caretakers. Child abuse in the state of California, for example, is defined as "any act of omission or commission that endangers or impairs a child's physical or emotional health and development. This includes: physical abuse and corporal punishment, emotional abuse, emotional deprivation, physical neglect and/or inadequate supervision, and sexual abuse and exploitation" (California Department of Justice, 1978, p. 1).

Incidence studies on abused children vary in terms of definition of abuse, geographical areas studied, and soundness of methodological studies (Head Start Bureau, 1978). Kempe and Helfer (1972) estimated that 380 children per one million general population were annually abused in the United States. An NIMH study in 1978 reported two million incidence of child abuse, stating that four percent of all children under age 17 were abused (Gorman, 1979). Generalizing from available State of California Department of Public Social Services statistics (1978) to a nationwide United States population, a shocking measure of parental abuse and impaired child-rearing practices is identified. Table 10-1 identifies the reasons for referral to the State Child Protective Services Bureau for the calendar year January–December, 1978.

The table reflects actual *families* referred, which often have more than one child involved in abuse and/or neglect. Recognizing public health figures that suggest that the actual incidence of any existing health pathology is at least five times that identified, there is substantial evidence that at least four million families within the United States during a calendar year are sufficiently at risk to require active Child Protective Services intervention. These data do not include statistics on deaths of children by nonaccidental, inflicted trauma, estimated to be 5 to 10 percent of all physically abused children.

Evaluation of incidence and sociological studies on child maltreatment (Gelles, 1973) indicates that child abuse is distributed among all cultures, irrespective of race, creed, color, or religion. However, examination of demographic data does identify high-risk subgroups of parents, in which socioeconomic and sociocultural factors such as unemployment, inadequate housing, substance abuse, broken families, domestic violence, unwed teenage parents, and rigid patterns of parenting and child rearing positively correlate with abuse and neglect of children.

Voluminous data exist describing numerous personal and familial characteristics of abusing parents (Paulson and Blake, 1967; Steele and Pollock, 1974; Spinetta and Rigler, 1972; Helfer and Kempe, 1976; Lourie, 1979). Abusing parents are repeatedly described as emotionally immature, hedonistic, dependent, overly rigid in disciplining, and having inappropriately high expectations for behavior beyond the child's emotional and physical developmental level. Role-reversal behavior of the parent has also been repeatedly identified, where the child is expected to behave in a highly adult manner in order to gratify infantile dependency needs of the parents (Morris and Gould, 1963). Pathognomonic of child abuse is a history of physical abuse and emotional trauma in the early childhood of maltreating parents. In terms of social learning, behavioral modeling, and identification with the agressor, it is theoretically and clinically understandable that children raised in an environment of rejection and hostility are predisposed (without intervention) to later adult violence, impulse impairment, projection of blame, and displacement of anger upon those emotionally and physically unable to defend or protect themselves.

Early writings on child maltreatment focused primarily on medical identification of abuse and effectiveness of psychotherapy for abusing parents, with specific reference to the emotional, social, and psychological characteristics of the abusing parents (Galdston, 1965; Elmer and Gregg, 1967; Paulson and Blake, 1969; Paulson and Chaleff, 1973; Paulson et al., 1974a; Morse, Sahler, and Friedman, 1970). Attention to and concern for the abused child were primarily in terms of medical indices and diagnosis of the battered-child syndrome. More recently, there has been a rededication of professional attention and fiscal expenditures, with a greater focus on primary prevention, identification of developmental disabilities, and effectiveness of treatment modalities for the abused child (Klaus and Kennell, 1970; Brazelton, 1974; Martin, 1976; Frommer, 1979). Secondary intervention with abused children and their parents can ultimately reduce the incidence and trauma of parental violence (Paulson, 1975, 1976, 1978a). However, equally necessary is the application of theory and the direction of human resources to primary prevention programs in order to reduce high-risk parenting and endangered homes to a level where emotional and physical trauma to children will not occur.

Primary Prevention Theories in Child Abuse Intervention

An interdisciplinary, multicausal, multitheoretical approach to the understanding and treatment of child abuse is providing increased awareness of the disturbing amount of parental violence toward children. Intervention must carefully examine the historical-cultural roots of family life in order to determine the most effective means of preventive intervention. Child abuse is not endemic to only one lifestyle; it is endemic to all societies of adults and children living together in a relationship requiring parental responsibility. There must, therefore, be defined and disseminated bodies of knowledge and theories that will enhance the prevention and treatment of child abuse.

Preventive intervention must draw upon many existing theories in order to mount a multi-faceted investigation of the etiology of child abuse. Such theories are the foundation stones upon which many societies of caring, nurturing families are rearing their children. The importance of the mother-infant relationship and its effect on later adult behavior and parenting practices have been carefully documented (Spitz, 1945; Erickson, 1963; Bowlby, 1969, 1973; Harlow, Harlow, and Soumi, 1971; Gewirtz, 1972; Martin, 1976). Concomitant with these writings was the pioneer paper of Kempe et al. (1962), which jarred the professional and lay community into realizing that parents do vary in the quality and degree of their child-rearing practices. Such variations extend from positive nurturing and affectional stimulation, to neglect, abuse, abandonment, and even willful infliction of death upon a child. If primary prevention is to be effective, we must first research the pathological roots of such severe parental discipline and abuse and examine the intertwining roles and contributions of environment, parent personality, and the target child to understand the etiology of child abuse (Sandgrund, Gaines, and Green, 1974; Friedrich, 1976; Paulson, in press; Garmezy, 1971).

Prematurity and low birth weight, for example, are associated with parental abuse (Elmer and Gregg, 1967). Klein and Stern (1971) reported that 12 percent of 88 abused children in one study were premature; in another study, 23 percent of 51 abused children had low birth weight.

Klaus and Kennell (1970) found a correlation between mothers separated from their newborn, and later abuse of the child. Parmelee et al. (1976) and Kass et al. (1976) reported that prematurity of birth correlated positively with early neurological and behavioral dysfunction of the young child. Mental retardation (Brandwein, 1973; Morse, Sahler, and Friedman, 1970), physical handicaps (Lynch, 1975), individual differences in behavior style (Soeffing, 1975; Green, 1978), and temperament of infants have also been identified as characteristics associated with high-risk, abused children (Thomas, Chess and Birth, 1968; Carey, 1972).

It is becoming increasingly evident that early infant-caregiver interaction strongly influences later emotional, social, and physical growth of newborns. Hofer (1975) described varying patterns of parental interaction in his examination of (1) mother-infant roles in monkeys; (2) patterns of human maternal behavior after delivery; (3) sensitive and critical periods of attachment and bonding; and (4) effects of infant-mother separation due to illness, trauma, or death. At the same time, Sameroff and Chandler (1975) emphasized the importance of family-based hazards, both physical and psychological, that impact upon and negatively affect the infant-caregiver dyad. Parmelee et al. (1976) described many prenatal and perinatal factors that determine in part the future infant growth and development; they found that for many vulnerable children such growth patterns were pathological.

An additional, important variable in planning programs for primary prevention of child abuse is recognizing the special role of the child itself. Researchers must examine all process-oriented dimensions of caregiver interaction—such as the intensity and nature of social stimulation within the family, quantity and quality of physical touching, and the nature of mother-infant interaction during the neonatal and postnatal periods. The importance of the presence or absence of such stimulus interaction has been noted by Klaus and Kennell (1970) and by Leifer et al. (1972), the latter stating that the amount of contact a mother has with her newborn may be associated not only with the quality of later mothering, but also with mother's satisfactions in social relationships outside of the family. Therefore, such infant-initiated activity as smiling, cooing, and reaching out to the mother are major variables that must also be carefully studied in understanding attachment theory relationships important in primary prevention of child abuse.

Recognizing that children identify with and model their behavior after their parents, it is important to realize that the difficult child, the slow-to-warm-up child, and the easygoing child possess observable behavioral and temperamental characteristics that can play a significant and contributory role in family and domestic violence. The maturational growth of a competent, normal infant or an infant at risk from prenatal, perinatal, and postnatal complications can be measured in terms of the specific contributions of the child and its role in the infant-parent relationship. Findings obtained in clinical and research studies can thus make for the preventive application of specifically needed primary care strategies by combined health delivery teams of pediatric and child care specialists in order to eliminate the epidemic of neglect and abuse of children.

Recognizing that even the normal, healthy child under the "wrong" family conditions can be a victim of violence and/or neglect, it is even more understandable that the premature infant must be considered "a child at risk." Korner

(1974) enumerates many increasing risks for the continually crying, nonsooth-
able child, especially with reference to the young, inexperienced mother, whose
feelings of incompetence and inadequacy as a caregiver are negatively reinforced
by such continual or sporadic crying. It is increasingly evident that the spectrum
of child rearing and child discipline, ranging from appropriate parental responses
to violent physical abuse and even death, are products of complex, personal-
social factors interfacing within and among the parent, the child, and the family.
For example, Beckwith (1976), in describing the caregiver-infant interaction and
development of the high-risk infant, states that prenatal and perinatal factors
may determine not only the probability of survival of newborns, but may also
put them at greater statistical risk during their childhood. Leiderman and
Seashore (1975, p. 213) concur on the importance of understanding the reciprocal social interactions between mother and infant, stating, "The study of mothers
of premature and full-term infants showed that the type and amount of social
interaction between the human mother and her infant in the immediate post
partum period can influence the mother's subsequent behavior and attitudes
towards the infant." Pasamanick (1975, p. 550) reviewed studies supporting the
hypothesis that premature children or those from abnormal pregnancies have
lowered irritability thresholds, the results of which can be a source of increased
pressure on the already physically and emotionally distraught mother. Lacking
material and affectional supports, having conflicting and ambivalent feelings
about the pregnancy and/or the newborn child, such a mother often becomes
the primary abuser of a newborn high-risk child.

Applied clinical findings have also substantiated the value of the attachment-
dependency theory as a means of predicting later parenting behavior. Using
movies of mother-infant interaction in the delivery room, Gray et al. (1976)
accurately predicted later parenting behavior. His filming of the birthing process
of several mothers showed varying patterns of acceptance and rejection of newborns by the mothers. A follow-up study of these families revealed a good degree
of correlation between early bonding behavior and later child-rearing attitudes
and parenting practices. For those mothers with positive early emotional out-
reaching to the newborn child, a psychologically meaningful and healthy attachment and child-parent closeness were noted later. For mothers more distanced
from their newborn, evidence of familial conflict and child-parent estrangement
was found.

A more recent but similar technique of videotaping of birthing by Schmitt
and the American Academy of Pediatrics (1979) also demonstrated varying
degrees and styles of parent-to-child outreach that can be used to identify
possible high-risk newborn infants and their mothers. Such immediate verbal
responses as "he's ugly, he doesn't look like me, I didn't want a boy" should be
regarded by the delivery room staff as indicators of maternal stress and potential
later rejection of the newborn. It is therefore important to explore the attitudes

of both parents to the newborn to see whether the present parental feelings and family environment can provide the necessary physical and emotional elements of caring, affection, and nurturance needed by the infant. If such necessary elements of adequate parenting are not present, immediate primary prevention should involve the following: (1) close postnatal observation of the mother-infant interaction, (2) infant-mother classes for positive parenting and understanding of developmental milestones, (3) inclusion of a parent aide or a family member as a support for the anxious, insecure parents, and (4) frequent home visits and regularly scheduled appointments to the well-baby clinic.

Who Are the High-Risk Children and Families?

There are multiple socioeconomic and sociocultural factors that predispose a child and its family to domestic violence. Successful intervention by health professionals in many communities is limited because of meager manpower resources. However, in the areas of education, service delivery, and applied research, much knowledge is available to both the lay and professional communities. This knowledge of resources, effectively applied and directed toward high-risk families and populations in greatest need, can result in a significant reduction in the incidence of parental abuse and neglect of children. Although available birth control methods have reduced the incidence of pregnancy in middle-income, young, unwed females, the increasing number of abortions and rising birth rate in lower-income families identify this population as a high-risk group. Absence of planned parenthood clinics and minimal sex education programs, especially in economically deprived minority cultures, are identified daily in almost every emergency room and obstetrics department of county hospitals, nationwide, as predictors of future high risk parenting. The following case history reflects many characteristics of such an abusing, high-risk, child-parent relationship.

A single, 16-year-old, white mother, separated from her parents, presented in the emergency room with an eight-month female infant that was in obvious medical and nutritional need. The child had two bruises on the buttocks, healing cigarette burns on the palm of one hand, and a swollen right forearm (later identified as fractured); her dress was filthy and she was infested with fleas. History revealed the mother to be living alone, unsupported materially and emotionally by the father of the infant, and engaged in prostitution and drug pushing in order to survive in a ghetto-type community. Skilled interviewing by the emergency room staff plus documented radiological and clinical findings substantiated the diagnosis of battered-child syndrome (Caffey, 1972). The infant was immediately placed in protective custody. After medical treatment, a juvenile court placed the infant in a suitable foster home for up to one year. The mother was required to undergo weekly psychotherapy and attend parenting classes, the expectation being that by the end of the child's temporary placement period the mother would gain a better understanding of the basic principles of child growth and development. The multidisciplinary hospital- and community-based team of health and Protective Services professionals felt that the child could later be safely returned to the biological mother.

While an important goal of child abuse intervention is, when possible, return of the child to its biological parents, the most important responsibility of the intervention professionals is to ensure the continued physical and emotional security and safety of the child. When these conditions cannot be met the child may be temporarily or even permanently removed from the home of the biological caregivers. Such an ultimate and well-considered decision by a professional staff should be made without guilt and with the conviction that the safety and welfare of the child must supersede the parent's right for the continued care and rearing of the child.

The premature infant is always a high-risk infant. The elements contributing to a premature birth frequently cause anxiety and pain for the expectant parents, shaping, at least temporarily, ambivalent or negative feelings and fears with regard to the newborn. After delivery, medically indicated mother-infant separation may interfere significantly with immediate and/or early attachment and bonding. The separation of an acutely ill premature infant from its mother delays the formative moment when the mother and, hopefully, the father can share the arrival of the newborn child. The lost or delayed opportunity to "regard" the newborn, to view for the first time the sex of the child, and to count its fingers and toes; the inability of the mother and father to hug each other and to share the joy as they look at their baby *en face* and accept the newborn infant as a lifelong, meaningful link in the family circle—all of these are opportunities and experiences whose absence can impair the development of healthy child-parent attachment, bonding, and trust.

What is the effect of short- or long-term interruption of the bonding process? Opinions vary. To understand the consequences, one must examine the theoretical positions in child development. Bonding—the experiencing of emotional and physical intimacy between infant and parent—is best understood by examining closely the theories of attachment, social learning, and child growth and development. Rutter (1974) provides a detailed and comprehensive reassessment of the literature on bonding, placing in perspective the opponents and proponents of bonding theory. The studies are exciting but incomplete. Continued research is necessary to establish more definitively the short-term and long-term effects of neonatal and early postnatal separation on mother and infant.

Who then are the high-risk infants and children? They are, to name but a few: the unwanted child; the child conceived out of wedlock; the child with a single parent; the physically or mentally handicapped child; the chronically crying and colicky child; the premature child; and the highly irritable, drug-dependent newborn with a substance-abusing mother. These are some of the high-risk infants (Bolton, Laner, and Kane, 1980). The special demands to properly nurse and care for such children are for many mothers frequently overwhelming. Compounding the risk to these children is the early hospital discharge of indigent mothers and newborns into an economically disadvantaged community with little or no available medical, psychological, and social welfare resources for the family (Kinard and Klerman, 1980).

The child with nonorganic failure to thrive (FTT) syndrome is invariably a product of inadequate nurturance and parental neglect. When falling below the third percentile by weight, an infant is by definition an FTT child. Acute emotional withdrawal, failure to respond to verbal and behavioral stimulation, physical emaciation, and delayed growth are observations characteristically noted upon medical examination. After only several days of in-hospital care, the nonorganic FTT infant will almost always have a significant weight gain and will reach out, responding to nursing care with noticeable behavior and emotional animation. This affectional response to such parent-surrogate stimulation can provide much of the temporary psychological bonding needed for normal growth and development. In many marasmus infants and children described by Spitz (1945), there was found a similar absence of early infant-parent stimulation, with extreme and chronic emotional deprivation. Early anaclitic dependence and attachment are at this immediate postnatal period essential ingredients of the infant-mother relationship, ingredients that are invariably missing in the nursing experience of the FTT child.

The sudden infant death syndrome (SIDS) has been studied with reference to possible child abuse, especially where coroner findings are obscure and suggestive of nonaccidental death. The occurrence of a SIDS death requires careful and sensitive professional exploration of the infant-parent relationship, for, in the great majority of such deaths, there is found no evidence of parental neglect or inflicted willful trauma. Insensitive interrogation and accusatory statements made by investigators to innocent family members arouse justifiable and intense rage and intolerable guilt within the parents. Unfounded accusations can lead to family withdrawal as a means of avoiding judgmental looks and insensitive inquiry from neighbors. Although only a very small percentage of the 10,000 SIDS deaths occurring annually in the United States are later identified as child abuse, neglect, or death by homicide, the pediatrician will occasionally be involved in the investigation and diagnosis of a SIDS death or a near-miss sudden infant death syndrome. Knowing the medical and psychological correlates of child abuse and SIDS, the physician can fulfill an important diagnostic role in making final determination of an unexplained infant death. In the rare case that a SIDS death is in fact a willful act of negligence, violence, or homicide, the authorized physician has a responsibility to make the necessary disclosure. When in such a family there exist other siblings, it is essential that early preventive medical-legal intervention be undertaken to protect the lives of the other children potentially at risk. For the vast majority of innocent, guilt-ridden mothers and fathers who are victims of medicine's incomplete understanding of SIDS, the physician and all members of the health intervention team can be of immense personal support, as they provide reassurance and understanding to the surviving family members.

With a still incomplete understanding of SIDS, it is hoped that the findings of Valdez-Dapena (1978) will provide an increased incentive for researching the ultimate causes of such undiagnosed deaths. She writes: "Despite the fact that anatomic, histologic, and physiological differences between groups of (SIDS) infants have been described in detail, there is not as yet a single one of these differences that can be employed before or after death, as a predictive or diagnostic criterion . . . nor is there as yet one positive criterion that the pathologist can use to identify the subject at autopsy."

Recent research in dwarfism and delayed growth responses has brought attention to an additional high-risk group of children who are potential victims of failure to thrive and/or child abuse (Money and Needleman, 1976). Associated behaviors accompanying impaired endocrine functioning in psychosocial dwarfism include unusual eating and drinking behavior, sleep deprivation, night roaming, social distancing, enuresis, encopresis, pain agnosia, elective mutism, defiant aggressiveness, tantrums and crying spells, compensatory hyperkinesis, retarded motor development and intellectual growth, and a history of pathological family relations, including physical and emotional neglect and cruelty. Subsequent to accurate diagnosis and laboratory analysis of pituitary growth hormone, and with both psychological and hormonal therapy, the syndrome of abuse dwarfism is reversible. The parent's own psychopathology must also be identified and treated in order to effect necessary changes in the family milieu (Money, 1977). Confirming Money's description of the Munchausen-like behaviors of several such patients (mendacious, deceitful, and expert at hoodwinking professionals) are the findings of Meadow (1977), who reported two cases of child abuse in which the histories as given by the mothers were deliberately and consistently falsified. Psychologically, both mothers were labeled as having hysterical personalities, being depressed, and using their children's illnesses and subsequent hospitalizations as a means of providing a sheltered hospital environment and friendly medical-nursing staff for their own dependency needs. Such parenting behaviors are classical examples of the role-reversal behaviors of abusing parents, as reported by Morris and Gould (1963).

The depressed or suicidal latency-age or early adolescent child should always be carefully screened and interviewed in order to elicit a possible history of earlier physical or sexual abuse (Paulson, in press). Clinical studies and follow-up research on earlier abused children show many adult sequelae, such an aggressiveness, alcoholism, divorce, mental retardation, plus physical and/or sexual abuse toward their own children. It is surprising, however, that in spite of such acute physical and emotional trauma, the child psychology and child psychiatry literature make hardly any reference to suicidal behavior of young children being related to ongoing or earlier violent abuse and maltreatment (Paulson and Stone, 1974, 1978). Paulson (in preparation), in a study of the relationship between child abuse and childhood suicidal behavior, examined three such cases, one of which is reported below.

A single, 40-year-old female was referred for psychotherapy following an unconsummated affair in which the size of the partner's erect penis precipitated a sudden acute terror, avoidance of penetration, and later, uncontrolled fears of wanting to scream when in a relationship of sexual intimacy. Subsequent history revealed that the patient had been molested and raped by her father beginning at the age of four years and, following his return to the home fives years later, was again raped at the age of 10. Shortly afterward, the father died under conditions that indicated probable suicide. Although the mother was aware of the earlier sexual abuse, the patient had been given no emotional support or psychotherapy to help her adjust to the inflicted sexual, and at times physical, abuse. The patient, at age 11, lacking any kind of family support, fearful of men, and experiencing massive and ambivalent feelings of love and hate toward her recently deceased father, purposefully ran in front of an approaching truck with intent to kill herself. The suicide attempt was unrecognized by the mother, and the patient was severely punished for being careless and "not looking where she was going." Subsequent successful psychotherapy identified the roots of her fears of screaming and of sex as related to the early experience of intercourse at age five, when she screamed from the pain and fear of her father's sexual penetration. Tragically, neither the mother, a nurse, nor the family physician were at that time aware of the twofold trauma: (1) the recurring rape and sexual molestation by the father and (2) the concomitant acute depression and guilt, in which the attempted suicide was the only perceived escape from the terror of sexual and physical abuse.

Case histories and clinical research have identified many pediatric conditions and categories of children whose idiosyncratic emotional and/or physical status places them at high risk for abuse, neglect, and maltreatment by their parents. It is imperative that the emotional and physical health of all pediatric patients be preserved. Only through the continuing vigilance and understanding provided by the pediatric and child health specialists will high-risk children be saved from purposeful or accidental maltreatment by abusing or abuse-prone parents (Kenny and Clemmens, 1975).

Techniques for Identifying High-Risk Parents

Understanding the ultimate goal of child trauma intervention to be effective and complete prevention, researchers stress that greater attention must be given to techniques for the early identification of "at-risk" parents and families. Frankenburg and Camp (1973) classified basic conepts in screening, establishing primary guidelines for future research, and identifying such high-risk parents. They state that any good screening instrument must possess "sensitivity" in being able to identify high-risk subjects and at the same time must have "specificity" in being able to identify low-risk subjects. Eisenberg (1973), however, cautioned that the identification of a potential behavioral problem may result in the actual creation of such a problem. Recognizing the epidemic nature of child maltreatment and the need for primary prevention intervention, Paulson et al. (1975a) developed an MMPI scale (Minnesota Multiphasic Personality Inventory) for identifying "at-risk" abusive parents; this was followed by later studies using psychometric profiles and statistical procedures for identifying abusive parents (Paulson, 1975, 1976). Subsequently, the Parent Attitude Research Instrument (PARI) was used to further examine clinical and statistical inferences valuable in understanding abusive mothers (Paulson et al., 1977).

Helfer et al. (1977) designed a 50-item questionnaire found experimentally useful in identifying parents who might have problems interacting with their children. However, in examining the potential risk in such early identification of unusual child-rearing practices, Helfer cautioned that the ability to distinguish a group that will physically abuse or seriously neglect one or more children will probably never be possible. He stated further that screening methods now available can only identify parents who may have a potential problem with parent-child interaction. What is possible, however, Helfer emphasized, is the ability to identify "at-risk" parents or future parents who themselves had unfortunate childhood experiences that may be manifested by unusual child rearing as they themselves become parents. Moreover, one of the most readily accessible times for inexpensive, efficient mass screening or mass intervention is when the pregnant woman comes in for prenatal care or delivery at a hospital. "Those who are most available to be screened are pregnant women coming to offices and clinics for prenatal care and subsequently going to hospital for delivery. . . . We have no good evidence that women who use private practitioners in hospitals have fewer problems with child rearing than those who are less well off financially and use public facilities. Care must be taken to assess all groups in the screening program" (Helfer, 1976, p. 187).

Gray et al. (1976, p. 389) express cautious hopefulness in reporting on the prediction of child abuse in their Colorado study, stating:

> Using interviews; questionnaires; and labor, delivery, and postpartum observations, a sample of 100 mothers was identified as 'high-risk' for abnormal parenting practices and placed in an intervention versus a non-intervention program. Results showed the following three outcomes: 1) A high-risk group was successfully identified by peri-natal screening procedures; 2) Five children in the non-intervention program were hospitalized with severe inflicted injury, but none from the intervention group or the low-risk, control group; and 3) Labor, delivery, and nursery observations provide the most accurate predictive information. Interview and questionnaires did not add significantly.

Hunter (1976) stated that the degree of risk for parental abuse or neglect can be predicted before the newborn child leaves the hospital. She identified eight family characteristics associated with high risk, such as a family history of abuse or neglect, financial problems, inadequate child care, childishly dependent parents, social isolation, nonacceptance of the pregnancy, apathetic maternal attitudes, and a major psychiatric diagnosis in at least one parent. The data were gathered while the mother and infant were still in the hospital. Follow-up one year later showed no abuse in the low-risk families, but episodes of abuse and neglect occurring in the high-risk families in spite of social and mental health intervention given when the high risk was first identified. Hunter also reported that high-risk infants were usually firstborn, tended to be more sickly than low-risk babies, their hospital stay was twice as long, and they were more apt to have congenital defects and other residual medical problems.

If health professionals generalize from Hunter's findings that "child abuse or neglect occurred to one out of six of the total number of infants involved in the study" (16 percent), then there is indeed a national crisis involving present-day parenting practices. Hunter concluded: "Ideally, high-risk for maltreatment should be identified pre-natally, but the striking lack of prenatal care of many of our high-risk mothers suggests that for the present, the time of delivery may continue to be the only opportunity."

The current status of research in the area of primary intervention and prediction through early identification is both controversial and limited. The delivery room observation studies of Kempe (Gray et al., 1976) and Schmitt (1979) are exciting, although expensive and not practical for the screening of large numbers of expectant mothers. Helfer's screening instrument is a promising scale, needing continued cross-validation on groups of high-risk parents from many socio-economic, cultural, and ethnic backgrounds. The psychometric scales and profiles derived by Paulson et al. (1974b, 1975a, 1975b, 1976, 1977) also require further cross-validation and application to a variety of subsamples of parents and caregivers. While highly valid and reliable prediction of future parenting practices is still to be achieved, awareness of its need and continuing interdisciplinary research collaboration will hopefully provide further answers. Parmelee et al. (1976), in studying biological factors associated with high-risk infants, similarly concluded that "the strength of prediction for a pregnancy or perinatal events has been very weak . . . especially for single events. . . . There is difficulty predicting the outcome even if an individual is considered at higher risk on the basis of pregnancy and perinatal problems."

Pediatric and child development specialists have identified high-risk child-rearing practices in abusive parents. Many pediatric conditions have also been documented that influence present and future growth patterns in children. However, minimal prospective data have yet been gathered that clearly identify and measure relationships of prenatal and neonatal parental attitudes to later normal and pathological milestone developments of the child. There is a moral and medical urgency, and a professional responsibility, for early identification of "at-risk" children and families. There is a need to validate existing and new procedures for screening, prediction, and prevention based not on pathologically labeled families, but on families who are a representative cross-section of America. Zigler (1976), in passing the torch of responsibility to the professional community, stated:

> Theoretical and empirical research efforts (in child abuse) remain primitive and rudimentary. . . . The knowledge base is much too limited to direct us to any socially acceptable and realistic intervention of far-reaching effectiveness. . . . Our ability to help individuals cannot outdistance relevant and valid information about them. If there is anything that must be done first and done correctly, it would be the development of the knowledge base that is prerequisite for cost-effective intervention. Our society is willing to engage in secondary intervention but is almost totally disinterested in primary prevention.

Zigler has given a challenge to society that can be accepted through continuing and persistent research in those clinical-theoretical areas of pediatric health sciences involved in the assessment and evaluation of biological and psychosocial concomitants of positive, effective parenting. He admonishes that if present and future generations of children and families are to be protected from inadequate parenting, then procedures for early identification and subsequent preventive intervention must be found. While preparation for positive parenting should ideally begin in the home and be carried on in meaningful programs of elementary and high school education, the reality is that for many health delivery professionals the first opportunity for recognizing future potential "at-risk" parenting is during the prenatal or neonatal examination.

Knowing that for an increasing number of disadvantaged families, parents, and parents-to-be there exists minimal opportunity for adequate prenatal and postnatal care, health care communities must work closely with affiliated resources, such as public health, the Red Cross Society, and local planned-parenthood clinics. Integrating lay workers and home visitors into the health team will provide opportunities for preventive health care for many high-risk mothers and families in both rural and urban centers.

SECONDARY INTERVENTION AND TREATMENT OF ABUSIVE PARENTS AND CAREGIVERS

Knowing that abuse and maltreatment of children is multicausal, it is important to recognize that no one therapeutic approach will be successful in treating any broad spectrum of abusing parents. In addition to recognizing the sociocultural and socioeconomic factors contributing to abuse of children (Gil, 1970; Gelles, 1973), any dynamic treatment program must also explore the following etiologic factors: (1) the family heritage of child abuse, in which the present maltreatment often is only one in a series of earlier, multigenerational abuses occurring within the family (Green, Gaines and Sandgrund, 1974); (2) the psychopathology of the relationship between the father and the mother and how such relationship conflicts affect the care and welfare of the child (Paulson and Blake, 1967; Paulson et al., 1974a); (3) the particular psychopathology of each of the parents with reference to impulse control, absence of conscience, intellectual retardation, psychotic or borderline ego functioning, and capacity for adapting to stress (Paulson et al., 1975a, 1977); (4) the particular nature of the child—mental, physical, social, and emotional (Martin, 1976; Green, 1978; Lewis and Rosenblum, 1974); and (5) the accumulated, immediate life events that occur at any moment and in conjunction with any or all of the above, predispose a parent at a moment of stress to suddenly act out frustrations by displacing negative, and at times violent, feelings upon a scapegoat child (Steele and Pollock, 1974; Spinetta and Rigler, 1972).

In using multiple therapy interventions, one must also recognize that not all individuals can or will benefit from treatment. Those parents motivated for help and willing to accept the need for change have a better prognosis. An admission of personal inadequacy and failure in parenting, a capacity for emotional insight, a willingness to risk self-exploration and confrontation from peers and therapists, and a determination to persist in an extended form of treatment (be it individual or group) are attributes that contribute to successful intervention. In contrast, denial of feelings; chronic projection of blame upon individuals, agencies, or society; and nonacceptance of the responsibility for inflicted injury or trauma are attitudes and behaviors that are countertherapeutic.

Psychotherapeutic Modalities

The last two decades of child abuse treatment have seen the application of multiple treatment modalities. The decade of the 1960s saw traditional case work intervention followed by varied techniques of group treatment, and, less frequently, individual therapy (Elmer and Gregg, 1967; Helfer and Kempe, 1974; Paulson et al., (1974a). Psychiatric studies of parents who abuse their children provided detailed descriptions of the psychopathology of both parents, whether they were active or passive abusers (Flynn, 1970; Helfer and Kempe, 1974). As clinical research of abusing parents expanded, there was increased use of questionnaires, inventories, and psychological assessment procedures, each designed to aid either in the description of the psychopathology of maltreating parents or in the early identification and prediction of high-risk parents (Frankenburg and Camp, 1973; Helfer, 1975, 1976; Paulson et al., 1974b, 1975a, 1975b, 1977; Paulson, Schwemer and Bendel, 1976).

The dysfunctional family was studied in terms of violence within the family (Steele, 1976; Helfer and Kempe, 1974); impairment in parent-infant bonding (Klaus and Kennell, 1970; Beckwith, 1976); family pathology (Ounsted, Oppenheimer, and Lindsay, 1974; Lynch, 1975; Paulson and Blake, 1969; Paulson, 1978a); early recognition and prevention of potential problems in family interaction (Helfer and Kempe, 1976); and perinatal assessment of mother-infant interaction (Parmelee et al., 1976). Each of these areas of study provided information and knowledge that, augmented by federal resources and trained community professionals, resulted in an explosion of research studies and findings in the decade of the 1970s.

For affluent individuals able to afford private-practice fees and motivated toward a long-term, intensive treatment program, individual psychotherapy is occasionally the therapy of choice. However, therapists' negative countertransference feelings and lack of experience in working with physically and sexually abusing parents often make for minimal referral resources, even in highly urban areas (Helfer, 1975). Increased professional responsibility regarding reporting of suspected abuse has resulted in a tremendous number of identified high-risk children and families being referred to mental health centers. Group psychotherapy was then seen as the expedient treatment, primarily because of the large number of referrals and the minimum treatment resources available. However, as the results of state and federally funded programs in child abuse intervention become known, it is increasingly evident that group therapy for the great majority of abusing parents is the treatment of choice not because of limited resources, but because it, as a modality of intervention, has a better success rate with regard to decrease of the incidence of abuse and remission of symptoms of parent and family psychopathology.

Lynch and Ounsted (1976), in reporting on a residential therapy approach to the inpatient hospital treatment of the entire family, describe positive outcomes gained from such a medical, ward-based, psychiatric-social assessment and treatment intervention. Adapted to the needs of each family member, such a therapeutic program provided for verbal release and catharsis of feelings, role modeling, admission of responsibility for the earlier abuse, and abreaction of emotions related to the family violence. Identifying attachment to the treatment center as a "liberating bond," the authors, in summarizing their success, state (Lynch and Ounsted, 1976, pp. 204-206):

> It (the residential center) is an open relationship, a new experience for these families, who have only known closed, destructive relationships. From this stable bond they are able to go on to make new bonds with their child, spouse, and other people in their lives. . . . An inpatient program that incorporates medical, psychiatric, social work, and legal expertise provides an accurate and comprehensive assessment of each family. In treatable cases, medical treatment, practical help, and the initiation of ongoing psychotherapy make it possible for these troubled families to be rehabilitated without prolonged separations.

In studying the curative factors in group psychotherapy in general, Yalom (1975, pp. 3-4) lists 11 primary concepts or categories. Each of these has direct relevance to the successful treatment of physically and sexually abusing parents. Applied along with treatment modalities involving male-female cotherapy in a parent-surrogate model (Paulson and Chaleff, 1973), these concepts offer, for the motivated family, increased hope for the elimination of abuse and the positive therapeutic rehabilitation of the family. These curative factors are:

1. Instillation of hope.
2. Universality of experience: recognizing that others also have similar behaviors.
3. Imparting of information and realistic understanding of problems.
4. Altruism: the giving and receiving of support and reassurance.
5. The corrective recapitulation of the primary family group, where in many groups, the male-female cotherapist team closely simulates parental configurations and interactions in the patient's earlier childhood.
6. Development of socializing techniques.
7. Incorporating of imitative behavior as an effective therapeutic force.

8. Interpersonal learning, such as insight, and working through of the transference.
9. Group cohesiveness: the analogue of "relationship" in individual therapy.
10. Catharsis: the purging of emotional experiences through abreaction and verbalization.
11. Existential factors: the philosophic acceptance of life and death and their relationship to ongoing life events, for which each parent must be personally and ultimately responsible.

Psychotherapeutic intervention for the child as victim of family violence and parental abuse has only recently become a priority area for secondary intervention (Martin, 1976; Kass et al., 1976; Lynch, 1975; Parmelee et al., 1976). For the preverbal child, the primary intervention modality, in addition to adequacy of medical care, is the establishment of an environment of affection, caring, and emotional bonding (Beckwith, 1976). For many professionals, the inadequacies of a foster home are still preferred to the violence within the parental home. Except in the case of extreme threats to the life and safety of a child, many juvenile court judges within the dependency courts, however, still return children to custody of high-risk parents, in spite of medical and psychological contraindications for such a return; the courts feel that such affectional closeness and parent-child interaction is preferred to family separation and dislocation. For the verbal-age child, a variety of treatment modalities are available from a skilled and resourceful therapist. Play therapy; the use of puppets; finger paints and dolls; individual therapy; group therapy with similarly victimized peers; and, for the older children, family therapy are modalities that for many motivated families become important techniques for rehabilitation. For those children severely scarred emotionally and needing inpatient psychiatric care, there is available a 24-hour treatment unit providing the following: (1) strengthening of interpersonal skills through daily living with peers; (2) providing individual prescriptive education in a structured and psychologically oriented school program; (3) mandatory individual and group psychotherapy with emphasis on individual difficulties and conflictual child-parent relationships; and (4) working with other peers in a safe, family-ward setting, which fosters increased communication and understanding. In addition, family therapy where possible and chemotherapy when needed are additional resources available to maximize the rehabilitation of the hospitalized, psychiatrically ill, maltreated child. For physically and emotionally abused children, the 11 curative factors of group psychotherapy (Yalom, 1975) are as applicable as they are to adults.

Emotional neglect and psychological abuse of children are more difficult to identify and prove in a court of law; yet their consequences can be even more long standing and devastating than occasional physical punishment. Excessive verbal assault, such as belittling and sarcasm; inconsistency in the administration of discipline; constant family discord and negative child-parent interactions; and depriving the child of feelings of being loved, wanted, worthy, and respected—all these are aspects of emotional abuse, deprivation, and affectional starvation, which in later adolescence and in adulthood are seen as contributory or causal elements in delinquency and criminal behavior (California Department of Justice, 1978).

Where and how can such psychological abuse of children be best identified? The most effective means of identifying such abuse is in the schools. Here, for five of the seven days in each child's school life, the teacher and/or school nurse has an opportunity to observe multiple emotional and behavioral responses of the child. Indications of apathy, depression, and withdrawal should be noted and investigated, along with evidence of "acting out" and other disruptive classroom behaviors. Rigid and overly conforming behavior may be an index of a family milieu that is marked by extreme parental authority, personal humiliation, and suppression of feelings within the home. Withdrawal from peers, unexpected decline in academic performance, frequent absences from school without reasonable cause, inappropriate seeking of affection and attention from peers and teachers and exaggerated fears—all these are behavioral clues that, in the absence of pathological physical findings, should alert school authorities to the possibility of emotional and psychological abuse of a child.

If such emotional abuse is suspected and affirmed by the child, sibling, or others, then immediate remedial intervention is necessary. The parents should be carefully and sensitively interviewed in order to elicit their own conflict areas and reasons for such parenting failures. Referral of the family to a mental health facility or child guidance clinic should be made, with the professional agency extending as much additional support to the family as needed. In situations of acute psychological abuse, temporary out-of-home placement may be needed, not only to protect the child and perhaps siblings from further emotional trauma, but to provide the child with a new family environment free from emotional stress, an environment in which the emotionally abused child can experience a caring, loving relationship with parent-surrogate, adult caretakers. Hopefully, during this interim separation, therapeutic intervention for the parents and the involved child(ren) will result in the elimination of family tensions, a growing capacity for the parents to provide increased emotional understanding and sharing, and the fostering of deep and positive affectional relationships between the child and its parents.

The Health Visitor in the Home

The health visitor concept (Kempe, 1976) provides an opportunity for both primary prevention and secondary intervention. Recognizing the need for periodic health assessment, the health visitor, as a trained lay worker, can provide additional paramedical services to the family and at the same time release other medical and allied personnel for more demanding kinds of intervention. A more positive child-parent relationship can be fostered through prenatal, perinatal, and postnatal observations in the physician's office, the prenatal clinic subsequent to delivery, and later within the home of the parents. Critical information can be gained regarding parental attitudes toward bonding and attachment, husband-wife relationships that impact upon the present and future quality of parenting, and the availability of support systems and resources within and outside the family. Kempe recommends regular and frequent health visitor appointments in the first few months of life of the child, and continuing visits every six months until the child has reached school age. He states: "Health visitors are fully capable of determining which children are at risk, whether they are thriving adequately or not doing well, whether the child is unloved or deprived, whether the mother's inexperience or the father's lack of support are interfering with the care of the child" (Kempe, 1976, p. 944). All children have the right to be protected emotionally and physically from trauma and have a right to adequate and comprehensive health care. Early periodic screening, diagnosis, and treatment, Kempe feels, can determine not only the baseline medical status of the child; but such screening must, in addition, be oriented toward an evaluation of the emotional growth and development of the child and implementation of remedial measures when child-parent stress is identified. Kempe concludes (p. 947):

> 1) When parenting is defective or blatantly harmful, prompt, effective intervention by society is essential. . . . 2) Universal, egalitarian, and compulsory health supervision, in the broadest sense, is the right of every child. . . . (3) Predicting and prevention of child abuse is practical, if standard observations are made early and . . . (4) the utilization of visiting nurses . . . or indigenous health visitors who are successful, supportive, mature mothers . . . is the most inexpensive, least threatening and most efficient approach for giving the child the greatest possible chance to reach his potential.

Cedar House: A Neighborhood Family Renewal Center Concept

While traditional programs of hospital- and clinic-based multidisciplinary treatment provide excellent rehabilitation for those highly urban areas adjacent to available medical center resources, most communities—urban, suburban, and rural—lack such opportunities. What then can a concerned community and dedicated professionals and lay persons do to provide the needed treatment for those families overwhelmed by parenting responsibilities who manifest their parenting failures by abuse and neglect of their children? Cedar House, in Long Beach, is a home-based, residentially located treatment center whose philosophy is that "treatment of abusing families is most successful if done in a non-threatening, domestic setting; that a multidisciplinary team approach is important in working with high-stress families inclined to violence and physical abuse; that 'saturation therapy' and other non-traditional treatment techniques developed at Cedar House . . . have been effective in reducing the incidence of abuse in families and in improving their level of functioning; that a treatment team must be reinforced by a strong volunteer system, good communication and strong ties between professionals and organizations that interface with the clients and good support from the community at large" (ICAN, 1980, p. iii).

Conceived by two dedicated and inspired social workers in 1974, Cedar House has now become a nationally recognized, community-supported treatment center that provides multiple resources for abused children, their parents, and the family. For the children, rehabilitation includes play therapy, individual and group treatment, peer group support, crisis nursery care for the infant, and child development programs for the parents. Treatment resources for the parents include individual and group psychotherapy, family and couples' counseling, crisis intervention, parent aide or lay therapy counseling, 24-hour hot-line counseling, and parent education classes. Where indicated, treatment services for the families also include individual therapy, family therapy, and, when necessary, psychiatric consultation and referral. Additional family supports are: homemaking services; free legal consultation; income and employment counseling; out-of-home care for a placed child; and multiple social reinforcements and supports, such as group outings, picnics, and peer socializing. Cedar House is now supported financially by a major industrial corporation and has been strongly endorsed by the Los Angeles County Interagency Council on Child Abuse and Neglect (ICAN). Such endorsements by the community and the many professional groups and individuals identified with child abuse intervention attest to the high regard and respect for Cedar House as a concept and as a functioning rehabilitative center. It is a model that should be emulated by communities large and small.

Children's Village, USA (CVUSA):
A Residential Treatment Program for Abused Children and Their Families

Founded and funded by International Orphans Incorporated (I.O.I.), Children's Village, located in Beaumont, California, just east of Los Angeles County, exists for several purposes: (1) as a pilot project demonstrating the rehabilitative value of a unique, residential treatment center; (2) as a training center for professionals and paraprofessionals working in the area of child abuse; (3) as a treatment resource for a limited number of abused children and their families;

and (4) as a research and resource center that will advance the art, the knowledge, and understanding of constructive family and child development theory and practice (Children's Village, 1979). Designed to accommodate up to 100 children, ages 2–12 years, Children's Village has an interdisciplinary staff consisting of behavioral, social, and medical scientists who provide for the children an array of services, including a therapeutic preschool and day care program, individual and group therapy, and educational and recreational therapy. An extensive community outreach network provides treatment resources for the abusive and neglecting parents who, temporarily separated from their child(ren), can receive rehabilitation from a treatment agency close to their home. Working within such a network, the parents can prepare themselves emotionally and intellectually for that day when the rehabilitation provided them and their children will allow the safe return of their child to a home now free from emotional, physical, and domestic violence.

For those children permanently removed from their parents by order of the court, Children's Village works with the adoptive or foster parents, preparing them for their new parenting responsibilities and providing follow-up services as indicated. For the children cared for by CVUSA, there is an opportunity to heal the physical and emotional wounds inflicted earlier by overwhelmed parents who were unable to cope with the responsibilities of parenthood. For those abusing parents receiving help, an opportunity is provided for emotional and educational relearning, in order to make them more effective and emotionally stable caregivers. Through an extensive in-service and outreach program provided by professional and paraprofessional therapists, Children's Village provides a model network and paradigm of treatment that can be adopted by metropolitan communities nationwide.

Self-Help Treatment Resources

Because many communities have limited professional and financial resources to offer those with problems in living, there have sprung up highly successful rehabilitative programs organized and conducted by the very persons who have the greatest need for help. Alcoholics Anonymous is an example of the rehabilitative failures of health professions, and the success of alcoholics themselves, in developing a program of recovery based upon mutual support, sustained and constantly available outreach, and a recognition that alcoholism is an illness, not a sin.

With increasing numbers of identified abusing parents being self-referred or referred by the courts, schools, and Protective Services agencies; and with insufficient resources for receiving needed treatment, there began in 1970, in California, a self-help group of abusing mothers and fathers (later identifying themselves as Parents Anonymous) who took the initative to develop their own program of recovery. Supported later by federal funds, Parents Anonymous

(P.A.) spread nationwide; they now have chapters throughout the world. Based upon the concept of "unconditional positive regard" for each other, members find a bond of affection, a unity of purpose, and a shared common tragedy that unites them into a potent rehabilitative force. The chairperson of each chapter is drawn from the membership in the group, and as such this person functions as the active leader, the authority figure, one who must avoid judgmental and punitive attitudes toward group members, and the one who must realize that what members say is not necessarily what they are actually feeling. Working with the chairperson is the P.A. sponsor, a professional person who is asked to lead without seeming to do so and who takes "a 'back-seat' in the group situation by allowing the parent-Chairperson to be the active leader of the chapter. P.A. asks that whatever the Sponsor's professional background and experience, he make the commitment to the parent-as-leader model. Without this, there can be no P.A. chapter. It may be therapy . . . but it's not P.A." (Parents Anonymous, 1975, pp. 9-10).

Like all successful self-help groups, P.A. provides multiple resources for families who, in need, turn to the chapter members for either momentary respite or long-term help, support, and insight. Recognizing that P.A.'s concept of group interaction is not suitable for every person, P.A. is quick to refer to a responsible agency those members who cannot benefit from it. The chapters stress anonymity and confidentiality; they exchange telephone numbers, provide a 24-hour hot-line for each other and for the community at large, and provide educational resources and parenting classes for those members in need of parent education and knowledge of growth and development of children. P.A. identifies parental failure in terms of physical abuse, physical neglect, sexual abuse, verbal abuse, emotional abuse, and emotional neglect. Working closely with local health centers and Protective Services, P.A. fully acknowledges its responsibility to report cases of abuse and neglect and at the same time provide a continuing support to those families whose parenting failures manifest themselves through abuse and/or neglect of children. P.A. is a viable and powerful deterrent to abuse of children. Recognized worldwide, and continuing to receive federal funds for the support of its chapters, P.A. stands high in the regard with which the professional and lay community respect this self-help group for "striving to be better" mothers and fathers.

LAW ENFORCEMENT, PROTECTIVE SERVICES, AND LEGAL ISSUES IN REPORTING AND INVESTIGATING CHILD ABUSE AND NEGLECT

Reporting of Abuse and Neglect

State procedures for legally mandated intervention in cases of child abuse vary. In many states the criminal justice system is involved only to a minor degree, with county departments of social service assuming primary responsibility for the investigation and disposition of cases of suspected or identified child abuse and/or neglect. In those states where such investigation is primarily under the authority of Social Services, many professionals feel there is greater potential for more effective rehabilitation of the abusing family. Parents are not viewed within a criminal-model philosophy, and, except in cases of extreme brutality or willful death of a child, there is seldom legal or criminal prosecution of the perpetrator.

In other states however, the process of child abuse investigation and intervention is more oriented toward a judicial process philosophy, one in which the act of abuse or neglect is viewed in terms of statutes defining procedures and penalties for assault upon an individual. Such an investigative and dispositional approach may be seen as countertherapeutic and oriented toward punishment rather than toward rehabilitation. Those supporting the process of criminal justice intervention feel that such "legal clout" allows for a more thorough investigation, the administration of deserved punishment, and greater participation in therapy for parents mandated to undergo rehabilitation. Additionally, law enforcement involvement in the process of child abuse investigation allows for immediate, 24-hour response to crisis situations that at any moment may involve a life threat to the child. Immediate accessibility to the scene of a suspected abuse is not possible in those cases in which a Protective Services investigation is conducted without police officer involvement.

All 50 states mandate specifically enumerated professionals to report cases of suspected abuse and neglect. Those reporting must do so by telephone and in writing within a specified period of time, usually 36 hours. In all states those persons responsibly reporting are immune from both civil and criminal liability, even if the suspicion of abuse is later nonsubstantiated. In many states, there can be criminal and/or civil liabilities assessed against those guilty of failure to report suspected abuse (Ramsey and Lawler, 1974; Light, 1973; Isaacson, 1975). Those persons mandated to report abuse and severe neglect should clearly recognize that they are reporting only *suspicion* of maltreatment; they do not have the responsibility for verifying or proving such suspicions. That needed information is gathered by those agencies or services subsequently delegated to the investigation of suspected abuse of a minor.

Almost all states have a repository for compiling statewide cases of suspected or identified abuse and neglect. For some, this reporting is made to the state Department of Social Services, while in other states it is the criminal justice department that has the responsibility for the establishment and functioning of such a central registry of child maltreatment. Mandated reporters should be aware that reporting in and of itself does not necessarily mean that civil or criminal proceedings will automatically be initiated against the parent or perpetrator. It does mean, however, that such a report will initiate investigation by either county Protective Services or a local law enforcement agency in order to affirm or deny the allegation or suspicion of abuse and child endangering.

Investigation of Child Abuse and Neglect

What happens when a suspicion of serious child abuse is reported? In those states where Protective Social Services is the principal intervention agency, an immediate or early home investigation will be made. If the child is seen in any danger of continuing abuse or severe neglect, it will, along with other siblings, be taken into protective custody and placed under the jurisdiction of welfare or the juvenile court, pending a preliminary hearing. Subsequent investigation and dependency court decisions will, if the initial report is substantiated, result in the child either being returned to the parental home under close supervision, with recommended therapy for the parents, or the child will be placed out of home until such time as the home and the parents can adequately care for the child, both physically and emotionally. In only the most severe cases of maltreatment are criminal charges filed, and, if substantiated, the perpetrator can be given a jail term or suspended sentence with probation.

In those states—California, for example—where suspected child abuse and neglect is viewed more as a criminal violation of the law, there is an initial patrol officer response, followed by, in many highly urban communities, an intensive investigation by a specially trained team of law enforcement child abuse officers who, from the very beginning, collaborate closely with the local Protective Services Bureau in all phases of the pretrial investigation. Copies of all written reports received by the local police authority and/or health and welfare departments are then forwarded to the Bureau of Identification of the State Department of Justice in the state capitol. The report is then entered into a statewide central index to determine whether there is evidence of prior abuse, neglect, or molestation of either the victim or of another minor within the same family. The reporting law enforcement agency, the local juvenile probation office, and/or the welfare department are then notified immediately if the Child Abuse Unit record reveals any previous report of suspected or actual infliction of physical injury, sexual molestation, physical pain, or mental suffering on another family member or on the present victim. Subsequent Juvenile Dependency Court rulings then determine the immediate and long-term custody, care, and control of the minor child pending the outcome of court-recommended treatment, counseling, and/or parent education for the parents. If criminal charges are later filed against one or both parents, such action may result in acquittal; probation, usually with mandated therapy; incarceration for a determinate or indeterminate period of time; and/or later restriction of postincarceration parental rights, and visitation with the minor child.

In those cases where the reported abuse is of a relatively minor degree and does not require immediate law enforcement response, the investigation may be conducted by the Protective Services unit of the Department of Public Social Services. The Protective Services worker will visit the home and the school, talk with neighbors, and attempt to obtain any information necessary to support or refute the allegation. Cooperating with and notifying the local law enforcement agency involved maximizes the interagency investigation. If the charges are found to be minor, most often the child is left within the home under the supervision of the Child Protective Services worker, and the parents are encouraged to participate in counseling or in a parent education program. If the evidence of abuse is more severe, a petition is filed with the Dependency Court seeking temporary placement either with responsible relatives or in a county-licensed foster home. Such placements are usually for one year, with the Children's Services worker supervising the family and providing periodic reports to the Dependency Court regarding progress by parents and child as a function of voluntary or mandated counseling. Hopefully, with successful intervention, the child will be returned home. If therapy is unsuccessful, the minor may be continued as a dependent child of the court as long as the home and/or parents are unable to provide the necessary safety, security, and emotional sustenance for the child.

Discipline Versus Abuse

Investigation of suspected child abuse invariably brings into focus the concept of "discipline versus abuse." Discipline is clearly defined by Federal Public Law 93-247, yet within almost every subculture there are historical, family, and personal attitudes toward child rearing that constantly influence the nature of child rearing and child disciplining. Numerous legal opinions have been expressed with regard to the rights of the parent versus the rights of the child (Fraser, 1977a). In many cases, medical opinion is needed to substantiate suspected abuse and/or neglect. But even here there is much ambiguity in interpretation. For example, what is the role of family corporal punishment? Is corporal punishment considered abuse, for example, when only reddened brusing is caused? Furthermore, what is the degree of bruising necessary to establish abuse? Are handprints on the buttocks of a 10-year-old child different from strap marks imposed by the same parent? Even though psychological abuse leaves no visible marks, it is evident that the emotional trauma of verbal violence upon a child can be as traumatizing as severe spanking. It is this dilemma in distinguishing between discipline and abuse that is constantly faced by judges, educators, day care workers, emergency room and pediatric personnel, and parents.

Consideration must also be given to those numerous instances of "institutional abuse" identified increasingly in schools, residential centers, foster homes, and day care treatment facilities. In addition to intrafamily dynamics, many cultural, ethnic, and religious values equally influence child-rearing practices. The role of all such cultural attitudes and biases must be considered carefully in differentiating "appropriate discipline" from abuse of a child.

For those professionals involved in child abuse intervention and identification, it is essential that they be knowledgeable about recent medical and legal opinions specific to child abuse and neglect. Katz et al. (1977) have examined legal opinions on child abuse regarding the philosophy that the individual has a right to raise his child according to his own personal dictates. Difficulties and limitations of legal research are explored by the authors with regard to the classification of abuse and neglect as a crime versus a civil wrongdoing. Criminal statutes are examined that permit prosecution of those identified as responsible for abuse. Juvenile and family court procedures are described in terms of their assets and liabilities in child abuse adjudication. Katz et al. (1977, p. 155) write:

> Criminal prosecution of parents is rare, and the whole process has been criticized repeatedly as being ineffective and even detrimental to the treatment and prevention of abuse and neglect. Criminal prosecutions are lengthy and final civil dispositions on the child's future are usually delayed until the criminal process is completed. The result is that the child either spends an extended period of time in foster care, or being left with the family, is subjected to unusual tension. . . . The criminal process, furthermore, seems to do little to rehabilitate the parent. It serves only to alienate him further from his family and from those who seek to provide treatment for them or reinforce the parent's sense of frustration and inadequacy. If a parent is acquited, he may feel his conduct is vindicated and may have his battering tendencies strengthed, although his ordeal may make him more subtle and cunning. If he is convicted, the whole family may suffer from the separation of imprisonment or the diminishment of the family income by a fine. . . . The literature is unanimous in recommending prosecution only in cases which result in death or serious injury to the child.

Until recently, legal intervention in child abuse has focused primarily upon the right of parents to discipline their child as well as the right of parents for legal representation in all courts of law. There has been minimal concern with regard to the rights of the child and its representation in such courts of law. Fraser (1977a) discusses the concept of independent representation for the abused and neglected child, postulating the appointment of a guardian *ad litem**

*The literal translation of guardian *ad litem* is *guardian appointed by the court*. The basis of guardian *ad litem* arose from the 1967 United States Supreme Court ruling that a child is entitled to constitutionally guaranteed safeguards when its liberty is endangered. One of the rights enumerated is the right to independent representation by counsel.

to represent a child's independent interests in ongoing legal and Protective Services intervention. He stresses that independent representation is the only real solution to adequately protecting the abused or neglected child's interests. Because juvenile rights and interests are often in sharp variance with those of the parents, the child, of necessity, should have such independent representation. Further, the representation responsibilities of the investigating social worker are at times obscure, often resulting in the worker representing the best interests of the Department of Welfare rather than the specific interests of the child.

Historically, in terms of common law, the parents' control over their children was virtually limitless, with parental rights viewed as rights of care, custody, and control. The parent could physically discipline his child; he could instill religious and political beliefs; he could educate his child as he saw fit; he was entitled to the child's earnings and he could grant or withhold medical care (Fraser, 1977b). This doctrine of parental control is vital in terms of differentiating abuse from discipline. Of equal importance in child care and child rearing is the awareness that physical punishment has little positive effect in changing behavior; yet an earlier Supreme Court ruling upheld the right of the public school system to inflict corporal punishment upon a child. It is, however, evident that recent judicial rulings are recognizing more and more the rights of the minor for equal protection under the law. The concept of *parens patriae* within the family is being legally reinforced not only because of judicial concerns, but because of greater awareness on the part of professionals and society that corporal punishment and overly severe discipline are ineffective, illegal, and psychologically damaging procedures for coping with family stress, child-parent conflict, and infant management frustrations in parents.

COMMUNITY-BASED, MULTIDISCIPLINARY INTERAGENCY COLLABORATION

Abuse of children, multiple in causality, cannot be successfully investigated, diagnosed, or treated by any one single discipline or agency. A multiple-impact program involving a combination of health professionals and community agencies is needed. Cohen (1977), in examining the interface between multidisciplinary teams and the community, describes the evolution of the multidisciplinary child protection team in terms of a need for prompt interagency communication among professionals working with child abuse and neglect. Such a multidisciplinary team assumes that each professional has some expertise in the field, that each is willing and able to work with other disciplines, that sufficient information is presented upon which to make decisions, and that there will be a purposeful follow-up shared among all agencies involved in family intervention of child abuse and neglect.

Interagency coalitions operate on a set of assumptions that each subagency alone, having its own goals, policies, and organizational patterns, is dependent upon a collaborative and joint effort to maximize effective intervention for the abused child and its family. Many times the success or failure of such a coalition is a function of the personalities of the members of each agency and the degree to which they make a purposeful and concerted attempt to share, rather than to act as rivals in an adversary situation. The value of a successful interagency group is in its positive impact on the service delivery of each of the individual agencies. With a well-coordinated, community-based coalition of agencies and a committed, cooperative team of multidisciplinary child protection specialists, maximum success in child abuse intervention is possible (ICAN, 1980).

A coalition of community agencies is in many urban areas now identified as the local child abuse council, one that has in its membership representation from all concerned agencies and disciplines that in any way, directly or indirectly, interface with abused children and their families. In a number of states there has developed a statewide consortium of child abuse councils whose membership comprises representatives from each local council within the state. The Child Abuse and Neglect Resource Center of the Southwestern United States (HEW, Region IX), for example, defines the objectives of its statewide child abuse consortium as follows (Directions, 1980, p. 1):

1) to develop a model network to serve as a state-wide communication forum on child abuse related issues,

2) To consult and provide technical assistance to local child abuse councils in order to improve their efforts in fostering multidisciplinary involvement in the prevention and treatment of child abuse.

3) To study and make recommendations as appropriate, to public and private service agencies responding to child abuse.

Membership in such an organization should include Social Services, law enforcement, education, the juvenile courts, as well as representation from day care centers, substance abuse councils, probation departments, public and mental health associations, counseling centers, and medical-hospital professionals. On a national level, the federally funded United States National Center on Child Abuse and Neglect has an office for national dissemination of information and for funding areas of child abuse prevention and intervention (Besharov, 1977). Although limited in its budget, the National Center has provided support for pilot studies, demonstration programs, professional education, and research. The effectiveness of interagency collaboration, whether it be among local, state, or federal agencies or whether it be within a specific community, lies in the degree to which individual members can share ideas and resources and provide personal and professional support for each other's activities and programs.

BURNOUT: A COUNTERTRANSFERENCE PHENOMENON

The psychiatric literature is replete with descriptions of the transference relationship, an essential part of any therapeutic modality. The transference relationship is most times readily accepted and understood by the psychologically mature and professionally skilled psychotherapist. Such feelings, whether they are positive or negative, are those of the patient, and whatever the roots of such feeling, they must be understood, but they need not be "owned" by the therapist. Countertransference feelings, however—those feelings felt consciously and/or unconsciously by the therapist toward the patient—are a source of greater emotional stress for the health provider. He or she must acknowledge that such feelings are within the corpus of the therapist, and the expression, direction, and consequences of these feelings must be accepted by the therapist. Greenson (1959, pp. 1413-1414) wrote as follows:

> Counter-transference is a transference reaction of the therapist to his patient. Since it is a transference reaction it means the counter-transference is based on the unconscious, neurotic conflicts in the analyst's past, which make him react to the patient as though the patient were a significant figure in the analyst's past. . . . The therapist may react to the patient neurotically because of some stress or another source which is secondarily displaced onto the patient. The analyst may make errors of judgment from fatigue, boredom, etc. . . . Since counter-transference interferes with the capacity to use good judgment and to maintain a sufficient distance from the patient, or since the fear of counter-transference reactions may interfere with the empathy of the analyst, it is imperative that they be recognized and analyzed within the psychoanalyst. . . . When they occur repeatedly and are not amenable to self-analysis, it is a signal that the analyst should, himself, have some further psychoanalysis.

Twenty years after this statement was written, the related phenomenon of "burnout" became an index of occupational apathy and exhaustion. Burnout is identified especially in those occupations involving personal and intimate one-to-one relationships with others, relationships that are invariably associated with a variety of intense feelings of both a positive and negative nature. Greenson has identified boredom and depression as manifestations of therapist anxiety, which can be resolved either through self-analysis or, if necessary, through intense psychotherapy and psychoanalysis. However, for the great majority of present-day professionals working in a human services delivery agency, there are neither the financial resources nor the available opportunities for therapeutically resolving such feelings within the therapist relative to his/her patient. Maslach (1976, p. 16) writes:

There is little doubt that burn out plays a major role in the poor delivery of health and welfare services to people in need of them. . . . It is also a true factor in low worker morale, absenteeism, and high job turnover . . . (along) with other damaging indices of human stress such as alcoholism, mental illness, marital conflict, and suicide. . . . For the social welfare workers, one of the major signs of burn out was the transformation of a person with original thought and creativity on the job into a mechanical, petty bureaucrat. . . . Burn out is inevitable when a professional must care for too many people. Like a wire that has just too much electricity, the worker emotionally disconnects. . . . Steps can be taken to reduce the occurrence of burn out because its causes are rooted not in the permanent traits of people, but in specific social and situational factors which can be changed.

How then can the individual and the agency concerned about the phenomenon of worker breakdown prevent the emotional overload of workers? There can be reassignment of responsibilities; rest and recreation; time off; rotation of duties involving heavy patient-therapist pressures; and, most important, a recognition by the administrative and supervisory personnel that burnout is not a phenomenon associated with "the shirker," but is highly correlated with the performance of a dedicated, personally involved, person-oriented employee (Gunning, 1977). Maslach (1976, p. 22) states further:

Burn out rates are lower in those professionals who actively express, analyze, and share a personal feeling with their colleagues. Not only do they consciously get things off their chest, but they have an opportunity to receive constructive feedback from other people as they develop new perspectives and understanding of their relationships with their patients/ clients. This process is greatly enhanced if the institution sets some social outlets such as support groups, special staff meetings or workshops. In general, we found that those professionals who are trained to treat psychological problems were better able to recognize and deal with their own feelings.

Most of the literature on burnout focuses on the emotional pressures, the heavy case load, the lack of staff morale, and the limited support from supervisors as dynamic factors in the development of professional exhaustion. While such occupational hazards do generate malaise, depression, and job dissatisfaction, there has been little attention directed towards the impact of *negative* countertransference feelings as a dynamic element in child abuse burnout. The severe neglect and sexual abuse of children, the battering of an infant, and the violation of a child's right by a power-driven parent stir within health workers rage, anger, frustration, and at times even a wish for retaliation against the abusing perpetrator. While such feelings may be seen as "normal responses" of any concerned citizen, they are, in the eyes of many professionals, often viewed as unacceptable, indicating the need for therapy on the part of that worker. While many mothers will say of their physically or sexually abusing partner, "Damn him; he should be emasculated," such feelings, attitudes, and expressions cannot be readily acknowledged by the therapist. Many times the continuing, thankless emotional investment in individual and/or group therapy of violent parents becomes even more exacerbated by the awareness of the violent emotional and physical trauma inflicted upon the infant. King (1976, p. 44) states: "Counter-transference-based responses are an integral part of the therapist's reaction to the patient; and in that sense they are inevitable. They should, however, be as limited and controlled as possible, and used to understand and work with the patient's emotional problems." King, in describing counter-tranference feelings in working with violence-prone youth makes conclusions that can appropriately be generalized to adults who inflict violence upon their children. She states (1976, p. 52):

> The double pull of attraction and repulsion to the antisocial drives of these youth raises severe problems in finding a viable approach for help. Most people, professionals, social workers, educators, are either caught up in a system of unhelpful, often inappropriate responsive behaviors and feelings to these kids, or they reject them altogether and so get rid of the problem. The psychoanalytic concept of counter-transference . . . provides a dynamic framework for cataloguing feelings and recognizing their interplay in the child caring, educative, and clinical process. . . . Acknowledgement and sharing of negative counter-transference . . . as well as realistic feelings evoked by the impact of a given situation can be most beneficial in treatment.

The wise supervisor, cognizant of the occupational hazards of professional burnout, must develop preventive and rehabilitative programs for those mental health and allied health professionals who are each day intimately involved in the identification, treatment, and prevention of child abuse by parents. Burnout prevention must recognize not only the relationship between stress and those therapist-patient factors that induce burnout, but it must also recognize the therapeutic and positive reinforcements of "time out," better pay schedules, increased support systems, and a positive supervisor-supervisee relationship as features to be implemented to counteract personnel exhaustion. There is much evidence that while any human services delivery system carries increased emotional pressures, there are also individual, personal, and work-ethic characteristics—such as overconscientiousness and highly dedicated concern—that predispose professionals to burnout. It is therefore incumbent that all agency heads take every opportunity to prevent burnout from becoming an occupational hazard for those working in the area of child abuse and neglect.

This paper was supported by Grant No. MC-R-060339, awarded by Maternal and Child Health, DHEW, and by Catholics of Motion Picture, TV, Radio, and Recording Industry.

REFERENCES

Beckwith, L. Caregiver-infant interaction and the development of the high risk infant. In *Intervention Strategies for High Risk Infants and Young Children*, T. Tjossem, ed. University Park Press, Baltimore (1976), pp. 119–139.

Besharov, D. U.S. National Center on Child Abuse and Neglect: Three years of experience. *International Journal of Child Abuse and Neglect, 1,* 173–177 (1977).

Bolton, F., Laner, R., and Kane, S. Child maltreatment risk among adolescent mothers: A study of reported cases. *American Journal of Orthopsychiatry, 50,* 489–504 (1980).

Bowlby, J. *Attachment and Loss: Attachment.* Basic Books, New York (1969).

———. *Attachment and Loss: Separation.* Basic Books, New York (1973).

Brandwein, H. The battered child: A definite and significant factor in mental retardation. *Mental Retardation, 11,* 50–51 (1973).

Brazelton, T. *Toddlers and Parents: A Declaration of Independence.* Delacorte, New York (1974).

Caffey, J. The parent-infant traumatic stress syndrome. *American Journal of Roentgenology, Radium Therapy and Nuclear Medicine, 114,* 218–229 (1972).

California Department of Justice. *Child Abuse: The Problem of the Abused and Neglected Child.* Information Pamphlet No. 8, Sacramento (1978).

Carey, W. Clinical applications of infant temperament measurements. *Journal of Pediatrics, 81,* 823–828 (1972).

Children's Village, USA. *Providing a Comprehensive, Interdisciplinary Program for Abused Children and Their Families.* Beaumont, Calif. (1979).

Cohen, A. Multidisciplinary teams or interagency coalitions? A comparative analysis. *Protective Services Resource Institute, 2,* 1–2 (1977).

Directions. HEW, Region IX, Child Abuse and Neglect Resource Center, *15,* (1980) pp. 1–10.

Eisenberg, L. On humanizing of human nature. *Impact of Science on Society, 23,* 213–223 (1973).

Elmer, E., and Gregg, G. Developmental characteristics of abused children. *Pediatrics, 40,* 596–602 (1967).

Erikson, E. *Childhood and Society.* W. W. Norton, New York (1963).

Flynn, W. Frontier Justice: A contribution to the theory of child battery. *American Journal of Psychiatry, 127,* 375–379 (1970).

Frankenburg, W., and Camp, B. *Pediatric Screening Tests.* Charles C. Thomas, Springfield (1973).

Fraser, B. Independent representation for the abused and neglected child: The guardian ad litem. *California Western Law Review, 13,* 16–45 (1977a).
———. The concept of a guardian ad litem. *Child Abuse and Neglect, 1,* 459–468 (1977b).
Friedrich, W. Epidemiological survey of physical child abuse. *Texas State Journal of Medicine, 72,* 81–84 (1976).
Frommer, E. Prediction/preventive work in vulnerable families of young children. *Child Abuse and Neglect, 3,* 777–780 (1979).
Galdston, R. Observations on children who have been physically abused, and their families. *American Journal of Psychiatry, 122,* 440–443 (1965).
Garmezy, N. Vulnerability research and the issue of primary prevention. *American Journal of Orthopsychiatry, 41,* 101–116 (1971).
Gelles, R. Child abuse as psychopathology: A sociological critique and reformulation. *American Journal of Orthopsychiatry, 431,* 611–621 (1973).
Gewirtz, J. *Attachment and Dependency.* Wiley, New York (1972).
Gil, D. *Violence Against Children.* Harvard University Press, Cambridge, Mass. (1970).
Gorman, W. A perspective on child abuse. *Arizona Medicine, 36,* 453–454 (1970).
Gray, J., Cutler, C., Dean, J., and Kempe, C. Perinatal assessment of mother-baby interaction. In *Child Abuse and Neglect: The Family and the Community,* R. Helfer and C. Kempe, eds. Ballinger, Cambridge, Mass. (1976).
Green, A. Self-destructive behavior in battered children. *American Journal of Psychiatry, 135,* 579–582 (1978).
———. Child abuse and neglect. *Journal of Child Psychiatry, 18,* 201–205 (1979).
Green, H., Gaines, W., and Sandgrund, A. Child abuse: Pathological syndrome of family interaction. *American Journal of Psychiatry, 131,* 882–886 (1974).
Greenson, R. The classic psychoanalytic approach. *American Handbook of Psychiatry,* Vol. 2. Basic Books, New York (1959), pp. 1399–1416.
Gunning, P. Burn-out: As apathy replaces empathy. *Connection, 2,* 1–3 (1977).
Harlow, H., Harlow, M., and Soumi, S. From thought to therapy: Lessons from a primate laboratory. *American Scientist, 59,* 538–549 (1971).
Head Start Bureau. *New Light On An Old Problem.* U.S. Department of Health, Education, and Welfare. DHEW Publication No. (OHIDS) 79-31108 (1978).
Helfer, R. Why most physicians don't get involved in child abuse cases and what to do about it. *Children Today, 4,* 28–33 (1975).
———. Child abuse and neglect: early identification and prevention of unusual child-rearing practices. *Pediatric Annals, 5,* 91–105 (1976).
Helfer, R., and Kempe, C., eds. *The Battered Child,* 2nd ed. University of Chicago Press, Chicago (1974).
———. *Child Abuse and Neglect: The Family and the Community.* Ballinger, Cambridge, Mass. (1976).
Helfer, R., Schneider, C., Hoffmeister, J., and Tardi, B. *Manual for the Use of the Michigan Screening Profile of Parenting.* Department of Human Development, Michigan State University, East Lansing (1977).
Hofer, M. *Parent-infant Interaction.* Ciba Foundation Series 33, Associated Scientific Publishers, Amsterdam (1975).
Hunter, R. *Predicting Child Abuse.* American Public Health Association Meeting, Miami Beach (October, 1976).

ICAN. *Cedar House: A Neighborhood Family Renewal Center. Descriptive Analysis and Evaluation.* ICAN Associates, County of Los Angeles (1980).

Isaacson, L. Child abuse reporting statutes: The case for holding physicians civilly liable for failing to report. *San Diego Law Review, 12,* 743–777 (1975).

Kass, E., Sigman, M., Bromwich, R., and Parmelee, A. Educational intervention with high risk infants. In *Intervention Strategies for High Risk Infants and Young Children,* T. Tjossem, ed. University Park Press, Baltimore (1976), pp. 535–543.

Katz, S., Ambrosino, L., McGrath, M., and Sawitzky, K. Legal research on child abuse and neglect: Past and future. *Family Law Quarterly, 11,* 151–184 (1977).

Kempe, C. Approaches to preventing child abuse: the health visitor concept. *American Journal of Disease of Children, 130,* 941–947 (1976).

Kempe, C., and Helfer, R. *Helping the Battered Child and His Family.* J.B. Lippincott, Philadelphia (1972).

Kempe, C., Silverman, F., Steele, B., Droegemueller, W., and Silver, H. The battered child syndrome. *Journal of the American Medical Association, 181,* 17–24 (1962).

Kenny, T., and Clemmens, R. *Behavioral Pediatrics and Child Development: A Clinical Handbook.* Williams & Wilkins, Baltimore (1975).

Kinard, E., and Klerman, L. Teenage parenting and child abuse: Are they related? *American Journal of Orthopsychiatry, 50,* 481–488 (1980).

King, C. Counter-transference and counter-experience in the treatment of violence prone youth. *American Journal of Orthopsychiatry, 46,* 43–52 (1976).

Klaus, M., and Kennell, J. Mothers separated from their newborn infants. *Pediatric Clinics of North America, 17,* 1015–1037 (1970).

Klein, M., and Stern, L. Low birth weight and the battered child syndrome. *American Journal of Diseases of Childhood, 122,* 15–18 (1971).

Korner, A. Individual differences at birth: Implications for child care practices. In *Infant at Risk,* D. Bergsma, ed. Stratton Intercontinental, New York (1974).

Leiderman, P., and Seashore, M. Mother-infant separation: Some delayed consequences. In *Parent-Infant Interaction,* M. Hofer, ed. Associated Scientific Publishers, New York (1975), pp. 213–240.

Leifer, A., Leiderman, P., Barnett, C., and Williams, J. Effects of mother-infant separation on maternal attachment behavior. *Child Development, 43,* 1203–1218 (1972).

Lewis, M., and Rosenblum, L. *The Effects of the Infant on Its Caretaker.* Wiley, New York (1974).

Light, J. Abused and neglected children in America; a study of alternative policies. *Harvard Educational Review, 43,* 556–598 (1973).

Lourie, I. Family dynamics and the abuse of adolescents: A case for a developmental phase-specific model of child abuse. *Child Abuse and Neglect, 3,* 967–974 (1979).

Lynch, M. Ill health and child abuse. *Lancet, 2,* 317–319 (1975).

Lynch, M., and Ounsted, C. Residential therapy—a place of safety. In *Child Abuse and Neglect: The Family and the Community,* R. Helfer and C. Kempe, eds. Ballinger, Cambridge, Mass. (1976).

Lystad, M. Violence at home: A review of the literature. *American Journal of Orthopsychiatry, 45,* 328–345 (1975).

Martin, H. *The Abused Child: A Multidisciplinary Approach to Developmental Issues and Treatment.* Ballinger, Cambridge, Mass. (1976).

Maslach, C. Burned-out. *Human Behavior, 5,* 16–23 (1976).

Money, J. The syndrome of abuse dwarfism (psychosocial dwarfism or reversible hyposomatotropinism). *American Journal of Diseases of Children, 131,* 508–513 (1977).

Money, J., and Needleman, A. Child abuse in the syndrome of reversible hyposomatotropic dwarfism. *Journal of Pediatric Psychology, 1,* 20–23 (1976).

Morris, M., and Gould, R. Role-reversal: A necessary concept in dealing with the battered child syndrome. *American Journal of Orthopsychiatry, 33,* 298–299 (1963).

Morse, C., Sahler, O., and Friedman, S. A three year follow-up of abused and neglected children. *American Journal of Diseases of Childhood, 120,* 439–466 (1970).

Ounsted, C., Oppenheimer, R., and Lindsay, J. Aspects of bonding failure: The psychopathology and psychotherapeutic treatment of families of battered children. *Developmental Medical Child Neurology, 16,* 447–456 (1974).

Parents Anonymous: Chairperson-Sponsor Manual. Parents Anonymous, Redondo Beach, Calif. (1975).

Parmelee, A., Sigman, M., Kopp, C., and Haber, A. Diagnosis of the infant at high risk for mental, motor and sensory handicaps. In *Intervention Strategies for High Risk Infants and Young Children.* T. Tjossem, ed. University Park Press, Baltimore (1976) pp. 289–297.

Pasamanick, B. Ill-health and child abuse. *Lancet, 2,* 550 (1975).

Paulson, M. Child trauma intervention: A community response to family violence. *Journal of Clinical Child Psychology, 4,* 26–29 (1975).

———. Multiple intervention programs for the abused and neglected child. *Journal of Pediatric Psychology, 1,* 83–87 (1976).

———. Early intervention and treatment of child abuse. *Psychiatric Opinion, 15,* 34–38 (1978a).

———. Incest and sexual molestation: Clinical and legal issues. *Journal of Clinical Child Psychology, 7,* 177–180 (1978b).

———. Identifying and helping the child abusing family. In *Psychosocial Aspects of Medical Practice: Children and Adolescents.* Robert O. Pasnau, ed. Addison-Wesley, Menlo Park, 61–75, 1982.

———. Relationships between experienced child abuse and later childhood suicidal behavior (in preparation).

Paulson, M., and Blake, P. The abused, battered and maltreated child: A review. *Trauma, 9,* 1–136 (1967).

———. The physically abused child: A focus on prevention. *Child Welfare, 48,* 86–95 (1969).

Paulson, M., and Chaleff, A. Parent surrogate roles: A dynamic concept in understanding and treating abusive parents. *Journal of Clinical Child Psychology, 11,* 38–40 (1973).

Paulson, M., and Stone, D. Suicidal behavior of latency age children. *Journal of Clinical Child Psychology, 3,* 50–53 (1974).

———. Suicide potential and behavior in children age 4–12. *Suicide and Life-Threatening Behavior, 8,* 225–243 (1978).

Paulson, M., Savino, A., Chaleff, A., Sanders, W., Frisch, F., and Dunn, R. Parents of the battered child: A multidisciplinary group therapy approach to life threatening behavior. *Life Threatening Behavior, 4,* 18-31 (1974a).

Paulson, M., Afifi, A., Thomason, M., and Chaleff, A. The MMPI: A descriptive measure of psychopathology in abusive parents. *Journal of Clinical Psychology, 30,* 387-390 (1974b).

Paulson, M., Afifi, A. Chaleff, A., and Thomason, M. An MMPI scale for identifying "at risk" abusive parents. *Journal of Clinical Child Psychology, 4,* 22-24 (1975a).

Paulson, M., Afifi, A., Chaleff, A., Liu, V., and Thomason, M. A discriminant function procedure for identifying abusive parents. *Suicide* (formerly *Life Threatening Behavior), 5,* 104-114 (1975b).

Paulson, M., Schwemer, G., and Bendel, R. Clinical application of the Pd, Ma and (OH) experimental MMPI scales to further understanding of abusive parents. *Journal of Clinical Psychology, 32,* 558-564 (1976).

Paulson, M., Schwemer, G., Afifi, A., and Bendel, R. Parent Attitude Research Instrument (PARI): Clinical vs statistical inferences in understanding abusive mothers. *Journal of Clinical Psychology, 33,* 848-854 (1977).

Paulson, M., Strouse, L., and Chaleff, A. Intra-familiar incest and sexual molestation in children. In *Children and the Law: Children's Rights and Children's Attitudes,* James Henning, ed. Charles C. Thomas, Springfield (in press).

———. Further observations on child abuse: An a-posteriori examination of group therapy notes (in press).

Ramsey, J., and Lawler, B. The battered child syndrome. *Pepperdine Law Review, 1,* 372-381 (1974).

Rutter, M. *The Qualities of Mothering: Maternal Deprivation Reassessed.* Jason Aronson, New York (1974).

Sameroff, A., and Chandler, M. Infant causality and the continuum of infant caretaking. In *Review of Child Development Research,* Vol. 4, F. Horowitz, E. Hetherington, M. Siegel, and S. Salapatek, eds. University of Chicago Press, Chicago (1975).

Sandgrund, A., Gaines, R., and Green, A. Child abuse and mental retardation: A problem of cause and effect. *Journal of Mental Deficiency, 79,* 327-330 (1974).

Schmitt, B. *Medical Management of the Sexually Abused Child.* A Videotape. American Academy of Pediatrics (1979).

Soeffing, M. Abused children are exceptional children. *Exceptional Children, 42,* 126-133 (1975).

Spinetta, R., and Rigler, D. The child abusing parent: A psychological review. *Psychological Bulletin, 77,* 296-304 (1972).

Spitz, R. Hospitalism. *Psychoanalytic Study of the Child, 1,* 53-74 (1945).

Steele, B. Violence within the family. In *Children Abuse and Neglect: The Family and the Community,* R. Helfer and C. Kempe, eds. Ballinger, Cambridge, Mass. (1976).

Steele, B., and Pollock, C. A psychiatric study of parents who abuse infants and small children. In *The Battered Child,* 2nd ed., R. Helfer and C. Kempe, eds. University of Chicago Press, Chicago (1974), pp. 89-133.

Thomas, A., Chess, S., and Birch, H. *Temperament and Behavior Disorders in Children,* New York University Press, New York (1968).

Valdes-Dapena, M. *Sudden Unexplained Infant Death.* DHEW Publication No. (HSA) 78-5255 (1978).

Yalom, I. *The Theory and Practice of Group Psychotherapy.* Basic Books, New York (1975).

Zigler, E. Controlling child abuse in America: An effort doomed to failure. Lecture presented at Meher Children's Rehabilitation Institute, University of Nebraska Medical Center, Omaha (May 25, 1976).

11

Theoretical and Clinical Issues
in Severe Depression and Latency-Age
Suicidal Behavior of Children

Morris J. Paulson and Dorothy Stone

Psychiatry as a profession and humanity in general have accepted that for many people the unknownness and uncertainties of death are preferred to the emotional and/or physical pain of living. In some cultures, suicide is the noblest act of sacrifice on the part of a concerned adult, but never is it a noble act when done by children. Statistics from coroners' offices worldwide affirm the increasing incidence of both adult and adolescent suicide. Conflict within the home, chronic demeaning family quarreling, death of a family member, unwanted pregnancy, alcohol and substance abuse, joblessness, academic failures, a sense of personal despair, helplessness, hopelessness, and guilt are recognized as etiologic factors in intentioned and unintentioned self-inflicted acts of personal destruction by adults.

Society, and health and education professionals, are only beginning to realize that the same pains of living experienced by adolescents and adults can also be experienced by preadolescent and latency-age children—and with the same fatal consequences. Even though most coroners do not classify suicide as a cause of death of children, there is much evidence that death-seeking behavior by young children does occur. It is also increasing. Tragically, there are still too many parents, teachers, health professionals, and pediatric and mental health specialists who fail to acknowledge that depression in preteenage children exists, or that such children can consciously seek to end their lives.

The decade of the seventies has seen a proliferation of theoretical papers on whether there is such a concept as childhood depression and, if so, how it resembles or differs from adult depression (Anthony, 1975; Anthony and Benedek, 1975; Carlson and Cantwell, 1979; Conners, 1976; Kovacs and Beck, 1977; Malmquist, 1977; Schulterbrandt and Raskin, 1977; Toolan, 1978; Cytryn, 1979). Definition, diagnosis, and treatment (Schulterbrandt and Raskin, 1977) are examined in terms of conceptual models, such as psychophysiological, neurobiological, learned helplessness, and cognitive theories of depression. Several clinical studies (Paulson and Stone, 1974; Paulson, Stone and Sposto, 1978; Carlson and Cantwell, 1980; Cantwell and Carlson, 1979; Pfeiffer, 1978) have recently provided demographic, clinical, and descriptive measures of the extent and nature of acute depression and suicidal behavior of young children and early teenagers. Because of the extensive theoretical literature that is already well documented, the present chapter will briefly discuss the major concepts and theories of childhood depression and the self-punishing and self-destructive suicidal behavior of young children.

REVIEW OF THE LITERATURE

Bosselman (1958), in studying self-destruction in terms of a suicidal impulse, described the inborn drives to live and to love, which are inseparable and necessary for survival. He states (p. 7): "The marasmic infant is a pitiful and dramatic illustration of a primitive kind of self-destruction. The infant dies because his inborn strivings for contact and emotional interaction with other people are thwarted. He can neither love nor fight . . . he cannot develop the feelings of self-value which emerge in interpersonal relationships . . . in a state of annihilation he wastes away . . . (this is) . . . an example of the earliest manifestations of suicide."

Campbell (1959), in reporting on school phobias and manic-depressive disease in children, felt that children with these disorders were suffering from endogenous depression. Agros (1959) studied seven children with school phobias and their relationship to family psychopathology, finding that six of the seven children (86 percent) had depressive symptoms manifested by frequent outbursts of weeping. Forty-three percent had both a fear of dying and a wish to die, with one of the seven making several suicidal gestures. A marked depressive constellation was seen in six of the seven families. While such studies show a correlation between school phobias and later severe depression and suicidal potential, educational and health professionals at that time gave little attention to these early correlates of childhood depression.

Harrington and Hassan (1958) described their investigation and treatment of 14 girls, ages 8 to 11 years, in the Royal Hospital for Sick Children, Glasgow, Scotland, finding that half were suffering from clinically observable depression manifested by weeping attacks, fear of the death of parents, diffuse pain, night terrors, enuresis, school phobias, depressed anxiety, severe headaches, and vomiting. The onset of illness in all 14 girls was of recent origin. They were all regarded by their teachers and parents as "good children" and all were above average in intelligence, yet none of them had ever had a "best friend." Self-depreciation and fears of death and injury were prevalent. Accidents and illness were the prominent trigger factors related to hospitalization and subsequent identification of depression in 50 percent of the children studied. The observed self-depreciation and ego weakness were understood in terms of failure in identification and splitting of the functions of mothering with the fathers in the first two years of life. This, the authors felt, hindered the formation of a strong early feminine identification.

Lourie (1966), in a study of suicide statistics in the United States, stated that suicide in the 15–19-year age group ranked fourth as a cause of death, and that well over 100 suicides per year were recorded for children between ages 10 and 14 years. In talking to 100 school-age children with emotional problems, Lourie found that 70 percent reported thoughts and wishes for their own death, 69 percent indicated they at some time had consciously wanted to die, while 54 percent consciously thought of killing themselves. In studying 40 other children, ages 3–14, with a ratio of five males to one female, Lourie found none with a chronic preoccupation with self-destruction, except for four psychotic children. Most suicidal attempts were based on pressures of the moment, in children with poor impulse control. The predominant psychodynamic determinants that Lourie identified were: (1) aggression, revenge, and spite toward one of the parents or the whole family; and (2) an attempt to escape from an intolerable situation or reality, where the child felt helpless, where dependency fulfillment was threatened or withdrawn, or where dire punishment was imminent and inescapable.

Annell (1971) in studying depressive states in childhood and adolescence reported a 1.8 to 25 percent incidence of depression in a series of studies. She asks (p. 12): "Are depressions in bereaved children always due to exogenous mechanisms, or are some of these children also hereditarily disposed to endogenous depression?" Her studies indicate that depression should not be divided into exogenous and endogenous in the traditional manner, but instead a unipolar and bipolar form of depressive disease. Annell points out that in addition to the manifest symptoms of overt depression in children, there are such nonspecific states as anxiety, inhibition, aggression, enuresis, sleeping difficulties, fatigue, guilt, psychosomatic symptoms, and suicidal thoughts. The inhibition and lack of self-confidence, she feels, are often factors influencing rowdy school behavior and academic failures.

Mendelsohn, Reid, and Frommer (1971) studied 210 patients under five years of age in order to examine factors associated with depression, anxiety, and aggressive behavior in disturbed children. They found that depressed children had the highest incidence of abdominal pain (42 percent) and maternal depressive illness (66 percent), but no identifiable precipitating events. The authors conclude: "Developmental and persistent behavioral disturbances in small children, *however young*, in the absence of organic disease, call for a close and thorough investigation of the family. . . . They respond most satisfactorily to treatment" (pp. 156–157).

Berner, Katschning, and Poldinger (1973) note that the terms "masked depression," "hidden depression," and "missed depression" have been appearing more frequently since Walcher (1969) published his monograph, *Die larvierte Depression,* describing those cases of endogenous depression in which physical signs and symptoms predominate. Berner et al. stressed that a distinction must be made between masking due to a psychic defense mechanism and masking due to a predominant presence of somatic symptoms; they concluded that "the term 'masked depression' should be restricted to those latter cases" (p. 90). The authors, however, focused on masked depression primarily as an adult phenomenon and made no reference at that time to such a phenomenon in children.

Frederick (1978) notes that the rate of suicide in the age group 10-14 has tripled since 1960, stressing that lack of communication between children and their parents forces the child to turn to peers, other parent surrogates, and teachers for support. Tragically, however, many depressed, suicidal children have no one to turn to and thus become at risk for self-inflicted, nonaccidental injury or death. Frederick lists a number of etiologic factors found in the suicide of young children. These are: loss of confidence, humiliation, traumatic family events, recent losses within the family, death of a loved one, and moving away from long-standing peer relationships. While clues to suicide can be verbal, behavioral, or situational, Frederick stresses the need for health professionals and child care workers to be constantly alert to those covert signs that mask depression and that many times are not identified. He states that "it is a mistake to believe that an individual must be clinically depressed in order to commit suicide" (p. 6). Depression and suicide are not isolated concepts, but are elements in a network of experience and attitudes that are influenced by the age of the child, the quality of communication within the parent-child relationship, and an absence of a sense of worth within the individual.

Anthony (1975) wanted to know how children come to understand and communicate feelings of depression and whether childhood depression is an emerging phenomenon of our time. Developmental psychologists also ask whether it is necessary to have experienced a primary depression in the first five years of life in order to develop a childhood, adolescent, or adult depressive disorder and whether there is a correlation between infantile anaclitic depression and later adult depression. Spitz and Wolf (1946) and Bowlby (1969) have not postulated any specific and meaningful correlations between infantile anaclitic depression and later adult depression. However, Benedek (1956) sees primary infantile anaclitic depression as a precursor to subsequent depressive experiences. Jacobson (1946) described primary depression of the oedipal-age child as a function of pessimism and apathy, stating that these were the core experiences of all later major depressions. Yet, even with such developmentally important statements, health professionals failed to recognize the entity of clinical depression in childhood. In fact, Rochlin (1965) refuted the concept of childhood depression on the grounds that clinical depression is a superego phenomenon involving aggression directed at the self, which cannot occur in children; therefore, there can be no such entity as clinical depression in children. Later, Anthony (1975) described in detail the primary, secondary, and tertiary manifestations of childhood depression, concluding that "the primary manifestations occur by themselves in the infantile period; that both primary and secondary manifestations are evident during childhood; and that primary, secondary, and tertiary manifestations can be observed sometimes together and sometimes alone during adult life. Childhood and adult depression are therefore clinically fairly distinct from one another, and the differences are based on both descriptive and dynamic aspects" (pp. 255-256).

Earlier, Sperling (1959) had affirmed the concept of a depressive equivalent, pointing out the high degree of depression in children who also manifest such bodily functions as sleep disturbance, anorexia, pruritus, migraine, motor retardation, and ulcerative colitis. She stressed that the diagnosis of clinical depression in children should be based on various combinations of behavioral and psychophysiological signs and symptoms that have been found empirically to cluster together.

Cytryn and McKnew (1972) and Cytryn (1979), in reexamining the classifications of childhood depression, refocused professional attention on the frequency of parental loss in the histories of depressed children—loss that was experienced by separation, divorce, or death of a parent; by rejection and decathexis of interest by one or both parents; and parental depression, which in turn made such parents unable to give affection and caring to the needy child. Malmquist (1977) found much evidence of undue parental demands for conformity on the part of the young child and a requirement that the child "earn his desired affection and love." This is an interesting example of "role reversals," where the parents expect the child to behave in an adult manner to satisfy the parents' need for affection. Here is the paradox. On the one hand, children need to experience and feel bonding, attachment, and affection in the child-parent relationship in order to avoid the later or immediate development of withdrawal, malaise, and feelings of depression. On the other hand, the parents described by Malmquist require a level of conformity or performance on the part of the child that often is not possible. This absence of conformity results in parental frustration and anger, which in turn leads to a lack of positive child-parent stimulation and affection sharing, a precursor to the experience of emotional famine by the child. The consequent feelings of rejection, loss, and depression make it increasingly difficult for the child to satisfy "role-reversal" demands for their own fulfillment of affection.

In contrast to the findings of Cytryn and McKnew and Malmquist are those of Lokare (1971), who feels that parental separation has minimal dynamic significance in understanding childhood depression. Lokare studied neuroticism, extraversion, and the incidence of depressive illness in 170 children. He concludes: "The overwhelming majority of 88 separated children and 90% of the children living with their natural parents were not depressed. . . . The findings also suggest a clear link between personality trait, as all the depressives of the study form a part of the group of neurotic introverts." Lokare's findings thus appear etiologically to focus less on the child-parent dynamics of separation and coercion and more on character traits as an explanation of childhood depression.

Nissen (1973), in his study of masked depression in children and adolescents, states: "Some authors have claimed that, during childhood, depressive conditions largely or exclusively take the form of masked depression, because they are predominantly characterized by behavioral disorders and somatic equivalents" (p. 133). Nissen refutes this, feeling that depressions are not masked but are primary forms of the disease. He quotes from his study on the incidence of masked depression among 495 nonselected children and adolescents suffering from psychic or somatic disturbances, concluding: "We did gain the impression that there is hardly any type of behavioral disorder and hardly any psychosomatic syndrome which cannot in principle also be regarded as a manifestation of masked depression or as a somatic equivalent" (p. 137). Nissen concludes that "the predominantly somatic forms in which depression manifests itself during childhood can be classified as 'masked depression' only if considered from the standpoint of adult psychiatry. But when viewed from the angle of developmental psychiatry and from the cross-cultural aspects, they must be assigned to the category of 'genuine' *primary* depressions, from which . . . the typical forms of adult depression, conditioned as they are by cultural influences, must be distinguished as *secondary* depressions" (p. 140). As health professionals and pediatric specialists, we must now ask if borderline behaviors, learning and school difficulties, behavior disorders, rebellion toward parents, and family conflict in general are also expressions of a masked childhood depression. If so, what primary and secondary interventions can we initiate in order to preclude the later development of severe clinical depression in young children?

What is the consensus of opinion among professionals with regard to the theoretically and clinically important question, "Does depression in children have to be manifested with the same symptomatology as depression in adults in order to be so diagnosed?" Toolan (1978) feels that infants, children, adolescents, and adults can all be diagnosed as depressed, "provided that we employ different criteria than those used for adults" (p. 243). Postulating that depression is a reaction to loss that diminishes self-esteem and enhances helplessness, Toolan describes varying consequences of loss as a function of the chronological time of experienced separation. This, in turn, dictates the treatment approach most effective in working through the experience of abandonment, loss, and separation. Toolan sees childhood depressive reactions as chronic in nature, often continuing into adulthood, and requiring specialized intervention programs. To the pediatric health specialist, Toolan expresses caution, saying, "The average pediatrician, guidance counselor, or mental health worker, in my opinion, is not competent to work with such youngsters. The shortage of adequately trained therapists for this type of treatment is one of the reasons that many clinics resort largely to medication, as they do in the case of schizophrenic patients" (p. 246). With such a strong admonition to therapists, it behooves all professionals involved in the identification, diagnosis, and treatment of depressed children to seek expert resources for the child manifesting either overt symptoms of depression, or behavioral, psychosomatic, and educational signs that may well be masking an underlying, severe, life-threatening depression or suicidal risk.

Toolan, in discussing therapy for depressed and suicidal children, identifies six groups of high-risk children, all of whom can be seen in the daily practice of most pediatric care centers. The following children presenting at a health care center should be carefully assessed: (1) anaclitic infants separated from mothers for long periods of time; (2) infants with depressed parents; (3) children of divorced parents who show apathy and withdrawal; (4) children with inhibition of intellectual activity; (5) children presenting with somatic symptoms such as headaches, gastric distress, malaise, fatigue, phobias, enuresis, and frequently minimal direct depressive symptomatologies; and (6) children with anorexia nervosa, more often seen in girls and manifested by a refusal to eat and a disturbed body image (Toolan, 1978, pp. 247-248).

It is doubly important for all health and educational specialists to recognize that while a variety of behavioral and organic symptoms may mask an underlying depression, the depression itself, overt or masked, may be symptomatic of equally acute and life-threatening feelings, such as suppressed rage, anger, and homicidal feelings. Treating the symptom through a behavioral approach may result in significant symptom reduction or removal. However, it is important that any program of intervention also direct itself to the underlying psychodynamics behind such symptom choice. The etiological roots, most often psychodynamic in nature, must be identified and treated. Chronic and acute depression in children, often going unnoticed by parents, teachers, neighbors, and health professionals, is a meaningful, painful emotional state that for too many children can portend a suicidal attempt or even death by self-inflicted means.

Heinicke (1973), in a study of correlates between parental deprivation in early childhood and predisposition to later depression, identified four types of parental separation that can predispose a child to later depression: (1) absence of any sustained parent-child contact from birth on, such as with an institutionalized child; (2) separation for periods of more than six months (for example, divorce); (3) deprivation not from separation, but due to inadequacies of parenting (for example, marasmus and failure to thrive); and (4) deprivation due to death of one or both parents. In a review of retrospective studies on the relationship between parental deprivation and later depression and of longitudinal studies on the impact of parental loss experiences, Heinicke concludes: (1) the greater incidence of adult psychiatric disturbances in children in general is associated with an early childhood experience of prolonged separation from the parents due to divorce or marital separation; (2) a greater incidence of depression is associated with a childhood experience of parental death; (3) patients who suffer from a severe—as opposed to mild—form of depression have more frequently experienced either parental death in childhood or an acutely inadequate parent-child relationship, or both; (4) patients who attempt suicide have more frequently experienced parental death in childhood; and (5) the incidence of parental death in the 0-5 and 10-14 age groups is higher for depressed patients (pp. 157-158).

Lefkowitz and Burton (1978), in a critique of the concept of childhood depression, ask whether childhood depression is really an independent clinical constellation of symptoms or whether it is a transitory, developmental phenomenon that appears over time and is per se not a precursor of later adult depression. The quandary of definition and classification is well presented by the authors, who state:

> In the extensive reviews of the symptomatology of childhood depression by Kovacs and Beck (1977) and Malmquist (1975), the list of feelings and behaviors observed in depressed children become so broad as to necessarily include, at one time or another during development, almost all children. When the masked symptoms and depressive equivalents such as hyperactivity, aggressive behavior, psychosomatic disturbances, hypochondriasis, delinquency (Cytryn and McKnew, 1972), temper tantrums, disobedience, truancy, boredom, and restlessness (Toolan, 1962) are added to this list, then virtually no child can escape the classification. In this regard, Weinberg et al. (1973) stated that they were "impressed by the relative frequency of depressive symptoms in pre-pubertal children' . . . and accordingly, 63% of their subjects were diagnosed as depressed. Cytryn and McKnew (1972) also found sad affect and depressive symptoms to be 'very common in children' (Lefkowitz and Burton, 1978, p. 718).

Following their lengthy, detailed, and analytical examination of many studies, the same authors conclude:

> Evidence adduced from the research literature to support the concept of a syndrome of early childhood depression is insufficient and insubstantial. . . . Diagnosis of this presumed condition in children would appear

to be premature and treatment unwarranted. The possibility of producing iatrogenic effects on the child, the risk of masking other problems, and the unknown effects of parents underscore the need for rigorous research of this question. . . . No reliable and valid method for assessing this putative condition has been developed. . . . Without supportive normative data, the notion of a syndrome of childhood depression rests largely on surmise (Lefkowitz and Burton, 1978, p. 724).

In contrast to such a highly cautionary position are the earlier findings of Toolan (1962) and the later ones of Malmquist (1971; 1975), who both feel that stages of childhood growth and development in great part determine the expression and manifestation of depression in children. However, in many depressed children and adolescents, phobic-obsessive symptoms, psychosomatic preoccupations, and behavioral disorders also appear to be primary manifestations of conflict, rather than mood disorders, guilt, and classical affect disturbances. Conners (1976), for example notes the double-bind conflict in differentiating true depression from masked depression or depression equivalents. He states: "If most or all of the symptoms and signs (of depression) are qualitatively different 'equivalents' from those found in adults, the concept of depression can be used to explain virtually all psychopathological expressions in childhood and adolescence" (p. 183). Conners's review of the literature identifies bereavement and loss as common causes of childhood depression and later adult depression. As noted earlier, these findings are in contrast to those of Lokare, who stated: "Children with depression as a whole show no greater liability than a group of control individuals to parental deprivation . . . nor early object loss and deprivation" (Lokare, 1971, p. 147).

Cytryn and McKnew (1972), confining themselves only to neurotic depressive reactions in children ages 6-12, postulate three classifications of depression: (1) masked depression, common among children from families having severe psychopathology, where the child's response includes hyperactivity, aggressiveness, psychomotor disturbances, hypochondriasis, and delinquent behavior; (2) a depressive affect dysfunction manifesting sadness, social isolation, psychomotor retardation, lack of hope, school failures, sleep and eating disturbances, and suicidal ideation and/or attempts; (3) a subdivision of point 2 above into acute and chronic states, where acute depression is associated with definite and definable object loss, while chronic depression is associated with multiple losses, family psychopathology, and a history of depression in family members (pp. 64-65).

Nissen's (1973) study supports the correlation between depression and family pathology. Nissen found that boys tend to show difficulties in establishing peer contacts, which, combined with learning inhibitions and irritability, lead to difficulties in school and social aggression, while girls tend toward brooding and quiet and inhibited behavior. "Perhaps the most important finding in Nissen's study was the fact that symptoms of brooding, dysphoria, day dreaming, inhibition of learning, suicidal attempts, 'vital sadness,' restlessness and mutism were prognostically highly unfavorable. 'Mood swings' seemed to be a sure sign of impending schizophrenia rather than depressive disorder of adult life" (Conners, 1976, p. 186).

Malmquist's (1977) examination of childhood depression from a clinical and behavioral perspective provides a clear and succinct integration of many issues. Noting the absence of the category of *childhood depression* in the 1968 *Diagnostic and Statistical Manual of Mental Disorders* (DSM-II) of the American Psychiatric Association, and the lack of a developmental perspective in understanding childhood depression, Malmquist directed his attention to 10 important clinical and research issues that provide guidelines for future research and a review of the theory and concepts historically relevant to depressive states of young children. Commencing with the studies of Levy (1937) and Burlingham and Freud (1943), he presents clinical evidence of the apparent seriousness of maternal deprivation, especially when occurring at a young age. Examining the concept of anaclitic depression (Spitz, 1946) and later writings on maternal deprivation (Bowlby, 1969; 1973), Malmquist cautions, "The concept is weighted in the direction of an over-emphasis on early infantile experiences leading to an unilateral outcome without sufficient cognizance of other significant variables in the child's life" (p. 39). Malmquist reviews the early psychodynamic formulations of depression, beginning with the works of Freud and Abraham and ending with the more recent object relations theories of Klein (1964), who postulated introjective-projective processes occurring from birth onward, which, concomitant with separation and loss during the 3-12 months of weaning, can lead to a "depressive position." Grief and mourning in infancy (Bowlby, 1969) are also examined in terms of loss of love objects, where "depression" is seen as one of the emotional states concomitant with the process of mourning. Recognizing that one of Bowlby's postulates is that loss of a mother figure between six months and three to four years of age has a high degree of pathogenic potential for subsequent personality development, Malmquist feels that close regard should be given to any incidence of parental separation and parent-surrogate loss in the etiology of childhood depression. In examining the composite picture of a depressed child, Malmquist identifies 15 descriptive characteristics (p. 51):

1. Sadness, depression, and unhappiness
2. Withdrawal and inhibition
3. Somatization (the depressive equivalents)
4. Discontent
5. Feeling unloved and rejected

6. Negative self-concept
7. Low frustration tolerance and irritability
8. Discontent with reassurance from significant others
9. Clowning and foolish provocative behavior to deny underlying depression
10. Denial of feelings of helplessness and hopelessness in order to avoid despair and disillusionment
11. Provocative behaviors toward others and difficulties in handling aggression
12. Passivity and passive-aggressive behaviors
13. Self-condemnation and harsh self-critical judgments
14. Obsessive-compulsive behaviors associated with regressive magical activities
15. Episodic acting-out behaviors as a defense against depression

In examining these 15 characteristics, it is interesting to note that Malmquist has not included any reference to suicidal behavior, suicidal ideation, or suicidal attempts. Malmquist states that "depressed children experience losses as the painful discomfort that makes up part of their depressive core. Their acting out is related either to anxiety about object loss (separation) or to sadness that can progress to despair if they feel the object or part-object will not be recovered" (p. 54). Why, though, did he not examine suicidal ideation, behavior, and actions as variables? If, as many believe, acting out is a primary defense against depression, then it is incumbent upon teachers, parents, and all individuals, lay and professional, interacting with latency-age children to be cognizant of the deeper meaning of "acting out." Like the "cry for help" from an adult suicidal patient, preteenage acting out in a child may often have a similar message. We must not fail to recognize that message.

Cantwell and Carlson (1979) reexamined the terminology of childhood affective disorders, saying that depression as a symptom need not be part of a depressive syndrome or a depressive disorder. To them, depression as a syndrome is a dysphoric mood combined with a number of other symptoms that occur regularly, including affective changes, cognitive changes, motivational changes, and vegetative and psychomotor disturbances. Depression as a disorder implies that there is a depressive syndrome causing some degree of incapacity and there is a characteristic clinical picture, natural history, response to treatment, and possible biological correlates (p. 252). Recognizing that childhood depression is not a univariate phenomenon but is a complex interrelationship of many factors, they emphasize that it is necessary to specify diagnostic criteria in order to plan methodically sound research studies on childhood affective disorders.

Carlson and Cantwell (1980) studied 102 children, ages 7–17 years, in an attempt to "unmask" masked depression. They conclude: "In some children with hyperactivity, aggressive behavior, and some anti-social behavior, a depressive disorder co-exists. Insofar as the behavior disturbance is most out-standing, it may be said to over-shadow the depression. To an alert clinician con-ducting a thorough interview, however, the depression will not be masked" (p. 449).

Review of the literature on both psychological and drug treatment of depres-sion in children is relatively sparse considering the prevalence of and theorizing on depression in childhood. Little concrete information is available on the use of antidepressant drugs as a treatment modality for depressed children. Annell (1971) was one of the first to demonstrate the positive effects of lithium car-bonate on children with mood disorders, sleep disturbances, night terrors, cata-tonic-like stupors, and dysphoric mood alternating with hyperactivity. Frommer (1968) and Weinberg et al. (1973) reported on the use of amitriptyline and imipramine in depressed children. Amitriptyline was found to be the drug of choice for depressed children with enuresis. Phenelzine was the drug of choice for uncomplicated depression, while imipramine was the drug of choice for children with endogenous depressions.

Connors, in summarizing the literature, states (Connors, 1976, p. 196):

> Regardless of the precise mechanisms involved (in childhood depres-sion), it seems reasonable to make the following distinctions in further research with depressive states of childhood and adolescence: acute vs. chronic, phobic-anxious vs. non-phobic, early vs. late onset, positive vs. negative family history, and if positive where there is bi-polar or uni-polar affective illness. These variables would seem to be natural markers for establishing clinical subtypes and might well account for much of the apparent disagreement in the literature regarding depressive states in children. Whether any subtypes are uniquely responsive to tricyclic anti-depressants, MAOI drugs, lithium, or other therapies has not been satis-factorily demonstrated, and it is precisely the failure to control the afore-mentioned variables that may cloud the picture of treatment specificity and response. . . . The relevance of these factors has repeatedly been shown in adult studies of depression and virtually ignored in the child-hood studies until quite recently.

CLINICAL STUDIES OF LATENCY-AGE SUICIDAL CHILDREN

Paulson, Stone and Sposto (1978):
"Suicidal Potential and Behavior in Children, Ages 4–12"

From a population of 662 children 12 years of age and under, seen at the UCLA Neuropsychiatric Institute over a four-year period, 34 children were selected who, on the basis of primary and secondary complaints, showed either severe depression, suicidal behavior, suicide attempts, suicide threats, suicidal ideation, severe self-abuse (nonpsychotic), death wishes, and/or danger to self. Demographic analysis of the families of the 34 children revealed the following data: 23 were boys and 11 were girls; 80 percent were white, 6 percent black, 12 percent Hispanic, and 6 percent others. Parent education ranged from grade seven to postgraduate education, with a median education level for both fathers and mothers being "high school completed." Most of the families were low income, semiskilled, with 14 percent on welfare. Fifty-three percent of the parents were either divorced or separated, and only 32 percent of the children were living with both biological parents at the time of admission to the Neuropsychiatric Institute. The fact that 35 percent of the sample was already known to or under the supervision of the Los Angeles County Department of Public Social Services reflects preexisting agency concern with regard to the existence of neglect and/or abuse conditions within the homes of over one-third of the sample.

In examining suicidal ideation, life threats, and suicide attempts by sex, age, and race, it was possible to make multiple comparisons about that five percent of the total sample of 662 children ($N = 34$) whose intrapersonal and interpersonal stress was so acute that suicide was considered or attempted by most (76 percent) as a means of escape from emotional pain. No sex-significant differences in the ideational violence were identified. Boys and girls as young as five years of age showed in fantasy and in behavior that physical assault upon the self and family members was not a sex-determined factor. There were many forms to the children's violence manifested by displacement of anger upon siblings through homicidal attempts and by body mutilations, stabbing, cutting, scalding, smothering, burning, purposefully running into moving vehicles, and jumping from high buildings. All of these acts of desperation were violent behaviors that exceeded by far the occasional attempts to die by more passive and nonviolent acts, such as drug ingestion. "A significant association was noted between the violence and the ideational processes, the mutilating assault upon the body, and the extreme chaotic, disorganized state of the family" (p. 233).

Table 11-1 shows the rank order and percent frequency of symptoms for suicidal ($N = 34$) and nonsuicidal mentally ill children ($N = 628$), 12 years of age and under, referred to the UCLA Neuropsychiatric Institute over a four-year period. A computerized screening program allowed for the tabulation of 41 discrete symptoms under six specific categorites of symptomatology *(Behavior and Socialization, Affect Disturbances, Physical Handicaps, Delayed Development, School Problems,* and *Psychophysiological Disorders).* Due to the large number of primary symptoms identified under the category of *Behavior and Socialization* ($N = 23$) and the small sample of suicidal children ($N = 34$), only the top 10-11 most frequent primary symptoms are reported for the suicidal mentally

Table 11-1

Rank Ordering (RO) and Percent Frequency (%)[a] of Primary Symptoms, by Sex, for Suicidal and Nonsuicidal Mentally Ill Children Aged 4-12

| | Suicidal (N = 34) | | | | Nonsuicidal (N = 628) | | | |
| | Males (N=23) | | Females (N=11) | | Males (N=444) | | Females (N=184) | |
Categories of Symptoms	RO	%	RO	%	RO	%	RO	%
I. Behavior and Socialization								
Peculiar mannerisms					20	0	7	1
Bizarre behavior	4	23			7	3	5	3
Stereotyped behavior					22	0	8	0
Infantile regressive behavior					11	1	7	1
Autistic					5	3	4	4
Withdrawn					8	2	3	4
Self-abusive	1	55	1	50	4	3	4	4
Temper tantrums	2	41	3	25	2	6	2	6
Hyperactivity	3	32	3	25	3	5	1	7
Physically aggressive	2	41	3	25	1	11	3	4
Verbally aggressive	3	32			14	0	8	0
Lying	3	32	4	17	15	0	9	0
Stealing			4	17	12	1	6	2
Rebellious	3	32	2	33	6	3	3	4
Destructive	2	41	4	17	9	2	5	3
Fire setting					16	0	7	1
Truancy, running away	4	23			17	0	7	1
Sexual problems					18	0	8	0
Drug abuse					23	0	9	0
Sleep problems			4	17	19	0	6	2
Eating problems			4	17	13	0	8	0
Enuresis, encopresis			2	33	10	2	7	1
Somatic complaints					21	0	7	1
Other					—	—	—	

II. Affect Disturbances								
Anxious	9	3	0	0	3	2	3	3
Fearful	14	2	0	0	4	0	4	1
Angry	45	1	2	25	1	11	2	8
Depressed	45	1	1	50	2	8	1	12
Other	—	—	—	—	—	—	—	—
III. Physical Handicaps								
Speech impairment			0	0	2	0	0	0
Hearing impairment			1	4	0	0	0	0
Motor dysfunction			1	4	0	0	0	0
Convulsive disorder	1		0	0	1	0	1	0
Other	4		—	—	—	—	—	—
IV. Delayed Development								
Speech	9	1	0	0	1	2	1	2
Motor incoordination	4	1	0	0	0	0	2	0
Toilet training	9	1	2	8	3	0	2	0
Other self-help skills	9	1	0	0	4	0	0	0
Socialization	9	1	1	25	2	0	0	0
Other	—	—	—	—	—	—	—	—
V. School Problems								
Short attention span	23	2	2	9	5	0	0	0
Disruptive behavior	32	1	2	9	1	9	2	4
General underachievement	23	2	1	18	2	7	1	5
Reading disability	9	4	2	9	4	0	3	0
School phobia	14	3	0	0	3	1	0	0
Other	—	—	—	—	—	—	—	—
VI. Psychophysiological Disorders								
Specify	—	—	—	—	—	—	—	—

[a] Rounded off to nearest percent.

ill children. However, because such a large number of nonsuicidal mentally ill children were studied (N = 628), the rank ordering of all 23 symptoms under *Behavior and Socialization* is presented in order to provide additional interesting characteristics about the larger population sample.

Table 11-1 shows that 55 percent of suicidal male children report self-abuse as the most frequent primary symptom, followed by temper tantrums, physical aggressiveness, and destructive behavior. It is evident that the concept of depression as internalized and displaced anger is strongly substantiated. The expressions of depression in terms of the depression equivalent, or masked depression, are further supported by the next most frequent symptoms: verbal aggression, lying, hyperactivity, and rebellion. Though less intense in terms of behavioral responses, they nonetheless show the many ways in which latency-age children externalize life-threatening feelings of acute depression and suicidal preoccupation. In the category of *Affect Disturbances,* suicidal boys show the highest frequency on anger and depression symptoms, followed by fearfulness and anxiety, two symptoms that for the child are more amorphous yet incapacitating.

For latency-age suicidal girls, self-abuse is the most frequently reported dysfunctional primary behavioral and socializing symptom, followed by enuresis and encopresis, social rebellion, temper tantrums, hyperactivity, and physical aggression. Lying, stealing, destructive behavior, and sleep and eating problems comprise the sixth to tenth most frequent symptoms.

For nonsuicidal emotionally ill boys and girls, the three most frequent behavioral symptoms are physical aggression, hyperactivity, and temper tantrums. One may ask why in the 10 most frequent primary symptoms for the 34 suicidal children there was no indication of psychotic symptoms such as peculiar mannerisms, stereotyped behavior, infantile-regressive behaviors, autism, and withdrawal, yet for the suicidal boys, 23 percent reported bizarre behaviors. Where in any chart the primary or secondary complaint had been "self-abuse," the authors examined these cases further to exclude those children where such identified "self-abusive" behavior was related to autism, childhood schizophrenia, mental retardation, and borderline or psychotic behavior. The intent of the present study was to examine depression and self-abuse in terms of an affect and/or behavior disorder, rather than a mental retardation or autism-like dysfunction (p. 230). However, examination of the fourth most important behavioral symptom for suicidal boys, bizarre behavior, in which 23 percent of the sample indicated this symptom, revealed that the behavior was not bizarre in terms of a psychotic manifestation, but unique in terms of its description of either the family, the community, or the traumatic quality of the suicide attempt. It is also interesting to note the absence of bizarre behavior for suicidal female children, yet they did show a significant number of eating, sleeping, enuresis, and encopresis problems.

Although much of the literature on the etiology of physical abuse of children emphasizes the contributory role of the "special child" as an added stress variable for the parent, the present data do not identify physical handicaps as a concomitant variable in childhood suicidal depression; yet delayed development and school problems are significantly associated with acutely depressed suicidal boys and girls. Disruptive classroom behavior and underachievement must be examined by parents, pediatricians, teachers, and child development specialists as clues to severe depression, especially when accompanied by self-abusive behavior and other internally and externally directed severe behavioral responses. It is interesting that while marked preoccupation with fire setting as a means of retaliating against family members and/or using fire as a means of self-immolation were identified in four of the 21 males (19 percent), but not in females, none of the charts of the 34 suicidal children identified fire setting as a primary symptom.

No psychophysiological disorders were identified as a primary symptom in the 34 suicidal children, mainly because the children were being referred to the Neuropsychiatric Institute for evaluation. However, in studying the referral sources, 26 percent were from private physicians and 15 percent were from the UCLA Hospital, Pediatric Clinic. This means that the physicians in 41 percent of our sample of 34 children recognized psychological concomitants in the child's existing pediatric medical condition. Moreover, all the parents of the medically referred children agreed with the referring pediatrician that their high-risk children should be brought to the NPI for further evaluation and/or treatment.

On the basis of this sample of 34 latency-age suicidal and acutely depressed children, it appears that depressed boys show a slightly higher percent of self-abuse than do girls; and they show a significantly higher percent of physical aggressiveness, temper tantrums, destructiveness, hyperactivity, verbal aggressiveness, and lying. Depressed girls, on the other hand, have a higher frequency of sleeping and eating disorders, as well as problems related to enuresis and encopresis. It is interesting that while the child psychiatry literature discusses the positive correlation between enuresis and fire setting in children, none of the four male children preoccupied with fire and self-immolation were identified as having enuresis, while 17 percent of the depressed girls, none concerned with fire setting, were identified as having either enuresis or encopresis.

In the 444 nonsuicidal mentally ill male children, the percent rank ordering of the seven most frequent primary symptoms of the 41 symptoms listed as follows: anger, physical aggression, disruptive school behavior, depression, underachievement at school, temper tantrums, and hyperactivity. For the 184 nonsuicidal female patients, the most frequent symptoms, in declining order, are: depression, anger, hyperactivity, temper tantrums, and underachievement at school; of equal frequency are autism, withdrawal, self-abuse, physical agression, rebelliousness, and disruptive behavior.

While Paulson and co-workers (1974, 1978) described many findings specific to those events precipitating suicidal behavior, they did not examine the precipitating events in terms of age, sex, and ethnicity. Table 11-2 identifies such data by increasing age for those 26 children out of 34 who were identified not only as acutely depressed, but for whom there was also an identified suicide attempt or acute suicidal preoccupation. The remaining eight children manifested many indications of "depressive equivalents," but for none was there identified any suicidal behavior or active suicidal fantasy.

The precipitating events for the younger suicidal children centered on real, perceived, or imagined abandonment by one or both parent figures. Such separation fears were associated with divorce, threats of divorce, temporary separation, fear of rejection, rivalry at the birth of a sibling, and the decision of a single mother to go to work. All these separations, real or imagined, were psychodynamically meaningful, representing deep personal loss to the child. Said one six-year-old boy, emotionally rejected by his working mother, "I want to die because nobody loves me." An eight-year-old girl said, "They don't like me. I wish I was dead." A 10-year-old physically abused boy, whose 13-year-old brother had committed suicide, said to his therapist, "Everyone kills and everyone dies. There is no escape" (pp. 234-235).

The family dynamics of these 34 children were frequently associated with acute and chronic family stress, verbal and physical violence, sibling rivalry and assault, and a history of suicide or suicide attempts in close family members. This family stress was directly related to findings that 40 percent of the children were having serious failings in school in spite of the fact that the mean I.Q. for the 34 children was 93. Violence within the families was expressed in many ways. Self-immolation and fire-setting behavior were found in 12 percent of the children, all males. Homicidal behavior toward peers or family members was identified in five boys and two girls, comprising 20 percent of the sample. Threats and attacks with knives and scissors and attempted strangulation of a three-year-old sister characterize the violent intentions of children whose pretreatment family life offered no hope for rescue, salvation, or emotional peace and tranquility.

The family history of suicide for our 34 latency-age children is similar to that for adolescents and adults. Nine percent of the children had a close relative who committed suicide, six percent had immediate relatives who made unsuccessful single or multiple attempts at suicide, and for another nine percent of the children there were family members labeled as suicidal. In all, 25 percent of the children had a family life that, in one way or another, was directly linked to suicidal behavior of family members. In addition to such indices of physical violence, there were many indications of chronic psychological and emotional abuse and neglect, multiple out-of-home placements, and emotional rejection by family members. A chronically rejected nine-year-old boy expressed a wish to kill himself, his mother, his sister, and his grandmother, each of whom he saw as a nonnurturing and rejecting female. Out of fear and despair in anticipating her own real or imagined dying, a 12-year-old girl suffering from cystic hygroma made three suicide attempts, two by stabbing and slashing herself and one by overdosing on her mother's pills. After purposefully drugging her three-year-old sister, this girl said, "I would be better off dead. Then no one will ever have to look at my ugly face again."

Follow-up studies on the effectiveness of psychotherapy for depressed children are rare. Three years subsequent to the end of this four-year data-gathering period, Paulson, Stone, and Sposto (1978) did a follow-up study. The time range since the earlier evaluation of 13 of the 34 depressed children who were locatable was from three to seven years, with a mean time length of 4.4 years after evaluation. All 13 parents located responded positively to the follow-up. The following are typical comments from responding mothers: "The training program (behavior modification) was excellent, very constructive, the direction was terrific; behavior modification helped me get better results with my kids . . . NPI put me on the right course." Individual private therapy and child guidance clinic treatment contributed to significant emotional growth in the children and relaxation of tensions in child-parent relationships. Comments with regard to such process-oriented treatment were as follows: "He's doing remarkably well now, there is no further talk of suicide." "She is doing well now academically; she is no longer in crisis." "There are no further problems; my daughter and I are getting along better. She's an 'A' student" (her I.Q. was 97 at the time of evaluation). Residential treatment outcomes for the more disturbed and out-of-control children varied with the type of setting. "He is now in a therapeutic foster home and doing well." "He has outgrown his violence, but still needs help for his schooling." With respect to other residential placements, the comments were: "There are no further attempts at self-abuse, but he has a poor relationship with his stepfather." "He's making good progress in the institution and he has no thoughts of self-hate."

Foster-home placements varied in effectiveness. Following the fourth marriage of her mother, and after two foster-home placements, the 12-year-old girl with three suicide attempts, suffering from cystic hygroma, was finally placed in a residential center and was discharged at age 15. At that time she was living with a man who, fortunately, encouraged her stay in school. She was on drugs, continued to be violent with her mother, and is presently having only marginal success in coping. Another child, the five-year-old, white female who threatened her mother and sister with knives and who attempted to choke her sister, had been placed in adoption. The first adoption lasted six months and was described by the social worker as "horrible." A second, later adoption was much more

Table 11-2

Events Precipitating Suicidal Behavior, by Age, Sex, and Race of Child ($N=26$)

Age	Sex	Race	Precipitating Events
4	M	White	Intolerable home environment. Family abandoned by father
4	F	White	Talked of death and preoccupied with dying of her imaginary friend
4	M	White	Catastrophic home. Observed family fighting with knives and razors
5	F	White	Learned her mother was pregnant, saying, "My mother doesn't want me"
5	F	White	Violent home. Saw father beating up mother
6	M	White	Saw mother beaten by violent, drunken father. Family separated and child wanted parents to get together again
6	M	White	Mother working and child felt no one loved him. "I want to die because no one loves me"
6	M	White	Child abandoned by stepmother
7	M	White	Parental violence, acute depression, unbearable stomach distress
7	M	White	Earlier violent stabbing attack upon himself and his pet dog. Also tried to suffocate baby brother, age 18 months
8	M	White	Mother tells child she doesn't love him anymore and he feels he will be given away
8	F	White	Extreme marital tension. Said, "They don't like me." Harnessed to bed by parents to control her behavior
9	M	White	Wanted to kill self, sister, mother, and grandmother. "Everyone at school hates me"
9	M	White	Acute parental and family tension. Attacked sister and mother with knife and rock
9	M	Latino	Stabbed friend with knife on two occasions, threatened to kill mother and brother and heard father say, "Go kill yourself." Mother afraid she will hurt the child
9	F	White	"I want to kill myself. I would rather die than be spanked. They want me dead"

Age	Sex	Race	
10	M	White	Older brother committed suicide. Feels parents don't want him. Said, "Everyone kills and everyone dies, there is no escape"
10	M	Black	Acute marital conflict. Patient felt rejected by father
10	M	White	Threatened to run away. Feels he was rejected by mother. Felt everybody was picking on him
11	M	White	Child felt rejected at time of separation of parents
11	M	White	Divorced family. Mother working. "It doesn't matter if I'm dead." Tried to jump out of car while on freeway
11	M	White	Preoccupation with death. Threatened to kill himself and family. Tried to jump in front of moving car
11	F	White	Broken home. Reprimanded for skipping school, then made suicidal attempt by overdosing
11	F	White	Caught holding knife to younger sister's throat after setting house on fire. Stabbed self with knife, then hospitalized
11	F	Latino	Sexual assault by father followed by father's rejection. Overdosed on 19 aspirins
12	F	White	Has cystic hygroma. Drugged 3-year-old sister. Patient said, "I would be better off dead. No one will ever have to look at my ugle face again"

successful, with the adoption worker reporting, "It's a success story. . . . She's having regular therapy . . . and I feel confident it will be all right."

It appears that in spite of the violence within most of the families studied, the great majority of the follow-up children had responded favorably to intervention. None had committed suicide. While one girl showed borderline social adaptation, all children, when placed in an environment of warmth, affection, and acceptance, benefitted from treatment. In spite of the absence of close attachments in their early life and in spite of a wish to die because the felt unloved, these children had developed basic ego resources that allowed them to cope more effectively, at least through the present period of follow-up. Only time will tell how continued foster-home or residential placement will contribute to the rehabilitation of these children.

This study of 34 depressed latency-age children affirms that hopelessness, helplessness, aloneness, fear of rejection, and internalized and externalized violence are aspects of family life that can make a child want to die. Children can experience the acute pain of depression. Many may mask their symptoms of depression by a variety of behavioral, physiological, and educational manifestations. However, health providers and caregivers must realize that young children can be "at risk" for suicide. We must be alert to the depth and meaning of childhood depression. We must recognize symptom substitution and the depressive equivalent. We must attend to accidental injuries and poisoning. We must be alert to the dynamics behind school failure, peer isolation, and violent behavioral eruptions within the home and the school. Being alert, we are in a better position to intervene in the identification, early treatment, and ultimate recovery of severely depressed children (p. 241).

Pfeiffer (1978): "The Suicidal Methods of Latency-Age Children"

The author reports a four-year study of suicidal behavior in hospitalized latency-age children at Bronx Memorial Hospital, New York. Noting that suicidal behavior and completed acts of suicide are increasing in the adolescent population worldwide, Pfeiffer states: "Men complete suicide more often than women, and women attempt suicide more frequently than men. Adult men use more aggressive means such as hanging, strangulation, firearms, jumping from buildings, while suicidal women in general select more passive, self-destructive methods such as overdosing and ingestion of poisons." Pfeiffer notes that latency-age boys also show more violent acts of intentional death-seeking behavior such as running into traffic, jumping from heights, hanging, strangulation, and drug ingestion.

The demography of the Pfeiffer study is as follows: subjects studied were children ages 6–12 years, all from a low socioeconomic background, with 40 percent blacks, 46 percent Hispanics, and 14 percent white. The children were all hospitalized for self-destructive behavior, uncontrolled aggression, or severe psychotic symptoms. Her sample of 146 hospitalized children was divided into two groups: 66 suicidal children and 80 nonsuicidal children. Although the ethnic mix of the two groups was similar, there was a greater number of boys in both the suicidal and the nonsuicidal subpopulations. The sex distribution for the suicidal group was 48 boys and 18 girls, while in the nonsuicidal group the sex distribution was 66 boys and 14 girls. The mean age of children in both groups was approximately nine years.

In the suicidal population, 44 percent made bona fide attempts, 44 percent threatened suicide, and 12 percent contemplated suicide. The types of suicide attempts included: jumping from high places (41 percent), drug ingestion (34 percent), hanging, running into traffic, electrocution, and burning. Although the incidence of boys and girls *attempting* suicide was almost equal, more than twice as many boys as girls *threatened* suicide. Pfeiffer concludes: "It would be an error to look for one determinant. . . . Each suicidal method is influenced by the contribution of multiple factors such as: 1) the child's exposure to recent death, accidental injury or suicidal actions by friends or family members, and subsequent identification with such actions or intentions of family members; 2) developmental failures including the child's level of cognitive and motor skills; 3) choice of available methods for self-intended death; and 4) quality of emotional communication and interaction with family members and significant others."

In many respects the nature of violence in the Pfeiffer study parallels that described by Paulson, Stone, and Sposto. Despite the significant ethnic differences between the two studies, there is a common quality of emotional isolation, family fragmentation, loss of affectional supports, and a sense of hopelessness that characterize the self-destructive acts of all the children under study.

Carlson and Cantwell (1980):
"Unmasking Masked Depression in Children and Adolescents"

From a sample of 1,000 children screened at the UCLA Neuropsychiatric Institute, 210 English-speaking children aged 7 to 17 years were selected. One hundred and two children and their parents agreed to take part in a systematic evaluation consisting of not only the Beck Children's Depression Inventory (BCDI), but also an intensive psychiatric interview with the parents and separately with the children. From this random sampling of 102 children, the following data were elicited. Ninety-three of the 102 children were given an Axis I DSM-III clinical diagnosis with the following percent distributions: behavior disorders (35 percent); emotional disorders (17 percent); physical disorders (11 percent); psychotic disorders (8 percent); affective disorders (27 percent); and the remainder (2 percent) classified as *undiagnosed, other,* or *no mental disorder.* The discharge diagnosis for 28 children having an affect disorder were as follows: depressive neurosis or manic-depressive psychosis (39 percent); feeding disturbances, such as anorexia nervosa (11 percent); adjustment reaction (14 percent); unsocial aggressive reactions (25 percent); personality disorder (7 percent); and encopresis (4 percent).

In examining the symptoms, syndrome, and disorder of depression in their population of 102 children, Carlson and Cantwell provide confirming evidence of the multiple concomitants of childhood depression. Of the 28 children from the initial sample of 210 who were given a diagnosis of an affective disorder, 14 (50 percent) had another diagnosis that preceded the onset of the depression. The earlier diagnosis of these 14 children were as follows: hyperactivity (25 percent), drug abuse (7 percent), anorexia nervosa (11 percent), learning disability (4 percent), and seizure disorder (4 percent). In retrospect, it would be very interesting to know whether those physicians making the initial diagnoses had an awareness of the underlying depressive disorder in the children. If they did not suspect depression, this would substantiate the fact that many health professionals are not alert to the existence of depression as an acute stress variable in children manifesting multiple behavior disturbances, drug abuse, anorexia nervosa, learning disability, and seizure disorders. The behaviors and symptoms demonstrate the existence of "masked depression."

Carlson and Cantwell conclude that depression as a presenting complaint—and even high scores on a depression inventory—while found significantly more often in children with depressive disorders, appears too often in other psychiatric conditions to be discriminating or specific for affective disorders. From the sample of 102 children, 60 percent had a depressive symptom, 49 percent had a depressive syndrome, and 28 percent met the DSM-III criteria for the presence of an affective disorder. The authors conclude (p. 449):

> 1) It is possible to diagnose children over age seven as having a major depressive disorder using adult research diagnostic criteria . . . 2) when children are interviewed systematically about their symptoms, a much higher incidence of depressive disorder is found than by the usual evaluation procedure . . . 3) some children who meet criteria for depression also meet criteria for other disorders, most often attention deficit disorders (hyperactivity), conduct disorders, and anorexia nervosa . . . 4) not all children with behavior disorders or anorexia nervosa are depressed. In fact, a majority of the children studied neither described depression nor appeared depressed; and 5) there are two differences between the behavior problems of children who are simply depressed and those who have diagnoses of both depressive and behavior disorders. In children with depression, behavior problems were seen as less severe, and postdated the onset of depressive symptoms. In children with both diagnoses and in children with behavior disorders alone, the behavior problems were chronic and of

greater magnitude. . . . Although we have not addressed ourselves to all types of masked depression, we conclude that in some children with hyperactivity, aggressive behavior, and some anti-social behavior, a depressive disorder co-exists. Insofar as the behavior disturbance is most outstanding, it may be said to overshadow the depression. To an alert clinician conducting a thorough interview, however, the depression will not be masked.

CASE HISTORIES

While demographic and tabular data provide insights into categorized groups of patients, they often lack the personal, experiential flavor of what constitutes the emotional environment of the individual under study. The following case histories (Paulson, Stone, and Sposto, 1978) have been included to give a representative picture of the depressed and suicidal child in terms of age, sex, family dynamics, and nature of the violent, self-destructive acts and fantasies of the child.

Case 1

Johnny (male, white, age nine) attempted to hang himself following an attack upon his mother with a knife and an earlier attempt to seriously injure his sister with a large stone. Johnny had been doing well in school and in little league baseball, but was struggling in a family overwhelmed by great tensions. Johnny's fantasy life, as revealed through psychological testing, showed fearful and angry preoccupations with obsessive ideas of violence, death, and destruction. Embedded in a web of parental anger, unable to escape from the frustrations of the parents, guilty over his violent attacks upon his mother and sister, Johnny saw suicide as his only escape from an oppressive home and overwhelming guilt; he attempted suicide by hanging.

Case 2

Mary (white, female, age 8) lived with parents chronically involved in a verbally hostile marriage. Finding no love in her home, Mary's negative behavior patterns were the only means by which she could find any degree of recognition and attention. Behavioral difficulties over a four-year period included lying and stealing (both food and money). Mary was never rewarded for doing well, but constantly punished for doing poorly. Harnessed to her bed at night to prevent further acting out, Mary felt overwhelmed and unable to escape the violence and

and marital tension within her home. In a moment of acute depression, she entered a shower and purposely scalded herself, receiving severe burns.

Subsequently hospitalized for this self-destructive act, Mary continued banging her head and furiously punching a stuffed doll. In one of her therapy sessions following a violent kicking and stomping of her doll, Mary took a toy phone pretending to call the police for help. The accident-prone nature of Mary further substantiates the self-destructive drives of this girl, who, full of guilt, hate, and anger, was unable to find an acceptable outlet for her aloneness, depression, and emotional deprivation.

Case 3

Carlos (male, Cuban, age 11), grieving over the earlier death of his grandmother, constantly punished because of expressed wishes to kill his family, and continually involved in violent fights with his brother and sister, told his older brother that he was going to throw himself in front of a car and kill himself so that his mother could become rich with insurance money. Disfiguring his face by violent self-beatings, preoccupied with matches and firesetting, Carlos, in a moment of despair, climbed out of an upper-story window and jumped to the ground.

In the past, his mother had threatened death to herself and her family because of violent arguments. The father, separated from the family, left Carlos, his mother, and siblings in a state of poverty and depression. In therapy Carlos talked about his angry feelings, his wish to kill all the people in the world, including his mother and his father, and again stated to his therapist that he would like to kill himself. Following lengthy hospitalization, return of the father to the home, and family therapy, significant therapeutic progress was made. Follow-up three years subsequent to Carlos's hospitalization indicated that he was doing well in baseball, had good peer relations, was progressing well at school, and no longer appeared depressed and suicidal. The father's follow-up statement was, "The boy is doing good. He's no more trouble."

THEORETICAL AND CLINICAL CONSIDERATIONS OF LATENCY-AGE SUICIDAL BEHAVIOR

Review of the literature on childhood depression indicates many theoretical positions; however, these are supported by relatively few solid clinical studies. There is a major need to define those emotional states that are: (1) both observable and nonobservable to parents and health professionals; (2) experienced and reported by children; and (3) identified in an increasing population of children who purposely seek to die because of the overwhelming pain in living in a family milieu lacking emotional supports and parental understanding. Anthony (1975) asks:

1. Is there a basic depressive affect or depressive mood?
2. Is there a depressive tendency?
3. Is there a primary depression?
4. Is there a depressive reaction of childhood?
5. Is the depression of childhood similar in its clinical manifestation to that of adult depression?
6. Can childhood depression and adult depression be considered within the same theoretical framework? If not, what is the nature of those theoretical frameworks that explain both childhood depression and adult depression?

For every question asked, there are concomitant answers, some of which are cautionary while others are strongly avowed and championed. Beck (1967), Anthony and Benedek (1975), Malmquist (1975, 1977), Schulterbrandt and Raskin (1977), Toolan (1974, 1978), and Carlson and Cantwell (1979, 1980) are only a few of the major references that provide multiple hypotheses and recommendations for further theoretical and clinical research into the questions posed by Anthony.

From a theoretical position as well as from the data presented by Paulson, Stone, and Sposto (1978), Pfeiffer (1978), and Carlson and Cantwell (1980), it is evident that the narcissistic needs of the very young child in an emotionally secure and giving family are gratified by the parents' willingness and ability to satisfy the anaclitic dependency of the newborn child. Absence of such gratification, however, may lead to marasmus, failure to thrive, and ultimately to death. Environmentally there are multiple factors associated with acute childhood depression and suicidal behavior. Some of these are: parental loss due to separation, divorce, death, or purposeful abandonment of the child, emotional rejection and parental indifference to the needs and wants of the child; rigid, emotionally frozen families unable or unwilling to share feelings and express affectional bonds such as touching, hugging, and listening; chronic and acute illnesses; and jealousy, loss of esteem, and anger at the pending birth of a sibling. Within the family of the depressed child are found such elements as familial mood disorders; narcissistic-oral parents whose "role-reversal" expectations and demands are so self-centered that such parents cannot in any way provide emotional nurturance to the growing child.

Spitz (1946), Bowlby (1969, 1973), and Heinicke (1973) have emphasized the effects of early infantile separation from the emotionally and biologically needed mother. Marasmus as a phenomenon is well understood in terms of object relations theory and object loss (Klein, 1964), where the infant's "depressive position" often becomes the forerunner for later adult depression. With or without such object loss, the later death of a parent may lead to a normal period of mourning; but unfortunately—and too often— it leads to a pathological state of chronic grief, where the internalized love object (the lost parent) unconsciously—and sometimes consciously—becomes identified as the person responsible for the loss of the child's narcissistic gratifications. The anger unconsciously felt toward the deceased or abandoning parent may be externalized, resulting in behavioral disturbances, severe sibling rivalry, and at times even homicidal feelings and actions directed at siblings and other family members. At other times the unconscious feelings of anger may be internalized, and, with the aggression turned inward, there may follow self-mutilating or self-destructive acts of personal violence. Body mutilation, self-immolation, and severe head banging are aspects of narcissistic injury repeatedly found in the acutely depressed and suicidal latency-age child.

The clinical findings of Paulson, Stone, and Sposto (1978) clearly indicate that childhood depression is not a univariate phenomenon arising from a single environmental stress. A history of chronic abandonment, a heritage of family suicide or suicidal behavior, loss of self-esteem as a function of perceived body-image inadequacies, and intrafamily violence were identified in almost every family. "Masked depression" and the "depressive equivalent" were found in a high percentage of children manifesting behavioral and socialization conflicts, school conflicts, and, to a lesser degree, delayed development. The most frequent behavioral and socialization defects were noted in terms of self-abuse, temper tantrums, physical aggression, hyperactivity, rebellion, and verbal aggression and lying. While suicidal boys and girls were equal in terms of the destructive nature of their fantasies and behaviors, there was a noticeable sex difference in terms of affect disturbance. Boys tended more toward anger as the primary symptom, while a greater percentage of girls showed depression as the primary symptom. In none of the acutely depressed suicidal boys were disturbances in sleep and eating or defects in elimination the primary symptoms. In contrast, these were major areas of distress for a significant percentage of the depressed girls.

All three of the clinical studies reported substantiate the presence of masked depression and depression equivalents as concomitants or later depression in children. Carlson and Cantwell, in a detailed psychiatric evaluation and classification of 102 children, aged 7–17, reported 60 percent with depressive symptoms, 49 percent with a depressive syndrome, and 28 percent meeting the DSM-III criteria for the presence of an affective disorder. There is a consensus in all three studies that depression in children is not easily recognized, that it is even more difficult to diagnose, and that within the multidisciplinary realm of mental and physical health specialties there is a substantial lack of agreement with regard to the theoretical bases of childhood depression (if it does exist); furthermore, there is a lack of agreement on whether the bases and techniques for assessing adult depression can be validly and reliably applied to the assessment of depression in young children.

The present paper has reviewed the extensive literature, not in detail, but sufficiently to allow the reader to formulate opinions with regard to the nature of depression as an experienced feeling and as a phenomenon masked under a multitude of behavioral and socialization stresses, physical handicaps, delayed development, school problems, and psychophysiological disorders. The clinical cases presented and the analysis of factors precipitating depression, suicidal ideation, and suicidal behavior provide a more personal insight into the experienced pain of living in those children ultimately referred for psychiatric evaluation and treatment. There are substantive data supporting the concepts of both primary and masked depression in children. The course of depression in many children begins early in infancy and extends through to adulthood. For some children the morbidity risk is high, and without intervention and treatment the risk of continuing chronic depression from childhood into adulthood is very real. The course and outcome of childhood depression is a function of: (1) how early the depression is identified; (2) how astute the professional is in looking beyond the evident symptomatology and seeking out the underlying primary area of focal stress; and (3) as Toolan cautions, what are the available skilled resources for providing the special intervention for emotionally and physically abused children whose primary, secondary, or tertiary symptomatology may or may not be depression?

Depression and suicide are as real for children as they are for adolescents and adults. We as health care practitioners may ourselves feel depressed when we read that "our prediction is that the diagnosis of clinical depression of childhood will be made with increasing frequency in the future" (Anthony, 1975; p. 273). However, we should feel professionally pleased and reassured that this increased identification is because pediatric, health care, and education specialists are willing to recognize that depression and suicidal wishes and actions are real and living experiences of children, and that when identified early, their treatment and intervention can be successful. The lay public and parents in particular must be aware of the consequences of emotional deprivation in the life of a child (and of adults also). It will be the wise, sensitive, and concerned parent who will seek out a health professional who is sensitive, astute, and skilled in assessing those children in whom family-peer-social-educational failures may be masking a deep-seated, life-threatening depression or suicide potential.

REFERENCES

Agros, S. The relationship of school phobia to childhood depression. *American Journal of Psychiatry, 116,* 533–536 (1959).

Annell, A. *Depressive States in Childhood and Adolescence.* Proceedings of the 4th U.E.P. Congress, Stockholm (1971), pp. 11–25.

Anthony, E. Childhood depression. In *Depression and Human Existence*, E. Anthony and T. Benedek, eds. Little, Brown, Boston (1975), pp. 231–277.

Anthony, E., and Benedek, T. *Depression and Human Existence*. Little, Brown, Boston (1975).

Beck, A. *Depression: Causes and Treatment*. University of Pennsylvania Press, Philadelphia (1967).

Benedek, T. Toward the biology of the depressive constellation. *Journal of the American Psychoanalytic Association, 4*, 389–427 (1956).

Berner, P., Katschning, H., and Poldinger, W. *Masked Depression*, P. Kielholz, ed. Hans Huber, Bern (1973), pp. 82–96.

Bosselman, B. *Self-Destruction: A Study of the Suicidal Impulse*. Charles C. Thomas, Springfield (1958), pp. 1–11.

Bowlby, J. *Attachment and Loss: Attachment*. Basic Books, New York (1969).

– – –. *Attachment and Loss: Separation*. Basic Books, New York (1973).

Burlingham, D., and Freud, A. *Infants Without Families*. Allen & Unwin, London (1943).

Campbell, J. Manic-depressive disease in children. *Journal of the American Medical Association, 158*, 154–157 (1959).

Cantwell, D., and Carlson, G. Problems and prospects in the study of childhood depression. *Journal of Nervous and Mental Disease, 167*, 522–529 (1979).

Carlson, G., and Cantwell, D. A survey of depressive symptoms, syndrome and disorder in a child psychiatric population. *Journal of Child Psychology and Psychiatry, 21*, 19–25 (1979).

– – –. Unmasking masked depression in children and adolescents. *American Journal of Psychiatry, 137*, 445–449 (1980).

Conners, C. Classification and treatment of childhood depression and depressive equivalents. In *Depression*, D. Gallant and G. Simpson, eds. Spectrum, New York (1976), pp. 181–204.

Cytryn, L. Current research in childhood depression. *Journal of Child Psychiatry, 18*, 583–599 (1979).

Cytryn, L., and McKnew, D. Proposed classification of childhood depression. *American Journal of Psychiatry, 129*, 63–69 (1972).

Frederick, C. *Adolescent Suicide*. Advocacy for Children. U.S. Department of Health, Education and Welfare, National Center for Child Advocacy, (1978).

Frommer, E. Depressive illness in childhood: recent developments in affective disorders. *British Journal of Psychiatry* (special publication), *2*, 227–236 (1968).

Harrington, M., and Hassan, J. Depression in girls during latency. *British Journal Medical Psychology, 31*, 43–50 (1958).

Heinicke, C. Parental deprivation in early childhood: a predisposition to later depression. *American Association for the Advancement of Science*, 141–160 (1973).

Jacobson, E. The effect of disappointment on ego and superego formation in normal and depressive development. *Psychoanalytic Review, 23*, 129–147 (1946).

Klein, M. *Contributions to Psychoanalysis*. McGraw-Hill, New York (1964).

Kovacs, M., and Beck, A. An empirical-clinical approach toward a definition of childhood depression. In *Depression in Childhood: Diagnosis, Treatment, and Conceptual Models*, J. Schulterbrandt and A. Raskin, eds. Raven Press, New York (1977).

Lefkowitz, M., and Burton, N. Childhood depression: a critique of the concept. *Psychological Bulletin, 85,* 716–726 (1978).

Levy, D. Primary affect hunger. *American Journal of Psychiatry, 94,* 643–652 (1937).

Lokare, V. Neuroticism, extraversion and the incidence of depressive illness in children. In *Depressive States in Childhood and Adolescence.* Proceedings of the 4th U.E.P. Congress, Stockholm (1971), pp. 142–148.

Lourie, R. Clinical studies of attempted suicide in childhood. *Clinical Proceedings, Children's Hospital, 12,* 163–173 (1966).

Malmquist, C. Depressions in childhood and adolescents. *New England Journal of Medicine, 284,* 887–893 (1971).

———. Depression in childhood. In *Comprehensive Textbook of Depression,* F.F. Flach and S. Draghi, eds. Wiley, New York (1975).

———. *Depression in Childhood: Diagnosis, Treatment, and Conceptual Models,* J. Schulterbrandt and A. Raskin, eds. Raven Press, New York (1977), pp. 33–68.

Mendelsohn, W., Reid, M., and Frommer, E. Some characteristic features accompanying depression, anxiety and aggressive behavior in disturbed children under five. In *Depressive States in Childhood and Adolescence.* Proceedings of the 4th U.E.P. Congress, Stockholm (1971), pp. 151–158.

Nissen, G. Masked depression in children and adolescents. In *Masked Depression.* P. Kielholz, ed. Hans Huber, Bern (1973), pp. 133–143.

Paulson, M., and Stone, D. Suicidal behavior of latency age children, ages 4–12. *Journal of Clinical Child Psychology, 3,* 50–52 (1974).

Paulson, M., Stone, D., and Sposto, R. Suicide potential and behavior in children ages 4 to 12. *Suicide and Life-Threatening Behavior,* 225–242 (1978).

Pfeiffer, C. The suicidal methods of latency-age children. Eleventh Annual Meeting of the American Association of Suicidology, New Orleans (April 6–9, 1978).

Rochlin, G. *Loss and Restitution, Grief and Its Discontents.* Little, Brown, Boston (1965), pp. 121–164.

Schulterbrandt, J., and Raskin, A. *Depression in Childhood: Diagnosis, Treatment, and Conceptual Models.* Raven Press, New York (1977).

Sperling, M. Equivalents of depression in children. *Journal of the Hillside Hospital, 8,* 138–148 (1959).

Spitz, R. Hospitalism. *Psychoanalytic Study of the Child, 2,* 113–117 (1946).

Spitz, R., and Wolf, K. Anaclitic depression. *Psychoanalytic Study of the Child, 2,* 313–342 (1946).

Toolan, J. Depression in children and adolescents. *American Journal of Orthopsychiatry, 32,* 404–415 (1962).

———. Depression and suicide. In *American Handbook of Psychiatry,* Vol. 2 Basic Books, New York (1974).

———. Therapy of depressed and suicidal children. *American Journal of Psychotherapy, 32,* 243–251 (1978).

Wealcher, W. *Die larvierte Depression.* Hollinek, Vienna (1969).

Weinberg, W., Rutman, J., Sullivan, L., Penick, E., and Dietz, S. Depression in children referred to an educational diagnostic center. Diagnosis and treatment—preliminary report. *Journal of Pediatrics, 83,* 1065–1072 (1973).

12

Teenage Pregnancy

Marianne Felice

> One of the main difficulties of being a teenager is sex, at
> once a great discovery, a great mess, a great pleasure, a
> great frustration, and an all around great muddle.
>
> (Daniel Callahan, 1976)

Teenage pregnancy in the United States is a complex problem that has reper-
cussions for all members of society. Pregnancy in this age group has medical,
psychological, social, and educational implications. Health professionals of
various disciplines are being confronted with requests for help from young pregnant patients or their parents. This chapter will provide guidelines for psychosocial care for health professionals who wish to respond to the special needs of
these young patients.

SUSPECT PREGNANCY

One-fifth of all births in the United States are to young women between the
ages of 10 and 19, resulting in approximately 600,000 births to teenagers each
year (Alan Guttmacher Institute, 1976; National Center for Health Statistics,
1976). Indeed, approximately one in ten adolescent girls becomes pregnant each
year; two-thirds of whom deliver an infant and one-third either miscarry or
choose to terminate the pregnancy (Alan Guttmacher Institute, 1976). Recent
statistics indicate that although the numbers of teenage births appear large, the
actual incidence of births to older adolescents (15-19 years) has decreased in the
past ten years. For younger adolescents (less than 15 years of age), the incidence
of teenage births is still rising (Baldwin, 1976), particularly to young, white
teenage girls.

In spite of these alarming figures, physicians still overlook the diagnosis of
pregnancy when confronted with vague or puzzling symptoms in an adolescent
girl.

Betty is a 16-year-old white high school student who presented to a special clinic for pregnant teenagers for her first prenatal visit at approximately 24–26 weeks' gestation. Betty relates that shortly after she missed her period, she began vomiting every day. Her mother took her to their primary care physician, who diagnosed viral gastroenteritis. The physician told Betty's mother that if the vomiting continued, he would schedule an upper GI series. The vomiting finally decreased, but about two months later Betty fainted at work at a busy fast-food restaurant where she worked parttime after school and weekends. The restaurant manager took her to a nearby emergency room where several laboratory tests were done, including a five-hour glucose tolerance test for suspected hypoglycemia. As Betty's blue jeans began to fit tighter, she finally confessed her suspicion of pregnancy to her boyfriend. In turn he discussed it with his older sister. His older sister took Betty to a Planned Parenthood Clinic, where pregnancy was confirmed and a referral for prenatal care was made. Betty was pleased to be pregnant and desired to keep the baby, which was fortunate, since she was too far along to have been considered for abortion. Betty's only remaining concern was how to inform her mother.

This case vignette demonstrates the frequency with which health professionals neglect to consider pregnancy as the etiology for the adolescent's symptoms. The younger the adolescent the less often it is considered, in spite of published statistics which report that sexually active adolescents are becoming sexually active at increasingly younger ages (Alan Guttmacher Institute, 1976; Sorensen, 1972; Vener and Stewart, 1974). Every adolescent should be seen privately and separately from her parents. The sexual history should be part of every patient's workup. Inquiry about menstruation provides an ideal entry into a discussion about sexual activities:

How old were you when you had your first period?
When was your last period?
Have you ever missed a period?
Have you ever been worried about your period, wondering if you might be pregnant?

Questions about sexual activity should be gently and tactfully asked. The health professional should provide a milieu in which the adolescent can be comfortable in discussing sexual issues without fear of scorn of breach of confidentiality. Establishing such rapport can be difficult and takes time. Even in ideal circumstances, adolescents can be afraid and cautious. Kim was such a patient.

Kim is a 15-year-old white adolescent girl who was sent to the adolescent clinic by her nurse-mother for evaluation of back pain and breast tenderness. While taking the history, the physician strongly suspected pregnancy. When asked about her last menstrual period, Kim readily blurted out a date approximately three weeks earlier and claimed it was a normal period. Upon further questioning, she staunchly denied the possibility of pregnancy. Upon completing the physical and pelvic examination, the physician was further convinced that Kim was pregnant, approximately 8-10 weeks. The physician explained her dilemma to Kim and asked permission to do a pregnancy test. Upon such confrontation, the patient burst into tears and admitted concerns about pregnancy. She was afraid that news about her pregnancy would spread through the clinic and embarrass her mother who had nurse friends who worked in the clinic. Kim calmed down considerably when reassured of confidentiality.

Both Betty and Kim knew they were pregnant when they went to the doctor. Betty kept hoping the physician would discover the pregnancy. Kim kept hoping the physician would not discover the pregnancy (although the ambivalence of both girls is obvious). Some adolescents, however, actually deny the pregnancy for quite some time. Such denial is a psychological defense mechanism; by denying the pregnancy perhaps it will "just go away." This attitude probably accounts for the fact that many adolescents present quite late for prenatal care (Nadelson, 1975). Other adolescents , however—particularly young teenagers— may not recognize the signs and symptoms of pregnancy through ignorance. This is particularly common in those adolescents who have just recently experienced menarche.

Wanda is a 12-year-old black girl who presented for her first prenatal visit at 28-30 weeks' gestation. Menarche had occurred at age 11½ and, apparently, Wanda became pregnant the following month. Wanda's mother, who had two older adolescent girls, was aware that Wanda had not had a period for several months, but attributed it to her immaturity. As she abjectly explained to the clinician, "I wasn't worried, because all my girls were irregular when they first began their periods." Wanda confided to the examiner that she didn't know she had missed a period because she wasn't sure how often to have them. When she noticed her breasts increasing in size, she thought it was part of "growing up." She never experienced nausea and vomiting.

THE CRISIS OF PREGNANCY

In general, the adolescent who is told that she is pregnany is an adolescent in crisis. Most teenagers receive the news that they are pregnant with fear, confusion, and, sometimes, panic. For this reason, the diagnosis of pregnancy should never be given over the phone. Instead, the health provider should inform the adolescent of the pregnancy in a private, quiet room where the adolescent's reaction can be observed and handled. Such a policy lessens the possibility of suicide attempts, which have been reported in the past (Whitlock and Edwards, 1968).

After notifying the teenager that she is pregnant, the health professional should explore with the adolescent the various options that are available to her: abortion, adoption, keeping the baby. Information should be given in a supportive, nonjudgmental manner, allowing the young patient time to reflect and ask questions. The session should be unhurried and sometimes will require two or three visits. The health provider should always bear in mind that the decision to keep or terminate a pregnancy belongs to the patient, not to the health professional. For further information regarding such counseling, the clinician is referred to the literature (Beresford, 1977; Kreutner and Langhorst, 1978).

Most states have laws that permit adolescents to receive medical care for certain problems without parental knowledge or consent. Such medical problems usually include: venereal disease, contraception, pregnancy, drug abuse, and abortion. Each health professional should become familiar with the laws in his state. If an adolescent does not wish her parents to know about the pregnancy, her desire for confidentiality must be respected. Oftentimes, however, an adolescent may wish to inform her parents of the pregnancy (particularly if she intends to continue the pregnancy), but is frightened to tell them. In those instances, the clinician can often be of assistance. One technique is to role-play with the adolescent, allowing her to "practice" telling her parents. Another useful tool is to invite the adolescent girl to bring her parents to the office and have her tell her parents in the clinician's presence. In this manner, the health professional can act as the young person's advocate as well as answer questions from the parents.

The physician should also inquire about the feelings of the father of the baby. Most girls become pregnant by a steady boyfriend as part of a meaningful relationship. Older adolescents are usually able to discuss the possibility of pregnancy with one another; younger adolescents are more commonly embarrassed and shy. The clinician can often assist the young adolescent in informing her sexual partner of the pregnancy, if the adolescent wishes to tell him.

COPING WITH THE PREGNANCY

All adolescents must proceed through a series of developmental growth tasks that have been well described in the literature (Erikson, 1968; Freud, 1975; Corey and Herrick, 1965). Most authors would probably agree that the psychological accomplishments of adolescence should include: (1) gradual development as an independent individual; (2) the mental evolvement of a satisfying realistic body image; (3) harnessing appropriate control and expression of sexual and aggressive drives; (4) integration of a value system applicable to life events; (5) the expansion of unisexual and heterosexual relationships outside the home; (6) transition from concrete to abstract conceptualization; (7) the construction of a realistic plan to achieve social and economic independence. Progression through the growth tasks is necessary as groundwork for healthy adulthood. Young adolescents may differ from older adolescents in focusing on different aspects of the tasks at different times (Felice and Friedman, 1978), but, in general, most adolescents grapple with all the growth tasks concomitantly.

Pregnant adolescents, like their nonpregnant peers, must also develop along the same psychosocial cognitive growth curves just described. However, pregnancy imposes certain adjustments that may accelerate or, at times, interfere with such growth. How an adolescent will react to pregnancy is dependent upon multiple variables, including her psychological maturity, her emotional stability, her relationship with the baby's father, the response of her family to the pregnancy, and the attitude of her subculture toward teenage pregnancy. Although one would expect that older adolescents would handle pregnancy more maturely than younger adolescents, one cannot generalize toward all adolescents.

Sharon is a 14-year-old black adolescent girl who was the oldest of five siblings. Her first and only sexual encounter resulted in pregnancy. Her widowed working mother was disappointed when Sharon was pregnant but admitted she welcomed the prospect of a grandchild, even if it meant that she would have to quit her job to care for the infant. Sharon felt quilty about the pregnancy, particularly because she felt no close ties to the baby's father and because her mother was talking about leaving work. She discussed abortion with the clinic nurse in three weekly visits. She finally concluded that she could not terminate the pregnancy because she opposed abortion on religious grounds. She briefly considered adoption, but her family strongly opposed such an action. Halfway through the pregnancy, she announced to the clinic staff that she had convinced her grandmother to watch the infant so that she could go to school and her mother could work. Furthermore, she had requested her school to transfer her to another junior-senior high school that had a day care center for babies over six months of age and taught about child care. After delivering a healthy, six-pound baby girl, Sharon requested birth control pills so that "she would not get pregnant again before she finished school."

Although Sharon was only 14 years old, she had remarkable resourcefulness. She carefully weighed her decision to continue the pregnancy. She independently made arrangements for infant care. Contraceptives were requested as insurance for the future, suggesting that Sharon intended to have sexual intercourse in the future but wanted to be prepared in advance.

Althea is a 17-year-old black adolescent girl who was the oldest of four siblings. She was considered one of the brightest girls in her high school senior class. It was assumed that she would be offered several college scholarships. She, too, became pregnant after her first and only sexual encounter. Upon receiving the news that she had a positive pregnancy test, she began to rant and rave in the clinic, staunchly denying the possibility of pregnancy. After discussion with the clinic staff, she demanded an immediate abortion. A referral was made to a nearby abortion clinic and an appointment was made for two days hence, but Althea never kept the appointment. Several weeks later she again appeared in the physician's office asking for another abortion referral. When asked about the other referral appointment, she replied, "I forgot to go." Althea was informed that she was now beyond the time for having an abortion, provoking another barrage of tears. The doctor asked if her parents knew about the pregnancy. Althea said no and asked the clinician to tell them for her. The physician declined the responsibility, but agreed to be present while Althea told them herself. Althea's family received the news about the pregnancy with surprise but warm support. The clinic staff was relieved to see a smiling Althea leave the clinic.

However, it became obvious that Althea's problems were not over. She attended all prenatal visits accompanied by relatives and often required their presence during physical examinations. She began wearing her hair in pigtails, and her clothes adopted a little-girl appearance. She had varied psychosomatic complaints throughout pregnancy. When asked about the future baby's name, she said her parents had not chosen a name. Althea and her parents required much concentrated intervention from the clinic staff.

These two vignettes demonstrate how two different adolescents of different ages coped with their pregnancies. Helping adolescents grow with the pregnancy should be an essential component of all prenatal programs designed for teenagers. For further information on this subject, the reader is referred to the literature (Adams et al., 1976; Davis and Grace, 1971; Marans, 1966).

PSYCHOSOCIAL IMPLICATIONS OF TEENAGE PREGNANCY

Teenage pregnancy has psychosocial implications for both mother and child, and ultimately for society as a whole. This topic has been reviewed in depth in the literature (Alan Guttmacher Institute, 1976; Baldwin, 1976; Frustenberg, 1976; Hollingsworth and Kreutner, 1978).

The most commonly reported negative consequence of teenage pregnancy that affects the young mother is school dropout. Some authors estimate that nine-tenths of girls who become pregnant at age 15 or less quit school (Alan Guttmacher Institute, 1976). Some authors even speculate that some girls become pregnant in order to leave school (Cattanach, 1976). Clearly, Furstenberg's six-year follow-up of a large group of pregnant Baltimore teenagers indicates that the younger the individual when first becoming a parent, the less the amount of formal education obtained (Furstenberg, 1976). This seems to be true for both boys and girls. Such young people should be encouraged to remain in school. School systems should be prodded to provide programs tailored to the needs of pregnant teenagers. Such programs should include desks that are comfortable for the gravid abdomen, classes in prenatal and postnatal care, and day care centers.

Pregnant girls who drop out of school are at high risk for becoming pregnant again while still in their teens (Trussell and Menken, 1978). Teenage girls who have not completed their schooling have a difficult time finding employment, particularly young adolescents. Such young women may become bored or lonely (or both) and attempt to have another baby to alleviate their own misery. In postnatal care, attention must be paid to contraceptive counseling. However, the health provider should not become discouraged if his or her contraceptive advice is not followed. Decisions concerning childbearing still rest with the individuals involved and not with the physician.

In this day and age, most teenagers do not give up their babies for adoption (Baldwin, 1976; Levkoff, 1978). In general, adolescents either have an abortion or choose to keep the infant. Some adolescent couples marry and attempt to raise the infant together. In such cases, both the young woman and young man may quit school—the teenage mother to care for the baby and the teenage father to find employment. They may not be emotionally or financially equipped for such an endeavor. It has now been well documented that such marriages are at high risk for failure, leaving both partners discouraged and disillusioned (Furstenberg, 1976).

Adolescent girls who do not marry generally bring the infant home to their own parents, and the baby is raised in the young mother's household. Different families adapt to the presence of a new baby in different ways. Different grandmothers participate in the infant's care in varying degrees. Some adolescents assume all responsibilities for their infant, requiring very little assistance or advice. Other teenagers relinquish all mothering chores to their own mothers and treat the infant as a sibling. Each family will handle the situation in a different way, but the health provider should be attuned to recognize households with difficulties.

Sara is a 15-year-old white girl who chose to raise her infant daughter in her widowed mother's home while she and her 16-year-old boyfriend finished high school. They then planned to marry after *both* had completed graduation requirements. Sara was the youngest of three siblings; her older brother was in college and her older sister was married. Sara's mother readily welcomed the baby and agreed to help Sara care for the infant. Sara was taking an extra class in parenting and child care and was eager to be a mother to her little daughter. She personally arranged well-baby appointments outside school time and carefully wrote down the pediatrician's and nurse's suggestions. Sara and her mother began to have arguments about when to introduce solid foods, how to treat teething, baby "shots," and other matters. Both Sara and her mother began to call the pediatric clinic asking the nurse to "choose who was right." Sara threatened to take her baby and run away from home.

Sara's mother was well intentioned and obviously relished the chance to care for an infant again. Sara, on the other hand, was a bright young woman who tried to assume as much responsibility as possible. She was also inexperienced and did not realize that there are many "right" ways to baby care. The situation was eased considerably after the pediatric staff held several sessions with Sara and her mother.

Linella is a 13-year-old black girl who also took her infant daughter home to her mother's house, where five brothers and sisters also lived. In the same neighborhood there lived an aunt, several cousins, and Linella's grandmother. The infant was born on November 30. While Christmas shopping two to three weeks later, Linella and her mother stopped in the clinic to show off the baby. Linella said she was tired but denied any problems. At her six-week postpartum checkup she was visibly sad. Upon gentle questioning, she burst into tears and reported that she had received *no* Christmas presents; all the presents had been for her baby. Furthermore, she no longer felt she could talk to her mother. Prior to the baby's birth, she and her mother spent much time together shopping or talking or cooking. Now, her mother had no time for Linella; she was busy caring for the infant.

Linella was a young 13-year-old and did not understand that her family could not afford presents for her *and* the baby. Unfortunately, her family was also insensitive to Linella's hopes for Christmas. Furthermore, Linella found herself in the awkward situation of competing with her own daughter for her mother's attention. Social work intervention helped Linella and her mother cope with a potentially tragic situation.

Much has been written about the infants of teenage mothers. However, the literature is conflicting and confusing. Most studies do not tease apart maternal age from race, socioeconomic status or the amount of prenatal care, which unfortunately skews the data. For example, pregnant adolescents are at high risk for having a low-birth-weight infant (Alan Guttmacher Institute, 1976; National Center for Health Statistics, 1976; Baldwin, 1976; Kreutner and Hollingsworth, 1978), particularly if the adolescent is young, poor, and black and receives no prenatal care (Menken, 1972). Low birth weight, of course, has been associated with various physical and mental handicaps (Drillien, 1969; Wiener et al., 1965; Clifford, 1964). But when adolescents receive consistent, intensive, multidisciplinary care, the incidence of prematurity can be significantly reduced (Perkins et al., 1978). Hence, the outcome to the infants of such young mothers will be greatly improved. Obviously, the age of the mother is a risk factor in the infant's development, but health professionals should refrain from generalizing until better research elucidates the picture.

One area that deserves extra attention for adolescent mothers and their children is cognitive and emotional development. Teenagers, like other new parents, are inexperienced and may not have the skills or knowledge to stimulate their infants. Programs designed to improve young parents' skills have been beneficial (Levkoff, 1978). Pediatric health professionals may also find it useful to spend more time with these young parents in anticipatory guidance. Adolescent parents sometimes have inappropriate expectations of their youngsters.

> Laura, a 17-year-old mother, brought her 18-month-old son, Martin, to the pediatric acute care clinic for "stomach pain." When the pediatric resident asked the young mother about the length of time of the symptoms, bowel pattern, vomiting, etc., she reported, "Ask Martin. He can tell you."

Laura was not being smart with the physician; she truly believed Martin was "old enough" to understand and respond to such questions. With time and gradual education by the clinic nurse, she was able to appreciate Martin's development as well as his limitations.

Much has been written in the lay press about adolescent child abuse. It is true that adolescent parents are often in a high stress situation, but it should be noted that, at this time, there are no published studies that truly support the theory that adolescents abuse their children more than older parents.

Pregnant teenagers often reach out to health professionals for help. Members of the health care team can assist these young people in various ways: by diagnosing pregnancy as early as possible, by collaborating with colleagues to provide prenatal care tailored to the adolescents special needs, and by encouraging the adolescent to progress along psychosocial growth curves. Most important, the health care provider must remember the pregnant teenager is an adolescent who happens to be pregnant, not a pregnant woman who happens to be an adolescent.

REFERENCES

Adams, B.N., Brownstein, C.A., Rennalls, I.M., and Schmitt, M.H. The pregnant adolescent—a group approach. *Adolescence, 11,* 467–485 (1976).

Alan Guttmacher Institute. *11 Million Teenagers, What Can Be Done about the Epidemic of Adolescent Pregnancies in the United States.* Planned Parenthood Federation of America, New York (1976), p. 57.

Baldwin, W. Adolescent pregnancy and childbearing—growing concerns for Americans. *Population Bulletin,* Vol. 31. Population Reference Bureau, Inc., Washington, D.C. (1976), No. 2.

Beresford, T. *Short Term Relationship Counseling.* Planned Parenthood of Maryland, Baltimore (1977).

Cattanach, T.J. Coping with intentional pregnancies among unmarried teenagers. *School Counselor,* 211–215 (1976).

Clifford, S.H. High risk pregnancy I. Prevention of prematurity the sine qua non for reduction of mental retardation and other neurologic disorders. *New England Journal of Medicine, 271,* 243 (1964).

Corey, S.M. and Herrick, V.E. The developmental tasks of children and young people. In *Readings of the Psychology of Human Growth and Development.* W.R. Baller, ed. Holt, Rinehart & Winston, New York (1965).

Davis, L.D., and Grace, H. Anticipatory counselling of unwed pregnant adolescents. *Nursing Clinics of North America, 6,* 581–590 (1971).

Drillien, C.M. School disposal and performance for children of different birthweight born 1953-60. *Archives of Diseases of Childhood, 44,* 562 (1969).

Erikson, E.G. *Identity, Youth and Crises.* W.W. Norton, New York (1968).

Felice, M., and Friedman, S.B. The adolescent as a patient. *Journal of Continuing Education in Pediatrics, 20,* 15–28 (1978).

Freud, S. The transformations of puberty. In *Psychology of Adolescence.* A.E. Esman, ed. International Universities Press, New York (1975), p. 86.

Furstenberg, F.F. *Unplanned Parenthood—The Social Consequences of Teenage Childbearing.* The Free Press, New York (1976).

Hollingsworth, D.R., and Kreutner, A.K.K. Outcome of adolescent pregnancy. In *Adolescent Obstetrics and Gynecology,* A.K.K. Kreutner and D.R. Hollingsworth, eds. Year Book Medical Publishers, Chicago (1978), pp. 249-275.

Kreutner, A.K., and Langhorst, D.M. Abortion and abortion counseling. In *Adolescent Obstetrics and Gynecology,* A.K.K. Kreutner and D.R. Hollingsworth, eds. Year Book Medical Publishers, Chicago (1978), pp. 79-119.

Levkoff, A.H. Biologic, emotional and intellectual risks in teenage mothers and their babies. In *Adolescent Obstetrics and Gynecology*, A.K.K. Kreutner and D.R. Hollingsworth, eds. Year Book Medical Publishers, Chicago (1978), pp. 277–291.

Marans, A.E. The psychological impact of pregnancy on the adolescent girl. In *Adolescent Gynecology*, F.P. Heald, ed. Williams & Wilkins, Baltimore (1966).

Menken, J. The health and social consequences of teenage childbearing. *Family Planning Perspectives, 4,* 45–53 (1972).

Nadelson, C. The pregnant teenager: problems of choice in a developmental framework. *Journal of Psychiatric Opinion, 12,* 6 (1975).

National Center for Health Statistics, DHEW (NCHS). *Vital* Statistics, of the United States–1974, "Natality" U.S. Government Printing Office, Washington, D.C. (1976).

Perkins, R.P., Nakashima, I.I., Mullin, M., Dubansky, L.S., and Chin, M.L. Intensive care in adolescent pregnancy. *Obstetrics and Gynecology, 52,* 179–188 (1978).

Sorensen, R.C. *Adolescent Sexuality in Contemporary America.* World, New York (1972).

Trussell, J., and Menken, J. Early childbearing and subsequent fertility. *Family Planning Perspectives, 10,* 209–218 (1978).

Vener, A.M., and Stewart, C.S. Adolescent sexual behavior in middle America revisited; 1970–1973. *Journal of Marriage and the Family, 36,* 728 (1974).

Whitlock, F.A., and Edwards, J.E. Pregnancy and attempted suicide. *Comprehensive Psychiatry, 9,* 1–12 (1968).

Wiener, C., Rider, R., Oppel, W., Fischer, L., and Harper, P. Correlates of low birth weight; psychological status at six to seven years of age. *Pediatrics, 35,* 434 (1965).

13

Early Identification of
Speech and Language Impairments

Chris Hagen

In the course of daily practice the pediatrician is called upon to identify, diagnose, and treat a wide array of childhood illnesses, injuries, diseases, and disorders. In addition, well-baby care and child development must be monitored; beyond all that, the pediatrician must respond to scores of parental questions and concerns. Such demands on the pediatrician's knowledge, skills, and time make it essential to establish priorities for the attention and concern to be allotted to the problems presented on a given day. Naturally, acute, life-threatening conditions must receive top priority. Existing or potential problems that may lead to life-threatening circumstances would be next in importance. The next priority would probably be conditions that are not life threatening but require early identification and treatment to prevent irreversible disabilities or disabling conditions. Speech and language disorders fall into this category. Such disabilities significantly affect a child's educational, emotional, and social development. If not identified and treated early, they may even affect futute vocational development. Further, the progression of speech and language disabilities is such that the earlier treatment can be instituted, the shorter it will be. This chapter has three purposes:

1. To describe the general characteristics of childhood speech and language disorders;
2. To present a rationale for the pediatrician giving a high priority to the identification of speech and language disorders;
3. To present assessment criteria and methods that the pediatrician can use to distinguish "normal" variations in speech and language abilities from speech and language impairments.

GENERAL CHARACTERISTICS
OF SPEECH AND LANGUAGE DISORDERS

Speech Disorder

Speech is the process of blocking or constricting the outflowing sound produced by the vocal cords as air is exhaled from the lungs. The lips, tongue, soft palate, and vocal cords block and constrict the sound in a manner that shapes and produces what the listener hears as a series of consonants and vowels. The accurate and clear production of these speech sounds depends upon the presence of normal bony, cartilage, and muscular structures of the face, oral cavity, pharynx, larynx, and respiratory system. Further, a normal central nervous system must provide the necessary muscle strength, coordination, sequencing, timing, and rhythm of movements and monitor the accuracy of the product (speech sound) via auditory, tactile, and/or proprioceptive feedback.

A speech disorder is characterized by one or a combination of the following symptoms:

1. Inability to produce consonants and vowels even though there is hearing and normal ability to understand speech;
2. Distorted, slurred, and/or scanning speech, although the child has normal hearing and understanding of speech;
3. Despite normal hearing and understanding, producing the first parts of words clearly, but with inappropriate sounds in relation to what is being described, and failure to produce the ending sounds of most words;
4. Connected speech characterized by multiple substitutions of one sound for another and distortion and omission of still others;
5. Ongoing connected speech accurate, except for the persistent misproduction of specific sounds;
6. Clear and accurate articulation characterized by repetition or prolongation of sounds at the beginning of words, severe struggle to produce a speech sound at the beginning of words, and/or a hesitant, halting, fragmented, and unrhythmical manner of talking (all of the foregoing are signs of stuttering).

Speech disorders may be caused by:

1. Paralysis, weakness, or dyscoordination of the facial tongue, soft palate, and/or respiratory musculature (dysarhtria);
2. Impaired tactile and/or proprioceptive sensation, feedback, or higher-level analysis of feedback from the speech production musculature;

3. Impaired analysis of auditory feedback;
4. Impaired ability to volitionally initiate and produce an ongoing sequence of oral-facial motor postures (dyspraxia);
5. Structural defects such as cleft lip and/or palate, aglossia, microglossia, macroglossia or micrognathia.

Language Disorders

Language is the neurophysiologically mediated and learned process of:

1. Receiving sensory information and relating it to objects and events that are occurring in one's environment;
2. Associating that which has been received or internally instigated with past learned experience and thereby grasping the "meaning" of the stimuli;
3. Integrating discrete "meaningful" stimuli into a whole idea or series of ideas;
4. Translating these ideas into appropriate vocabulary and sentence structure;
5. Volitionally facilitating and sequencing the speech production musculature in the manner necessary to produce the sequence of consonants and vowels that compose the words of the sentences.

A language disorder may result from a breakdown in one or a combination of these neurologically mediated processes. Consequently, not all language-disordered children present the same clinical characteristics. One child may have difficulty *receiving* or recognizing sensory information (when spoken to he gives no indication that he has heard what was said). Others may be able to receive information but are unable to interpret its meaning (the child may attend to instructions or may repeat the instruction but fail to do what was requested or respond inappropriately in relation to the original instruction). Some are able to understand and express language at a simple level related to physically present objects or events, but are unable to use language to integrate and formulate an idea about something in the past or future. Many language-disordered children are able to receive and interpret information, but are unable to sequence words appropriately within a sentence.

Thus, unlike the speech-disordered child, the language-impaired child often fails to grasp the meaning of spoken speech and frequently lacks the vocabulary and sentence structures of similar-age children. The language-disordered child's expressive language, while often meager in amount and confused in structure, is typically clearly articulated. It is, however, entirely possible, given the proximity and interrelationships of the neurological structures that mediate speech and language, for a child to present both a speech and language disorder.

A RATIONALE FOR THE ROUTINE SCREENING
FOR SPEECH AND LANGUAGE DISORDERS

Clearly the pediatrician must routinely screen patients for possible disabling conditions. Speech and language impairments represent significant disabling conditions and meet three basic criteria that justify routine screening for early identification: (1) their incidence is high; (2) they will not remit without therapeutic intervention; and (3) they hold the potential for present or future harm if not recognized and treated as early as possible.

INCIDENCE OF SPEECH AND LANGUAGE DISORDERS

In a review of a number of studies Milisen (1971) concluded that 12 to 15 percent of five-to-eight-year-olds and four to five percent of those 9 to 18 years of age presented with some type of handicapping communicative disorder. The 1955 White House Conference on Children produced data suggesting that 10 percent of all school-age children have a communicative impairment (Milisen, 1971).

When one considers the tremendous increase in the population within these age ranges in recent years, the significant increase in our knowledge of communicative disorders, and the increased ability to recognize and identify such problems, these estimates seem very conservative. A recent study conducted by the Perinatal Research Project of the National Institute of Neurological Diseases and Stroke (NINDS) Subcommittee on Human Communication and its Disorders (1972) found that from 12 to 15 percent of children show neurological abnormalities by one year of age. Such children were also found to be extremely vulnerable to receptive and/or expressive language impairments. On the basis of their data it was estimated that 1,500,000 children in the United States suffer from handicapping language disturbances. However, Irwin and Michael's estimate of 8.7 million is probably more accutate, since they include all etiologies (Irwin and Michael, 1972).

But if we took only the NINDS estimate of language disorders in children with positive neurological signs, it is probable that one out of every 170 children entering a pediatrician's office suffers some type of language impairment. When one includes all of the possible hearing, speech, and voice disorders as well, the probability that a communicatively impaired child will be brought to a pediatrician's office increases significantly. Taken as a whole, these data suggest that the incidence of communicative disorders warrants the pediatrician's time and effort in routine screening of all children under his management. As Mac Keith (1977) has pointed out, communication disorders are more common in children of three years and younger than any other conditions for which a pediatrician routinely screens a preschool child.

SPEECH AND LANGUAGE DISORDERS
DO NOT REMIT WITHOUT THERAPEUTIC INTERVENTION

It has long been recognized and accepted that children with speech and language disorders secondary to such conditions as cleft palate and cerebral palsy or such acquired conditions as meningitis, head trauma, or anoxia, necessitate speech and language evaluations and treatment in order to maximize their communicative abilities. However, this same understanding has not been extended to speech and language problems that occur in the absence of observable structural or neurological abnormalities. Our reluctance in this area stems from the fact that children develop speech and language at different rates, and what may appear as a problem at one office visit is absent at another visit six months later. The majority of children present with speech and language deviations rather than disorders, and, since the deviations tend to disappear, the pediatrician frequently views any difference from the norm as manifestations of a transitory phase of normal development. From this has grown the belief that children will "outgrow" their impairment. The data indicate otherwise (Milisen, 1971).

Studies of the incidence of speech and language disorders provide an excellent means of determining whether children outgrow their communication impairments. If children do in fact move spontaneously from disordered speech and language to normal communication, one would expect to find a complete absence (with the exception of such problems as cleft palate and cerebral palsy) of communication disorders after a certain age.

Milisen (1971) reviewed a number of incidence studies and drew the following conclusions: (1) approximately 12 to 15 percent of children between five and eight years have serious speech and/or language disorders; (2) four to five percent of 9- to 12-year-olds have similarly serious problems; and (3) approximately four to five percent of those 13 years and older remain similarly afflicted. The incidence in the age range of adolescence and above reported by Milisen may, however, be low. Morris (1939) reported that 16.8 percent of a random sample of 178 high school sophomores manifested speech impairments. Blanton (1921) found that 18 percent of 2,240 members of the University of Wisconsin freshman class had speech problems. In a more recent study, Calnan (1976) found that 16.5 percent of 11-year-olds studied presented with communication impairments. The seeming increase in speech and language problems in the older age ranges compared to the younger age groups is probably reflective of the assessment criteria used. Many of these studies included any abnormal speech or language patterns, while the studies of the younger age groups focused only on "serious" impairments. Thus, it is probable that the incidence of handicapping communication impairments in adolescents and young adults is less than 6 to 8 percent. Other studies shed additional light on the question of whether children outgrow their communicative impairments. Menyuk (1964) compared normally speaking three-year-olds with language-disordered six-year-olds. She found few significant differences between the two groups. She interpreted these results as indicating that after the language-disordered child reaches a certain stage in language development (around three years), abnormal language skills become fixated, and further development does not occur without speech and language therapy. Morehead and Ingram (1973) found that it takes language-disordered children three times longer than normal children to initiate and acquire basic sentence patterns. Another study (Ackerman, 1977) assessed language development in a group of two-year-olds who were "at risk" at birth and a control group of normal children. The results indicated that by age two normal children were significantly better in language comprehension and expression. De Hirsch (1975) found similar results in a longitudinal study of children born prematurely.

These data indicate that all children do not outgrow their communication impairments. To the contrary, a significant percentage of children enter school with such problems. One may argue that the sharp decrease in the incidence of problems after age eight suggests that a significant percentage eventually outgrow their problems. These children were identified in kindergarten, however, and the majority began receiving treatment at that time, so that the decrease probably represents the effects of treatment.

While all children do not "outgrow" their speech and language problems, it is also true that not all children whose speech and language is different from the norm have impairments. The implication of these data is the importance of distinguishing between normal speech and language delay and abnormal delay or speech and language disorders. Children who fall into the first category will outgrow their problems. Those in the latter two categories will not. The section of this chapter on screening criteria and signs will present a means of differentiating between these three categories.

A SPEECH OR LANGUAGE DISORDER HOLDS THE POTENTIAL FOR PRESENT AND FUTURE HARM IF NOT TREATED EARLY

Is the treatment of a speech or language disorder an elective procedure or a necessity? Does it pose a significant threat to an individual's ability to lead a normal and productive life? One's answer to this question will probably be determined by the individual definition of quality of life. If one defines quality of life in relationship to its physical parameters, one may say that it is an elective procedure. For such individuals the absence of physical disease and illness represents the highest quality of life. On the other hand, if the concept of quality of life is extended to include the educational, emotional, social, vocational, and avocational aspects of life, then the treatment of communicative disorders would be a necessity.

The ability to communicate is a faculty central to educational, emotional, social, and vocational development. Pause a moment and reflect upon the degree to which your ability to communicate (understand and express ideas, feelings, and needs) is critical to your professional and personal life. Reflect further on the role it has played in bringing you to where you are now. Your ability to communicate has been and is quite important. Now reflect a little further. What would your life be like if for some reason (stroke, brain tumor, head trauma, progressive neurological disease, cancer of the larynx, loss of hearing, etc.) you sustained an impairment in your ability to communicate? You would be physically alive, but what of the quality of your life? To what degree would you be able to pursue your career? Your family and social life? On reflection, you may find that the impact of communication disorder is not in the physical realm but that it affects one's ability to interact with others intellectually, emotionally, socially, and vocationally.

Clearly, a child's present and future quality of life is related to educational, emotional, social, and vocational development. The ability to communicate is inextricably interwoven into a child's ability to advance in all of these areas. Thus, while a communicative impairment does not threaten a child's physical life, it functions as a significant barrier to their highest educational, emotional, social, and vocational attainments.

Failure to identify, diagnose, and treat a child's speech or language disorder also holds the potential for harm from a neurophysiological standpoint. Most experts agree (Lenneberg, 1967; Menyuk, 1964; Moorehead and Ingram, 1973) that the preschool years are the optimal time for acquiring language. The older the child gets, the greater the therapeutic effort required to overcome the deficit. Menyuk's study indicates that untreated language-disordered children do not eventually "catch up" with normal children. They remain fixated at a particular disordered language level and the language abilities gap between them and normal children increases. Why does this occur? If speech and language is simply a behavior learned from parents and independent of organs of the body, we would expect that in time the parents continued talking would bring the child to a normal level of functioning. This does not occur, clearly underscoring the fact that speech and language are behaviors learned and mediated by components of the central nervous system. As such, their acquisition and utilization are dependent upon the development and integrity of that system.

Evidence strongly suggests an intimate and reciprocal relationship between speech and language development and brain maturation.

It has been clearly established (De Crinis, 1934; Gesell and Amatruda, 1947; Mecham, 1958) that language and speech do not develop in a random or capricious fashion. On the contrary, the information presented in Table 13-1 reveals that it develops in a chronologically timed, orderly, and sequential chain of events. Since language and speech evolve on a universal schedule, we know that their development is not solely related to environmental learning and/or social-emotional drive.

A number of investigators (Garoutte, 1967; Lenneberg, 1967; Luria, 1966; Mysak, 1961) have demonstrated the existence of a parallel between the rate and timing of brain maturation and that of language and speech development. Lenneberg's (1967) work indicates that the neurophysiological growth curves of brain development are strikingly similar to the onset and sequential stages of language and speech development.

A considerable amount of brain development occurs prenatally (neuronal, dendritic and axonal growth); however, it continues for some time after birth (Lenneberg, 1967; Garoutte, 1967; Flechsig, 1901; Luria, 1966; Schade and Groenigan, 1961). The actual number of individual neurons does not increase substantially through infancy, although the mean size of the neurons increases between birth and two years of age (Schade and Groenigan, 1961). Dendritic elaboration, which allows for increased synaptic connections, continues to approximately 13 years of age (De Crinis, 1934), with the most accelerated dendritic growth occurring between birth and three years (Lenneberg, 1967). Myelinization continues up to early adolescence. Again, however, the most accelerated growth occurs between birth and five years. Thus, there would appear to be a growth spurt in brain maturation between birth and five years. A similar growth spurt in speech and language development occurs during this same period.

When the maturation of brain and language and speech development is considered in detail, there is a striking parallel between language and speech abilities at the various ages and the degree of brain development.

The infant develops the rudiments of receptive and expressive speech and language between birth and two years. The language developed during this period is quite functional with respect to sensorimotor events in the present or immediate past, but it is not an elaborative or highly specific communication system at this time. This level of language and speech abilities is consistent with the neurological development that has occurred up to this point. Specifically, the major growth has been in the areas of increased neuronal size, but has been slower in the areas of dendritic growth and myelinization. Growth in both of these areas is necessary to support more elaborate and specific language and speech abilities.

The child's language and speech abilities become more complex and skilled between the ages of two and three years. As indicated earlier, this is also the period of the most accelerated dendritic growth. There is a similar relationship between accelerated myelin growth between birth and five years and the development of the highly refined and skilled articulatory abilities that occur during this same period.

The parallel between brain and language development is also found in the myelogenetic and dendrogenetic studies of Flechsig (1901), De Crinis (1934), and others (Lenneberg, 1967; Luria 1966). According to these investigators, the cortex develops in a heterogeneous fashion, with certain areas of the cortex maturing at different rates and at different times. Luria (1966) divides these various cortical areas into primary, secondary, and tertiary zones with respect to rate and timing of maturation. There is a striking relationship between the rate and timing of maturation in these three zones and the chronological sequence of language and speech development.

The primary projection areas of somesthesis, audition, and vision mediate the reception and discrimination of tactile proprioceptive, auditory, and visual stimuli, respectively. The primary motor zone mediates the stimulation of muscle movement. These primary zones are the most functional of the three zones at birth. While they continue to mature until age five, their most accelerated rate of growth occurs between birth and the age of two. The functions mediated by the primary zones and the rate and timing of maturation within these zones are consistent with the language and speech behaviors developed between birth and one year with respect to sensory functions, and between birth and five years with respect to articulatory abilities.

The secondary zones lie immediately adjacent to the primary zones. While the primary zones receive and discriminate among sensory stimuli, as well as mediate muscle movement, the secondary zones mediate the temporal and spatial organization of sensory stimuli and motor movement across time. The secondary zones begin to become functional around six months and reach full maturity at approximately seven years. The most accelerated growth of these zones occur between six months and three years, and the beginning of meaningful verbal expressions occurs at around 18 months.

The structural makeup of the posterior and anterior tertiary zones allows for the mixing and correlation of sensory information and the maintenance of exploratory (goal-directed behavior) activity, respectively (Luria, 1966). The tertiary zones become functional around age one. They continue to mature up to adolescence, with their most rapid period of growth between one and five years. The maturation of these zones is consistent with the rapid growth of language abilities between 18 months and three years.

The parallel between language and speech development and brain maturation holds important implications relative to early identification of communicatively impaired children. It is admittedly difficult to identify communication disorders in early infancy. However, the unmistakable parallel between the rate and timing of brain maturation and that of language and speech development would suggest that we should attach more significance to a child's failure to reach a certain milestone at an expected time than we presently do. We have long recognized that delays in such motor skills as sitting, standing, and walking are often early warning signs of muscular or neuromuscular dysfunction. Speech and language delays are also often indicative of underlying dysfunction.

SCREENING FOR COMMUNICATIVE IMPAIRMENTS

Pediatricians are usually the first professionals to see children who may have present or potential speech and/or language disorders. They are in an excellent position to identify such children quite early. The following screening methods and criteria are not oriented toward the determination of the specific type and nature of a communicative disturbance. Rather, they are directed toward helping the pediatrician to decide whether a child should be referred to a speech-language pathologist for a complete workup.

Signs of existing or potential speech/language impairments can be derived from at least five sources: (1) the presence of identified aberrant congenital structural, neurological, and/or genetic conditions; (2) medical conditions that place the child at risk for central nervous system impairment; (3) significant deviation from speech and language development norms; (4) aberrant behavioral characteristics; (5) persistent parental concerns regarding speech and language development.

Aberrant Structural, Neurological, and/or Genetic Conditions

Speech or language impairments have a high correlation with a number of observable physical and neurological conditions. Consequently, the presence of cleft palate, aglossia, microglossia, micrognathia, motor movement disorders that fall within the broad category of cerebral palsy, infantile hemiplegia, other neurological signs suggestive of central nervous system impairment, and frank signs of mental retardation are all signals that the child should be evaluated by a speech-language pathologist.

Medical Conditions that Place the Child at Risk for Central Nervous System Impairment (Ackerman, 1977; Children's Hospital and Health Center, 1980; Fiedler et al., 1971)

1. Prenatal period
    a) Rh incompatibility
    b) Signs of fetal anoxia
    c) Maternal bleeding, especially during third trimester
    d) Maternal infection, toxemia, anemia
    e) Chronic medical disease
    f) History of trauma
    g) Mother over 35 or under 18 years of age
2. Labor and delivery
    a) False labor
    b) Fetal heart irregularities

    c) Premature rupture of membrane

    d) Abnormal, prolonged, or rapid delivery

    e) Breech birth

    f) Strangulation by umbilical cord

3. Perinatal period

    a) Prematurity/low birth weight (37 weeks gestation or less; birth weight, 2,500 grams or less; small for gestational age [SGA], by Lubchenco criteria)

    b) Perinatal asphyxia (indicated by Apgar score below 5 at one minute, or 7 at five minutes, and/or resuscitation after delivery)

    c) Respiratory distress syndrome

    d) Neonatal jaundice (term babies, 20 mg percent total bilirubin level; premature babies, 15 mg percent total bilirubin level)

    e) Confirmed neonatal infection (sepsis/meningitis)–viral, bacterial, parasitic

    f) Neonatal neurological abnormalities, including seizures

    g) Neonatal drug addiction

    h) Hypoglycemia requiring intravenous therapy

    i) Infants with major congenital anomalies

    j) Large for gestational age (LGA) (birth weight, 4,500 grams or more)

    k) Prolonged hospitalization beyond neonatal period (28 days)

    l) Convulsions

    m) Poor sucking ability

4. Acquired childhood problems

    a) Head trauma

    b) Brain tumor

    c) Cerebrovascular anomalies or accidents

    d) Infectious diseases leading to encephalitis or meningitis

The occurrence of these prenatal, perinatal, and postnatal problems does not always hearld the advent of a speech and/or language disorder. However, their presence can be used to distinguish between normal variations in language development and the existence of speech and language impairments. Thus, a child's failure or extreme slowness to progress through the early speech and language development at stages (described in the next section) in conjunction with these problems is sufficient cause to assume that a particular child is at risk for a speech and language disorder and should be referred for a diagnostic evaluation. The following are illustrative cases.

Case 1

Sean was seen for a speech and language evaluation at 3½ years of age. At the time of the evaluation his only mode of communication was gesture and pointing. When he attempted to talk he was able only to emit a prolonged vowel-like sound. On the other hand, his ability to understand the meaning of spoken speech was normal for his age. In general, he presented as a child with a severe oral-motor apraxia.

Medical History. Sean's mother reported that she had miscarried her four previous pregnancies and that her pregnancy with Sean was 10½ months. Medical records indicate that he was cyanotic at birth and required resuscitation. He was also found to be hypoglycemic as a newborn. A neurological examination conducted at two years of age concluded that the patient had a seizure disorder secondary to a perinatal hypoxia.

Case 2

Martin, referred for speech and language evaluation at age four, had an expressive language vocabulary of approximately 20 words and could understand only basic commands such as "No," "Don't," "Come here," "Time for bed," etc. He was diagnosed as having severe receptive/expressive aphasia.

Medical History. The mother was 41 years of age at the time of pregnancy. Labor was induced at eight months of pregnancy upon discovery of an Rh incompatibility. Three days after delivery Martin became jaundiced, and transfusion was performed. He was readmitted to the hospital at one month for further transfusions, at which time he experienced heart failure with concomitant respiratory distress syndrome.

Case 3

Alden was referred for speech and language evaluation at age five. His speech was found to be completely unintelligible.

Medical History. Alden's mother experienced prolonged vaginal bleeding during the second and third months of pregnancy and was expected to miscarry. The pregnancy, however, went to term, culminating in a precipitous delivery. Several hours after delivery, Alden was noted to be a bluish purple color and to have stopped breathing. Resuscitation measures restored normal breathing patterns, which were thereafter sustained independently. An EEG recording at age three was read as "abnormal." At that time he was only using three to five spoken words, all of which were grossly distorted.

Case 4

Carin was referred for speech and language evaluation at age two. She presented with mild impairment in understanding speech and severe expressive language impairment. She could only use two words consistently: "Mama" and "Dada." She attempted speech frequently, but could only produce an "uh"-like sound accompanied by gestures.

Medical History. Carin was the product of a 42-week pregnancy. At delivery she was noted to have nuchal cord x 1 with a true knot in the cord. Her face was contorted and she had a shoulder dislocation. At one and five minutes her Apgar scores were 8 and 9. Hyperbilirubinemia was noted on the third day. A neurological exam at four months of age found her to be hypotonic.

Case 5

Christopher was referred to a speech and language evaluation at three years. At the time of evaluation, he could only inconsistently understand commands related to activities of daily living and made no attempts to communicate verbally with those around him. He was diagnosed as having a severe receptive aphasia.

Medical History. The mother experienced spotting throughout her pregnancy, and she was delivered at seven months gestation. The delivery was breech. The mother had three miscarriages prior to this premature delivery.

In all of the cases noted above the children manifested significant delays in reaching early speech and language developmental milestones, and in some instances they had not developed any language. Their symptoms, plus the medical history, indicate that they could have been referred for evaluation much earlier without a significant risk of a false positive early identification of a speech or language disorder.

Significant Deviation from Speech and Language Development Norms

Since speech and language develops in a sequential, orderly and timed manner, significant deviations from the expected pattern of development stand as a major indicator that a child is at risk for a speech or language problem. While there is some variation among normal children with respect to the acquisition of certain subskills within a given stage, children without a speech or language problem generally progress through the various stages at a similar age.

Consequently, a delay of six months or more in manifesting the expected behaviors of a given stage of development, the complete failure to develop or progress beyond a given stage, or the regression to a lower, previously acquired stage are all indicative of the need to follow a particular child closely with respect to a potential speech or language impairment.

Table 13-1 shows the normal stages of speech and language development from birth to five years. The presence, delay, or absence of the various behaviors can be used as a method of screening. It is important to review all areas lsited for each stage (i.e., receptive and expressive abilities, when individual speech sounds begin to appear, the size of the child's vocabulary, general spontaneous communicative behavior and/or degree of speech intelligbility).

It is from the review of all of these factors that a total communicative profile of a child emerges that allows for objective differentiation between normal variation and disorder. Because an infant or young child does not always cooperate with examination procedures directed toward eliciting speech and language responses, it is sometimes difficult to differentiate between uncooperativeness and an actual problem. For this reason, a major portion of this information may have to be obtained through parent interview.

If this approach is taken, the various items within each developmental stage can be presented as questions to the parents. Care should be taken to elicit not merely a yes or no response. Information is necessary as to the quality, speed, and consistency of the child's behavior relative to a particular expected ability. The presence of an expected behavior does not necessarily rule out a problem. Sometimes the parents may respond in the affirmative when the behavior in question had only occurred once or twice, is quite inconsistent, or does not occur spontaneously but only in relation to repeated stimulation. Thus, one should assess the quantity as well as the quality of the child's speech and language abilities.

Case 1

Bobby was seen for a speech and language evaluation at age 3½ years. At that time his speech was almost unintelligible. His typical verbal expression consisted of a pronoun at the beginning of a sentence, followed by a series of random consonants and vowels. His understanding of spoken speech was normal for his age. His primary manner of communication was through the use of pantomime. His mother provided an excellent example of this. She reported that on the way to the appointment it had begun raining. Bobby began swinging his forearm back and forth in front of his face in an arc-like fashion, pointing with the other hand to the appropriate knob on the dashboard and simultaneously making a swishing noise.

Table 13-1

Normal Speech and Language Development

A. 0-6 Months

Receptive Abilities	Expressive Abilities
Alerting (1 mo.)	Cooing (4 mos.)
Orient to voice (4 mos.)	"Ah-goo," gurgles, laughs
Orient to bell (5 mos.)	(5 mos.) (6 mos.)

Appearance of individual speech sounds: some distinguishable vowels and consonants toward sixth month.

Size of vocabulary: 0

General communication behavior: reflexive; self-stimulated pleasure; the emergence of purposeful movement and manipulation of speech production musculature and coordination of respiration, phonation, and articulation

Percent of speech intelligbility: 0

B. 6-12 Months

Receptive Abilities	Expressive Abilities
Continues previous-level abilities	Continues previous-level abilities
Orient to bell II (7 mos.)	Produces speech-like sounds
Orient to bell III (9 mos.)	Reflexively babbling (7 mos.)
Imitates sounds (10-11 mos.)	Imitates some sounds or parts of
Responds to name (10-11 mos.)	noun words (10-11 mos.)
Responds to "bye-bye" (11-11½ mos.)	Expresses Dada/Mama appropriately
Imitates words ("Dada" "bye-bye")	(12 mos.)
(12 mos.)	Uses one to two words, sometimes
Follows simple instructions with an	meaningful, sometimes not
accompanying gesture (12 mos.)	(12 mos.)

Appearance of individual speech sounds: seven vowels, five consonants, and babbling in the first part of this level; ten vowels and nine consonants by the end of this level

(continued)

Table 13-1
(continued)

B. 6–12 Months
(continued)

Size of vocabulary: one to two words toward end of level (nouns)

General communication behavior: self pleasure; beginning of using speech to interact with others

Percent intelligibility: 0 at beginning of level and 10 percent toward end of level

C. 1–1½ Years

Receptive Abilities

Continues previous level of abilities
Can identify some familiar objects
  when named
Understands inhibiting commands
  such as "no, no," "stop," etc.
Can repeat simple words
Can identify hair, mouth, ears, and
  hands when named
Can follow simple one-step
  commands

Expressive Abilities

Continues previous level of abilities
Immature jargoning
Repeats words—some with meaning
Mature jargoning
Uses single-word sentences

Appearance of individual speech sounds: p, b, m, h, and w

Size of vocabulary: 10 to 20 words (nouns and verbs)

General communication behavior: purposeful babbling, lalling, and echoing for pleasure and social interaction at beginning of level; getting others' attention, conveying wants and states of being by leading another to that which meets need, and pointing accompanied by jargon and some meaningful words

Percent intelligibility: 20 to 25

Table 13-1
(continued)

D. 1½–2 Years

Receptive Abilities	Expressive Abilities
Continues previous levels of abilities	Continues previous levels of abilities
Can identify major body parts	Uses names of familiar objects
Can identify five familiar pictures when named	meaningfully
Can follow simple instructions using one or two prepositions	Talks in two-word sentences using noun + noun ("bye-bye," "all gone")
	Talks in two-word sentences using subject and predicate ("Daddy go," "me like," "me up")

Appearance of individual speech sounds: continued refinement of p, b, m, h, and w

Size of vocabulary: 10–20 words (nouns and some verbs) at beginning of level; 50–250 words (nouns, verbs, and adjectives) by end of level

General communication behavior: attention getting and meeting basic needs by pointing accompanied by jargon and some words at beginning of level; meaningful social control (causing others to do things for him/her) and requesting things by end of level

Percent intelligibility: 40–50

E. 2–2½ Years

Receptive Abilities	Expressive Abilities
Continues abilities of previous levels	Continues abilities of previous levels
Can identify at least 10 common objects or pictures when named	Can name at least 10 common pictures
Can follow simple commands without accompanying gesture	Asks for another
	Uses pronouns, I, me, you, but often inappropriately
	Talks in three-to-four-word sentences

(continued)

Table 13-1
(continued)

E. 2-2½ Years
(continued)

Appearance of individual sounds: continues development of previous sounds

Size of vocabulary: 250-400 words (nouns, verbs, pronoun "I")

General communication behavior: carries out long monologues describing things and events personally involved with for purpose of meaningful social interaction, attention, and control

Percent of speech intelligibility: 50-70

F. 2½-3 Years

Receptive Abilities	Expressive Abilities
Can identify at least 15 common pictures when named	Can name most common objects
Can identify action in pictures when named	Can name one color
	Verbalizes toilet needs to another
Can retain two digits or one to two objects named	Appropriate use of pronouns I, you, me, and plurals
Can follow two-part commands	Talks in four-word phrases and longer sentences

Appearance of individual speech sounds: t, d, n, k

Size of vocabulary: 400-500 words

General communication behavior: continues to develop speech as a social interactive tool to explain self-interests to others and control others. Also, child's behavior can be controlled by speech of others.

Percent of speech intelligibility: 75-90

Table 13-1
(continued)

G. 3-4 Years

Receptive Abilities	Expressive Abilities
Continues previous levels of abilities	Continues previous levels of abilities
Can point to at least 25 pictures when named	Can name most common pictures
Can retain three digits or two to three objects when named	Can say full name
Continues to be able to follow increasingly complex commands	Relates personal experiences
Can understand social conversation related to ongoing activities in which the child is involved either as participant or observer	Can recite short poem/sing song from memory
	Names all colors
	Speaks in complex sentences

Appearance of individual speech sounds: y, f, v first, then sh, zh, th (closer to four years)

Size of vocabulary: 800-1000 words (nouns, verbs, pronouns [you and me], plurals, adjectives, past tense)

General communicative behavior: talks a great deal, relates experiences, exaggerates, boasts; keeps conversation going by asking many questions; listens to others' experiences and explanations; increasing span of interest in listening to stories, records, TV, etc.

Percent of speech intelligibility: 90 (does not have mastery of l, r, s, z, sh, ch, j, and th yet)

H. 5 Years

Receptive Abilities	Expressive Abilities
Continues previous levels of abilities	Continues previous levels of abilities
Can identify all common pictures when named	Can name all common pictures
Can identify pictures of most common opposites when named	Can count to ten
	Names penny, nickel, dime
	Uses "please" and "thank you"

(continued)

Table 13-1
(continued)

H. 5 Years
(continued)

Receptive Abilities (continued)	Expressive Abilities (continued)
Can retain four digits or objects	Askes the meaning of words
Understands most conversations related to daily activities even though the child has not been involved	Relates fanciful tales
	Uses complex sentences in an ongoing conversational style of speaking

Appearance of individual sounds: s, z, th, r, ch

Size of vocabulary: 1000+ (nouns, verbs, adverbs, adjectives, future tense)

General communication behavior: Relates experiences of daily activity in considerable detail; interested in using new and larger words; seeks information by asking questions; makes up fanciful stories; listens to others' experiences and shares ideas and experiences related to what was heard

Percent of speech intelligibility: 95–100 (some distortion of r, s, and blends— i.e., bl, cl, st, etc.)

Developmental Profile. Bobby reached and progressed through the various gross and fine motor developmental stages within the expected age range. However, his speech and language development did not follow a similar profile. His perceptive language abilities progressed normally. His expressive language progressed normally through the babbling and jargon phases but did not progress further until 2 years and 10 months of age, at which time he began to speak approximately five crudely pronounced words. He had not made substantial progression from this level at the time of the evaluation.

Case 2

Robert was seen for a speech and language evaluation at age four. At the time of the evaluation he could only understand simple two-to-three word one-stage commands and his expressive language was completely unintelligible. His primary means of communication was through pointing and repeating an "uh" sound.

Developmental Profile. Gross and fine motor development was normal. Robert did not begin to understand single-noun words, such as bed, shoe, etc. until the age of two and could understand a few simple commands by age three. He did not attempt to speak until age three. His speech attempts from that age on have been meager and unintelligible.

Case 3

Gerhard was seen for a speech and language evaluation at age 4½ years. At the time of the evaluation he did not respond to general conversational speech, though his hearing was normal. When spoken to, he would continue his random activity around the room, giving no indication that he had heard what had been said to him. Gerhard exhibited no spontaneous spoken language.

Developmental Profile. Gerhard progressed normally in receptive language up to about eight months, but did not avdance beyond this level. His expressive language progressed through the babbling and cooing phase, and he began the jargon phase, but ceased all speech production attempts at about 11 months.

Case 4

. Norman was seen for a speech and language evaluation at age five. At that time his receptive language abilities fluctuated between verbatim repetition of what was said to carrying out simple, one-stage commands after repeating the instruction four to five times. Norman's expressive language consisted of a core vocabulary of approximately 25 nouns and a few adjectives. With these, he could name a number of objects and periodically put together a two-word sentence.

Developmental Profile. Norman did not begin to respond to spoken speech until approximately 10 months of age. By age two he could repeat parts of what had been said but did not understand the meaning. By age four he was beginning to comprehend some simple commands if they were repeated frequently, but could not understand conversational speech. Norman began to use three to four single words at two years, and by age three had only progressed to the point of using a few two-word sentences to express basic wants. His expressive language abilities had not advanced beyond this level at the time of the evaluation.

Case 5

Paul was seen for a speech and language evaluation at age five. At that time he tested above his age level in receptive and expressive language abilities but his speech was 80 percent unintelligible. Assessment of his oral-motor abilities revealed severe discoordination of movement on both isolated and rapid alternating movements of his facial and oral musculature. An attempt to protrude and retract his tongue in a continuous fashion produced a movement that was coarse, jerky, and decreased in motion. Typically, his lips would surround his tongue and act as a guide and stabilizer when attempting to protrude it. He had considerable difficulty in raising and lowering the tip of his tongue. When attempting to perform this muscular movement, he would initiate a rapid chewing motion that involved not only his tongue, but his lip and jaw musculature. A similar chewing motion was noted when he attempted to move his lips from a pursed to smiling position in a continuous fashion.

Developmental Profile. Paul progressed through the various receptive and expressive language developmental milestones at the expected ages. His speech intelligibility did not progress beyond the 12-to-18 month level.

These case histories are illustrative of the fact that early significant deviations in expressive and/or receptive language abilities herald the emergency of a speech and/or language disorder.

The eventual evolution of verbal language and speech abilities is dependent upon the appropriate development and mastery of the requisite preceding nonverbal and verbal language and speech processes. While all children do not reach the various developmental milestones at the expected time, the degree of variation among normally developing children is not great (Blanton, 1921; Calnan and Richardson, 1976). Thus, a delay of four months or more in the development of language and speech processes is cause for concern. Certainly the failure of a child to manifest or progress beyond the early nonverbal language and speech development milestones should be considered significant. A delay in or outright failure to develop these earlier behaviors does not unequivocably indicate the presence of a pathological state. The occurrence of developmental deviations of four months or more, however, represents a means of identifying children who should receive a differential diagnostic workup as early as possible.

Aberrant Communicative Characteristics

A child who is at risk for a speech and language disorder can also be identified on the basis of a number of general characteristics. The following are general signs of a potential communication disorder:

1. Failure to manifest receptive and/or expressive abilities characteristic of the first 18 months of development.

2. Inconsistent manifestation of receptive and/or expressive abilities characteristic of the first 18 months (i.e., exhibiting expected behaviors for a brief period of time, lack of those behaviors for one or two months, subsequent reemergence of abilities with no progress beyond them).

3. No progress beyond the abilities acquired at any given level of development.

4. Receptive and/or expressive abilities decreasing from a previously acquired level.

5. A delay of six months or more in the acquisition of the receptive and/or expressive abilities expected by the end of a given developmental level.

6. A stadily increasing gap between the child's chronological age and the child's speech and language age level (i.e., six months' delay at one year of age, 12 months' delay at two years of age, 18 months' delay at 2½ years of age, etc.).

7. Normal progress through the receptive abilities expected at the various age levels but no normal progress in the acquisition of expressive abilities.

8. Speech consisting of mostly vowels or vowel-like sounds after one year of age.

9. Using no meaningful spontaneous expressive speech by age two.

10. Responding more consistently by age two to gestures, vocal inflection, and vocal loudness than to the meaning of the spoken message.

11. No attempt to communicate in any manner by age three.

12. By age three, communicating primarily by taking a person to what the child wants and/or using pointing and gesturing accompanied by vocal inflection or a series of unintelligible sounds or partial words to indicate want or need.

13. Not using three or more words to form a sentence (e.g., "Me up," "Me want," "Go Dada," etc.) by age three.

14. Inability to identify most familiar objects and follow simple commands without gestures by age three.

15. Naming most familiar objects but inability to elaborate or provide additional information about them by age three.

16. Inability to comprehend complex instructions and conversational speech related to self or familiar activities and events of daily living at age four.

17. Ability to express ideas about physical self or objects and acitvities currently engaged in, but inability or difficulty in expressing ideas about past or future objects or activities that the child has been or will be involved with.

18. By age four, expressing ideas about the physical aspects of daily living but considerable difficulty in expressing abstract ideas and feelings (e.g., cause-effect relationships, inferred relationships between associated relationships).

19. Difficulty in comprehending who, what, when, where, why, and how questions related to familiar objects, activities, and events between four and five years of age.

20. Vocabulary quite meager by age four.

21. Vocabulary usage inappropriate to topic at age three.

22. Speech 60 percent or more unintelligible at age three.

23. At age three, speech can be understood only by parents.

24. By age two, consistently leaving off the ends of most words.

25. Persistent hoarse and/or breathy voice quality.

26. Hypernasal voice quality.

27. Noticeable struggle to produce speech with ease (stuttering, stammering) between four and five years of age; noticeable and frequent struggle to pronounce the first sounds or syllables of words; moments when no sound can be produced at all when intending to say a word (may be associated with other signs of muscle struggle such as closing or blinking of the eyes and lowering, raising, or turning of the head); awareness of the struggle to produce sounds and embarrassment or other upset about speaking difficulty.

Some of these characteristics can be identified by monitoring the child's pattern of speech and language development, and others through direct observation and/or parent interview. The following questions can be helpful in obtaining corroborating information from parents:

1. Does your child turn toward you or others when you talk to him/her?

2. Does your child appear to listen to you or others talking to him/her?

3. Does your child seem to listen to music, TV, radio?

4. Does your child appear interested in his/her surroundings, toys, other objects, and people?

5. Does your child understand the meaning of your words?

6. Can your child hand or bring to you toys or other objects when you name them?

The differentiation between the child whose language and speech development is within normal limits and the one whose delay indicates the presence of an underlying pathological state is most difficult. We are justifiably reluctant to make this distinction in early childhood for fear of a false positive diagnosis. An erroneous identification of a child unquestionably risks causing emotional distress for both the child and his parents. However, if we allow the passage of time to make the diagnosis for us, we run the risk of even greater consequences for the child with a communication disorder. The continued lag in or failure to develop language and speech functions at three to four years of age makes it easier to distinguish between the child who has a problem and the one who does not. However, by this time the child is past a critical language and speech development time period. From the standpoint of brain maturation, the potential for learning is lessened throughout the remaining time. Each year there is a decrease in the adaptability and reorganization potential of cortical structures (Lenneberg, 1967). When one considers these parameters, the delay of appropriate treatment until four or five years of age presents both the child and the speech pathologist with a most difficult task. The earlier the diagnosis is made, the greater will be the probability of taking advantage of the maturational sequence of brain development. In turn, there will be a greater probability of achieving the maximal results in the shortest time.

Failure to identify a speech or language problem early increases the complexity and length of treatment because:

1. Disturbance in one link of the developmental sequence impairs the acquisition of succeeding phases of development. As a result, the child not only has the primary organically based disorder but secondary disorders caused by the inability to acquire the speech or language abilities dependent upon the impaired ability.

2. Disturbed speech or language rapidly becomes a mislearned behavior. Thus, what was originally the spontaneous manifestation of an organic disorder becomes the child's learned form of communicating. Just as the normally developing child learns normal speech and language, the abnormally developing child learns abnormal speech and language.

3. The child rapidly develops emotional and cognitive mechanisms to cope with and compensate for the emotional/social effects of a speech or language problem. For example, the child may withdraw completely from attempts to communicate; he may interact only in situations where communication is easy for him, or he may adopt acting-out behavior in an attempt to cover up his problems. Any of these mechanisms will compound the underlying disorder by denying the child the opportunities to increase his skills. Cognitively, the child might adopt abnormal sentence-structure strategies to circumvent the disorder. He might decrease the length of his utterances in order to decrease the likelihood of being misunderstood, or he may learn to substitute words or whole phrases for those he is unable to master. These mechanisms act to cover up the disorder and consequently decrease the opportunities to deal directly with the problem.

Thus, if a speech or language problem is not identified early, it rapidly becomes a complex disorder comprising (1) the basic problem that is directly related to the organic impairment, (2) the mislearning of abilities that follow and are dependent upon the impaired skill, (3) emotional coping mechanisms, and (4) cognitive coping mechanisms. All four of these elements soon become mislearned behaviors. Early identification will allow treatment to begin when the speech or language problem is still only a spontaneous manifestation of the organic impairment.

Because of this:

1. Treatment can be oriented exclusively toward the specific disorder rather than having to deal with mislearned behavior and coping mechanisms.
2. Treatment can focus on the disordered speech or language ability at or close to the time that these particular skills would normally be acquired neurologically and developmentally.
3. Treatment can function to modify ongoing central nervous system maturation toward normal rather than abnormal behavior.
4. Treatment can take advantage of ongoing central nervous system maturation.
5. Treatment can decrease the probability of the child's mislearning of speech or language skills and of learning abnormal compensatory and coping mechanisms.

REFERENCES

Ackerman, J.A., Lewis, M., and Driscol, J. Language Development in two year old normal and risk infants. *Pediatrics, 59,* 982–986 (1977).

Blanton, S. Speech defects in school children. *Mental Hygiene, 5,* 820–827 (1921).

Calnan, M., and Richardson, K. Speech problems in a national survey: Assessments and prevalences. *Child Care Health and Development, 2,* 181–202 (1976).

Children's Hospital and Health Center. *Children's Hospital and Health Center Neonatal Risk Criteria,* Department of Neonatology, San Diego, California (1980).

De Crinis, M. *Aufbau und Abbau der Grosshirnleistenigen und ihu anatomischin Grunde.* Krager, Berlin (1934).

De Hirsch, K. Language defects in children with developmental lags, *Psychoanalytic Study of Children, 30,* 95–126 (1975).

Doll, E.A. *Vineland Social Maturity Scale,* Minneapolis Educational Test Bureau (1947).

Fiedler, M.F., Lenneberg, E.G., Rolfe, U.T., and Drorbaugh, J.E. A speech screening procedure with three year old children. *Pediatrics, 48,* 268–276 (1971).

Flechsig, P. Developmental (myelogenetic) localization of the cerebral cortex in in the human subject. *Lancet,* 1027–1029 (1901).

Garoutte, B. Cerebral development anomalies and disturbances of language. *Journal of Neurological Science, 4,* 339–347 (1967).

Gesell, A., and Amatruda, O.S. *Developmental Diagnosis,* Paul B. Holber, Harper Bros., New York (1947).

Human Communication and Its Disorders: An Overview. Monograph No. 10; National Institute of Neurological Diseases and Stroke, Bethesda, Maryland (1972).

Irwin, J.V. and Michael, M. *Principles of Childhood Language Disabilities.* Appleton-Century-Crofts, New York (1972).

Lenneberg, E.G. *Biological Foundations of Language.* Wiley, New York (1967).

Luria, A.R. *Higher Cortical Functions In Man.* Basic Books, New York (1966).

Mac Keith, R. Children who are not speaking at three years of age. *Developmental Medicine and Child Neurology, 19,* 573 (1977).

Mecham, J. *Verbal Language Development Scale.* American Guidance Service, (1958).

Menyuk, P. Comparison of the grammar of children with functionally deviant and normal speech. *Journal of Speech and Hearing Research, 7,* 109 (1964).

Milisen, R. The incidences of speech disorders. In *Handbook of Speech Pathology and Audiology,* L.E. Travis, ed. Appleton-Century-Crofts, New York (1971).

Morehead, D.M., and Ingram, D. The development of base syntax in normal and linguistically deviant children. *Journal of Speech and Hearing Research, 16,* 330 (1973).

Morris, D. A survey of speech defects in Central High School. *Quarterly Journal of Speech, 25,* 262–269 (1939).

Mysak, E.D. Organismic development of oral language. *Journal of Speech and Hearing Disorders, 26,* 377–383 (1961).

Schade, J.P., and Groenigan, W.B. Structural organization of the human cerebral cortex; maturation of the middle frontal gyrus. *Acta Anatomica, 47,* 74–111 (1961).

14

Occupational Therapy: A Process of Exploration and Adaptation

Mary Kawar

> In human capacities for play lie the developmental roots of competence, and therefore a major resource for endeavors to remedy human deficits.
>
> —M. Brewster Smith

The child with a disability or health problem risks the possibility of regression and lessened ability to realistically perceive his situation when placed in a medical arena. In such a crisis the imagination and innovation of an occupational therapist can elicit an adaptive response from the child through a process of "doing." She selects an inviting therapeutic activity that compels the child to constructively channel his ability, energy, and attention. In "doing" this activity, the child draws upon his inner resources to impact his immediate environment, thus reaffirming his self-esteem and potency as an individual. His ability to successfully adapt to a threatening environment will thereby have been significantly expanded.

Mandy provides a good illustration of how the occupational therapist develops treatment objectives which facilitate adaptation.

At age three, Mandy was sent to a prosthetist to be fitted for a below-the elbow prosthesis. Her mother was so stressed in approaching this experience that she told Mandy they were on their way to buy a dress for Mandy. When the prosthetist started wrapping her stump for the mold, Mandy became hysterical. She thought that he was going to remove the rest of her arm. It is not surprising that Mandy refused to wear her new prosthesis once it was completed. The only thing that she would willingly do with it was hide it under her bed. At this point, she was referred to an occupational therapist. It took two sessions to obtain Mandy's cooperation in placing objects in the terminal device of the prosthesis while it was lying on the table. Ronny, a five-year-old amputee, volunteered to help with Mandy's problem. The therapist invited the two of them to a tea party in occupational therapy. Ronny had a history of being very aggressive and sometimes destructive with his prosthetic "helper," but on this occasion his behavior was exemplary. Mandy could not take her eyes off Ronny because he used his "helper" during the tea party as though it were a part of his body. Once Mandy got home, she asked her mother if she could try her "helper" on. After two more therapy sessions, Mandy was wearing her "helper" regularly and becoming a skillful user. Ronny also benefitted from this therapeutic experience. The positive feedback he received from being a role model for Mandy motivated him to significantly improve his behavior at school.

The tea party seems so simple that one might question why it is called therapy. Occupational therapy at its best has a spontaneous, familiar quality while addressing issues of health and function. It is a dynamic process in which the patient, therapist, activities, and environment are purposefully interwoven in order to achieve the treatment objectives. Each of these components deserves a closer look in order to appreciate the subtle complexity of this process.

THE THERAPIST

The therapist is a change agent who gathers the essential facts, develops the plan of action, implements the process, and terminates the relationship when the desired goals are achieved. In this process, she utilizes her theoretical and practical knowledge of neuromuscular development, sensory integration, and psychosocial and cognitive development. She also relies on her expertise in skill development, task analysis, and environmental adaptation. Parents frequently view her as a role model when they are struggling with parenting and behavior management skills. She collaborates with the physician, the parents, the teacher, and the other health professionals who are working with the child. Human helping qualities that have been researched and developed in the field of psychology contribute to her effectiveness with the child. These include her ability to:

1. Accurately perceive what is going on within and around the child and share this insight in a manner that will expand the child's awareness of himself and his circumstances.
2. Set reasonable limits in a firm, caring manner.
3. Respect the child's uniqueness, his strength to master the challenge that he faces, and his freedom to make choices.
4. Take risks, such as confronting the child or his parents with critical issues at the appropriate time and in a manner that will facilitate their growth.

5. Evoke feelings of security and trust.
6. Display warmth, spontaneity, and flexibility.
7. Demonstrate harmony between words and action.
8. Nurture a relationship that is "present-oriented" and that enables the child to become "inner-directed."

The therapist uses her sensitivity to perceive the child's changing needs and moments of readiness. Her insight creates a springboard for stimulating the child to direct his own actions and thereby interact with initiative and purpose, exploring his potential while coping with his problems or disability.

THE CHILD

The patient referred to a pediatric occupational therapy service could range in age from a premature infant to a teenager. The general types of problems manifested by these children include: (1) congenital defects, (2) emotional adjustment problems, (3) acute or chronic disease processes, (4) developmental delays, (5) traumatic injuries, and (6) learning disabilities. The physician referral is usually prompted by the recognition of some form of restriction on the child's ability to perform developmentally appropriate activities and the accompanying need of the child for guidance in adapting to change.

A thoughtfully completed developmental history is essential to a comprehensive fact-finding process when the child is being evaluated by an occupational therapist. In a hospital, one has immediate access to the medical history, but information related to self-care skills, play interests and abilities, daily routine, sensory experiences, developmental progression, school performance, and relationships with family and friends must be actively sought. Often this information will help the therapist in planning her intervention strategy, and it may add clarity to her clinical observations of the child. Sometimes it will serve to reduce the significance of a test score in the occupational therapy assessment battery that is not representative of the child's usual performance.

Cultural influences are extremely important to the therapist when delineating objectives for the child.

Lupe came to the hospital from an impoverished home in Mexico during the Christmas season. She was not at all interested in making a Christmas stocking to put on her bed in preparation for Santa's visit. She became ecstatic when the therapist modifed the plan by showing her how she could use the same material to refurbish her beloved, tattered *piñata*, which was her only link with home.

The types of toys and games, the stories, the music, and even the humor have cultural implications. Social systems influence perceptions and behavior, potentially causing ineffective cross-cultural exchanges if care is not taken in discovering these subtle differences.

The infant or child who is stressed will have physiological symptoms, as well as psychological reactions, that significantly alter his ability to cope. His ability to rebound, compromise, or change will be influenced by many premorbid factors, such as his individual strengths and weaknesses. The therapist seeks answers to many questions. Does he handle fear or pain by withdrawing, crying, or fighting? What does he value and what does he need? How can he be motivated to initiate positive action? She also determines the available external resources and the adjustive demands that are being placed on the child before launching into a plan of intervention.

The therapist includes parents or caretakers when working with children. Even very highly functioning parents are stressed when their child has a problem, and can profit from participating in the care plan. It is not unusual for them to manifest their stress by discussing irrelevant issues, being over protective, falsely reassuring, angry, passive, or inconsistent. Eliciting their trust and support is crucial to the therapist before she can facilitate their effectiveness in relating to and managing their child's changing needs. If the parents are not generally effective, other members of the health care team will often be of further assistance in helping them while the therapist addresses the child's functional needs.

THE ACTIVITIES

Clark (1979) summarizes the philosophy for contemporary occupational therapy practice as "human development through occupation." Occupation in this context includes a broad range of purposeful activities, which can be classified under self-maintenance, play, and work. These activities are an essential part of human existence, providing media for exploration, discovery, and adaptive change. At the simplest level, activities can ensure survival, promote subsistence, and enhance the potential for coexistence (Cynkin, 1979). They are the tangible link between the individual and his environment. Skill acquisition, interpersonal relationships, and self-actualization all evolve through participation in a variety of experiential activities. It is no wonder that developmental assessment scales utilize a hierarchy of purposeful activities as the criterion with which to evaluate growth, achievement, and potential.

Many of the activities of infancy and childhood are classified as play. Until recently, little emphasis was placed on the meaning and significance of play. This attitude was reflected in comments such as, "He is just playing." Reilly (1974) describes play as a process of exploratory learning that creates a sense of mastery and the ability to cope successfully with the demands of the environment. Learning by doing—whether it be for the purpose of self-care, play, or work—evokes the collaborative energies of our body and mind. In the course of engaging in activities, we utilize our sensory systems to perceive time, space, objects, and people; we mentally plan our movements and then practice and reinforce these motor acts; we conceptualize, solve problems, make choices, and interact with others; we integrate what we are learning with past experiences, and discover the potential for applying what we are presently learning in new ways. When we are enjoying what we are doing, we are apt to be curious, creative, and able to easily remember what we have experienced. These pleasant experiences create a sense of enthusiasm for new learning adventures.

A child is deprived of his familiar daily rhythm and activity routine when he sustains a traumatic accident or develops a medical problem. He becomes the subject of concern, with the focus being very medically oriented (i.e., explain the pathology, control the disease process, alleviate the symptoms, repair the damage). Reorganization of his behavior through reestablishment of familiar activities should not be left to chance. The occupational therapist addresses the situation by engaging the child in familiar, purposeful activities in a systematic way. She may find it necessary to modify the activity itself or the tools being used, or even change the method of instruction. Her goal is to have the child transform his dysfunctional behavior into an adaptive ability that is appropriate for his developmental level and immediate circumstances. Talking with the child about doing something is not nearly as effective as putting him into an active situation where he experiences his adaptability and potential.

THE ENVIRONMENT

Occupational therapy may be performed in a variety of settings, which are chosen on the basis of the patient's needs and medical status at the time.

Sue, a 13-year-old who became a quadriplegic from a diving accident, first received occupational therapy on a circular electric bed in her room on the rehabilitation unit. As her medical status stabilized and she began to progress toward independence, there were a variety of areas designated for therapy. These environments ranged from the bathroom to the gift shop, depending on which aspect of self-care was being addressed (problem solving, adapting tools or techniques, and developing proficiency in the various tasks). Prior to discharge, Sue made a home visit with her occupational therapist to make environmental modifications that would ensure maximum self-sufficiency. Having the wall telephone lowered, modifying the television tuning knob, and adapting the sliding glass door handle are some examples of these efforts.

Wherever the therapy space, it should be used in a flexible, creative way, so that the environment will be as realistic as possible in order for the child to rehearse developmentally appropriate life tasks and roles. In order to help the child cope effectively with the human and nonhuman aspects of his world in spite of his disability or problem, the therapist needs to be something of an environmental specialist. As such, she identifies and modifies critical elements in the child's immediate surroundings that are interfering with or adversely influencing his performance. She augments other environmental factors in such a way that his development and functional ability are enhanced. For example, when working with a neonate in an intensive care nursery, she finds ways to reduce the adverse effects of constant bright lights and strange equipment noises, while providing normalizing sensory experiences with touch and movement.

The environment can have a profound positive or negative influence on behavior and learning. Ayers' (1972) comprehensive research and development of sensory integration theory, diagnosis, and treatment have laid the foundation for using sensory input to ameliorate disordered sensory processing as well as to promote normal sensorimotor development and function. The therapist assumes responsibility for "feeding" the child appropriate sensory information from the environment; this ensures that central nervous system development, motor performance, and higher cognitive functions are optimally nurtured. Such feeding requires knowledge of the needs and general state of the child at the time, so as to inhibit undesirable reactions and facilitate appropriate responses.

The environment can be considered therapeutic when it:

1. facilitates pleasurable participation and makes reasonable demands on the child's abilities;
2. stimulates the child's curiosity so that he explores, solves problems, and makes choices;
3. motivates the child to persevere in spite of pain, fear, or dysfunction;
4. provides a means of developing self-esteem, confidence, and social skills;
5. promotes learning that will be applicable in other situations;
6. develops the child's ability to concentrate, exercise good judgment, and assume responsibility for his actions;
7. helps the child to develop a sense of value for time and the ability to balance his periods of work, play, and rest (Meyer, 1922).

CONCLUSION

The dynamic interplay of the child, therapist, activity, and environment helps each child to enjoy what he is, rather than feeling remorse for what he is lacking. In so doing, occupational therapy mobilizes the "wellness" of the child. When the child has a physical dysfunction, the need for occupational therapy is obvious and the results of the therapeutic intervention are tangible.

Six-year-old Julie received a peripheral nerve injury of her right arm from running through a closed sliding glass door. Her occupational therapist constructed a series of hand splints which protected her wrist and hand during nerve regeneration and facilitated redevelopment of hand usage while she was engaged in graded therapeutic activities.

The benefits that Julie derived from occupational therapy were very obvious compared to Todd, who was referred at 2½ years of age because of a developmental delay. Much of his immature performance appeared to stem from a vestibular processing disorder, limiting his ability to adapt to the demands of gravity. He was readily disorganized by self-imposed as well as environmentally induced movement. His method of coping with this problem was to become a sedentary spectator of the life around him. Even though the colorful ball, the bolster swing, and the scooter board in the clinic looked inviting, Todd would not even attempt to engage in therapeutic movement for several weeks. After six months of weekly therapy and an accompanying home program, Todd spontaneously initiated gross motor play, while maintaining his balance in most experiences. His newly acquired confidence in playful movement allowed him to turn his attention to language acquisition and cognitive development. These somewhat subtle gains were attributable to maturation and helpful, caring parents as well as to occupational therapy intervention.

Thus, the occupational therapy process, whether subtle or obvious, tangibly facilitates "doing" and "becoming."

REFERENCES

Ayres, A.J. *Sensory Integration and Learning Disabilities.* Western Psychological Service, Los Angeles (1972).

Clark, P.N. Human development through occupation: A philosophy and conceptual model for practice, part 2. *American Journal of Occupational Therapy, 33,* 577–585 (1979).

Cynkin, S. *Occupational Therapy: Toward Health Through Activities.* Little, Brown, Boston (1979).

Meyer, A. The philosophy of occupational therapy. *Archives of Occupational Therapy, 1,* 1–10 (1922).

Reilly, M. *Play as Exploratory Learning.* Sage Publications, Beverly Hills (1974).

Smith, M.B. Forward. In *Play as Exploratory Learning,* M. Reilly, ed. Sage Publication, Beverly Hills (1974), pp. 7–8.

INDEX

INDEX

Abdominal pain
  functional, 133-136
  recurrent, 36
Abuse, child, *see* Child abuse
Academic underachievement, 21
Acute illness, 19-21
Addicted newborn, 152-153
Anorexia nervosa, 39-40
Anticonvulsant medications, 29
Anxiety, 20, 96-99
Aphasia, 116-119
Aphonia following encephalitis,
  120-122
Arthritis, septic, 92-94
Asthma
  cases, 90, 130-132
  psychiatric aspects of, 31-32

Behavior
  changes in, 21
  diabetes mellitus and problem, 94-96
  explosive, 86-88
  hyperactive, 116-119
  immature, 130-132
  manipulative, 130-132
  oppositional, 126-132
  seizure and problem, 101-104
  self-abusive, 222
  sullen, 92-94
  temper tantrums, 92-94
  withdrawn, 92-94
Behavior therapy, 71
Bleeding disorders, 33-34
Body image, 25-26
Bonding process, interruption of
  abuse of child and, 172-173, 176
  suicidal behavior and, 233-234
Brain contusion, 116-119
Brain maturation, speech and language
  development and, 258-259
Brain tumor, rapid deterioration with,
  104-106

Burnout, child abuse and, 163-164,
  198-201
Burns, 26

Cardiac disease, 30
Cedar House, 188-189
Cerebral concussion, 126-129
Cerebral palsy, 122-123
Child abuse, 169-201; *see also* SCAN
  team
  attachment-dependency theory of,
    174
  burnout and, 163-164, 198-201
  Cedar House, family renewal center,
    188-189
  child itself in, role of, 173
  Children's Village, residential treat-
    ment center, 189-190
  coalition of community agencies and,
    196-197
  countertransference and, 198-201
  definitions for, 169-170
  depression and suicidal behavior and,
    179
  discipline vs, 194-196
  dwarfism and, 178
  emotional neglect, 186-187
  etiologic factors in, 183
  failure to thrive and, 177
  follow-up for, 81
  guidelines for medical management
    of, 148-149
  health visitor in home for, 187-188
  high-risk children, 154, 173-183
  incidence of, 170-171
  intervention for, 183-191
  investigation of, 193-194
  legal aspects of, 191-196
  low birth weight and, 172
  parents who commit, *see* Child
    abusing parents
  physical, 150-151